Emerging Trends and Translational Challenges in Drug and Vaccine Delivery

Emerging Trends and Translational Challenges in Drug and Vaccine Delivery

Editors

Vibhuti Agrahari
Prashant Kumar

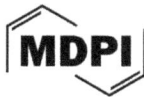

Basel • Beijing • Wuhan • Barcelona • Belgrade • Novi Sad • Cluj • Manchester

Editors
Vibhuti Agrahari
Department of
Pharmaceutical Sciences
University of Oklahoma
Health Sciences Center
Oklahoma City
United States

Prashant Kumar
Vaccine Analytics and
Formulation Center (VAFC)
University of Kansas
Lawrence
United States

Editorial Office
MDPI
St. Alban-Anlage 66
4052 Basel, Switzerland

This is a reprint of articles from the Special Issue published online in the open access journal *Pharmaceutics* (ISSN 1999-4923) (available at: www.mdpi.com/journal/pharmaceutics/special_issues/X66H8Y1DQC).

For citation purposes, cite each article independently as indicated on the article page online and as indicated below:

Lastname, A.A.; Lastname, B.B. Article Title. *Journal Name* **Year**, *Volume Number*, Page Range.

ISBN 978-3-7258-0812-0 (Hbk)
ISBN 978-3-7258-0811-3 (PDF)
doi.org/10.3390/books978-3-7258-0811-3

© 2024 by the authors. Articles in this book are Open Access and distributed under the Creative Commons Attribution (CC BY) license. The book as a whole is distributed by MDPI under the terms and conditions of the Creative Commons Attribution-NonCommercial-NoDerivs (CC BY-NC-ND) license.

Contents

About the Editors vii

Preface ix

Prashant Kumar and Vibhuti Agrahari
Emerging Trends and Translational Challenges in Drug and Vaccine Delivery [†]
Reprinted from: *Pharmaceutics* 2024, *16*, 98, doi:10.3390/pharmaceutics16010098 1

Zhe Wang, Xinpei Wang, Wanting Xu, Yongxiao Li, Ruizhi Lai and Xiaohui Qiu et al.
Translational Challenges and Prospective Solutions in the Implementation of Biomimetic Delivery Systems
Reprinted from: *Pharmaceutics* 2023, *15*, 2623, doi:10.3390/pharmaceutics15112623 4

Musaed Alkholief, Mohd Abul Kalam, Mohammad Raish, Mushtaq Ahmad Ansari, Nasser B. Alsaleh and Aliyah Almomen et al.
Topical Sustained-Release Dexamethasone-Loaded Chitosan Nanoparticles: Assessment of Drug Delivery Efficiency in a Rabbit Model of Endotoxin-Induced Uveitis
Reprinted from: *Pharmaceutics* 2023, *15*, 2273, doi:10.3390/pharmaceutics15092273 37

Tuong Ngoc-Gia Nguyen, Cuong Viet Pham, Rocky Chowdhury, Shweta Patel, Satendra Kumar Jaysawal and Yingchun Hou et al.
Development of Blueberry-Derived Extracellular Nanovesicles for Immunomodulatory Therapy
Reprinted from: *Pharmaceutics* 2023, *15*, 2115, doi:10.3390/pharmaceutics15082115 58

Ying Luo, Xiaoxiao Li, Yawei Zhao, Wen Zhong, Malcolm Xing and Guozhong Lyu
Development of Organs-on-Chips and Their Impact on Precision Medicine and Advanced System Simulation
Reprinted from: *Pharmaceutics* 2023, *15*, 2094, doi:10.3390/pharmaceutics15082094 83

Rahul G. Ingle and Wei-Jie Fang
An Overview of the Stability and Delivery Challenges of Commercial Nucleic Acid Therapeutics
Reprinted from: *Pharmaceutics* 2023, *15*, 1158, doi:10.3390/pharmaceutics15041158 111

Axel H. Meyer, Thomas M. Feldsien, Mario Mezler, Christopher Untucht, Ramakrishna Venugopalan and Didier R. Lefebvre
Novel Developments to Enable Treatment of CNS Diseases with Targeted Drug Delivery
Reprinted from: *Pharmaceutics* 2023, *15*, 1100, doi:10.3390/pharmaceutics15041100 131

Renée S. van der Kooij, Martin Beukema, Anke L. W. Huckriede, Johan Zuidema, Rob Steendam and Henderik W. Frijlink et al.
A Single Injection with Sustained-Release Microspheres and a Prime-Boost Injection of Bovine Serum Albumin Elicit the Same IgG Antibody Response in Mice
Reprinted from: *Pharmaceutics* 2023, *15*, 676, doi:10.3390/pharmaceutics15020676 156

Hafsa Shahid Faizi, Lalitkumar K. Vora, Muhammad Iqbal Nasiri, Yu Wu, Deepakkumar Mishra and Qonita Kurnia Anjani et al.
Deferasirox Nanosuspension Loaded Dissolving Microneedles for Intradermal Delivery
Reprinted from: *Pharmaceutics* 2022, *14*, 2817, doi:10.3390/pharmaceutics14122817 179

Hong Liang, William R. Lykins, Emilie Seydoux, Jeffrey A. Guderian, Tony Phan and Christopher B. Fox et al.
Formulated Phospholipids as Non-Canonical TLR4 Agonists
Reprinted from: *Pharmaceutics* **2022**, *14*, 2557, doi:10.3390/pharmaceutics14122557 . . . . **197**

Ke Peng, Mingshan Li, Achmad Himawan, Juan Domínguez-Robles, Lalitkumar K. Vora and Ross Duncan et al.
Amphotericin B- and Levofloxacin-Loaded Chitosan Films for Potential Use in Antimicrobial Wound Dressings: Analytical Method Development and Its Application
Reprinted from: *Pharmaceutics* **2022**, *14*, 2497, doi:10.3390/pharmaceutics14112497 . . . . **213**

About the Editors

Vibhuti Agrahari

Vibhuti Agrahari is an assistant professor at the University of Oklahoma College of Pharmacy. She received her Ph.D. from the University of Missouri-Kansas City (UMKC) and joined the BJD School of Pharmacy, Shenandoah University as an assistant professor of biopharmaceutical sciences. Her research focuses on novel nanotherapeutic development for ocular/otic delivery, and she is credited with two US patents. She has co-authored more than 35 peer-reviewed articles and 6 book chapters, and has been appointed as a special theme issue editor for various scientific journals. Dr. Agrahari received several awards and honors such as the American Association Colleges of Pharmacy (AACP) New investigator Award (2023), BJD faculty research award (2018), AAPS Biotechnology Graduate Student Symposium Award (2016 and 2015), AAPS-Ocular Drug Delivery Disposition Focus Group (2015 and 2014), Ronald MacQuarrie Fellowship (2015), Judith Hemberger Graduate Scholarship (2014), Scholar of PFF-SGS (2014–2016), and meritorious scholar of GAF Women's Council (2014–2017), at UMKC and Research fellowship by the Ministry of Human Resource Development, India (2005). Dr. Agrahari is an educator, mentor and active member of professional organizations, and has served in various leadership roles, including the Co-Chair and Scientific Committee Chair, Pharmaceutics Graduate Student Research Meeting (2016); AAPS SPOD Committee (2016); Secretary/Treasurer Controlled Release Society (CRS) – Ocular Drug Delivery Focus Group (2017); Council of Faculty - Junior Faculty Community Leadership Group- AACP (2018); Ambassador, CRS - Young Scientists Committee (2018–2020); AAPS Nomination Committee (2019); Track Leader, Formulation and Delivery/Biomolecular Committee, AAPS PharmSci 360 (2020); AAPS Strategic Planning Task Force (2020-2022), AAPS Horizon Planning Committee (2021–2023), UMKC SOP Alumni Board of Directors (2023–2025) and UMKC Women's Council Board of Directors (2023-2026).

Prashant Kumar

Prashant Kumar, PhD, is a Scientific Assistant Director at the Vaccine Analytics and Formulation Center (VAFC) at the Department of Pharmaceutical Chemistry, The University of Kansas, USA. His work focuses on the analytical and formulation development of low-cost and stable human vaccines to extend global access and compliance, especially in low- and middle-income countries. He has experience in developing several vaccine candidates, including an AAV-based COVID-19, sIPV, combination vaccine, Measles and Rubella, Shigella and Rotavirus (RV3-BB, and NRRV) vaccines, most of which are in phase 1-3 clinical trials. Dr. Kumar's multidisciplinary background in bioprocessing, formulation development, analytical and biophysical characterization coupled with the statistical design of experiments (DOE) and tech transfer experience has helped him in efficient process development and cost minimization necessary for the success of these projects. Dr. Kumar has been an invited speaker and chair for scientific conferences. He serves on the editorial board of various journals, and has several scientific papers and book chapters to his credit.

Preface

Drug and vaccine delivery are continuously evolving and have received significant attention in recent years to enhance safety, efficacy, and targeted and delayed delivery, as well as ease cost in order to enhance access to everyone. The evolution of therapeutics from small molecules to more complex macromolecules and conjugates has imposed additional challenges for the development of novel therapeutics from proof-of-concept lab-scale investigations to final large-scale applications. This reprint is a collection of efforts by several researchers engaged in the field to advance drug and vaccine delivery systems. The presented research and review articles are valuable for the scientific community focused on drug delivery research.

Vibhuti Agrahari and Prashant Kumar
Editors

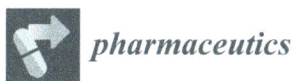

Editorial

Emerging Trends and Translational Challenges in Drug and Vaccine Delivery †

Prashant Kumar [1,*] and Vibhuti Agrahari [2,*]

1. Department of Pharmaceutical Chemistry, Vaccine Analytics and Formulation Center, University of Kansas, 2030 Becker Dr, Lawrence, KS 66047, USA
2. Department of Pharmaceutical Sciences, University of Oklahoma Health Sciences Center, 1110 N. Stonewall Avenue, Oklahoma City, OK 73117, USA
* Correspondence: prashant.kumar@ku.edu (P.K.); vibhuti-agrahari@ouhsc.edu (V.A.)
† This article belongs to the Special Issue Emerging Trends and Translational Challenges in Drug and Vaccine Delivery.

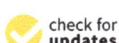

Citation: Kumar, P.; Agrahari, V. Emerging Trends and Translational Challenges in Drug and Vaccine Delivery. *Pharmaceutics* 2024, *16*, 98. https://doi.org/10.3390/pharmaceutics16010098

Received: 9 January 2024
Accepted: 9 January 2024
Published: 11 January 2024

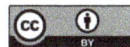

Copyright: © 2024 by the authors. Licensee MDPI, Basel, Switzerland. This article is an open access article distributed under the terms and conditions of the Creative Commons Attribution (CC BY) license (https://creativecommons.org/licenses/by/4.0/).

Drug and vaccine delivery have received considerable attention in recent years. Many rationally designed innovative approaches are being explored to address the challenges related to safety, efficacy, patient compliance, and cost-effective means for existing and new therapeutics. The extensive assessment of drug delivery involves pre-formulation and physicochemical characterization, mechanistic biochemical pathways at the molecular level, pharmacological and toxicological evaluations, and detailed preclinical investigations. Recent advancements have evolved to address the limitations that emerged with the evolution of novel therapeutic modalities from simple small molecules to more complex macromolecules, including nucleic acids, peptides, proteins, antibodies, and conjugates [1]. There's immense interest in exploring the in vitro and in vivo behavior of drugs and vaccines to overcome biological barriers to reach target sites, and in expeditious translation from the lab to a manufacturing scale [2]. This Special Issue on "Emerging Trends and Translational Challenges in Drug and Vaccine Delivery" is the collection of those efforts by several researchers to address the unmet need of advanced drug and vaccine delivery systems. The studies published in this Special Issue are summarized below and are valuable for the readers of Pharmaceutics and the scientific community working in the field of drug and vaccine delivery.

The first paper in this collection by Alkholief et al. demonstrated the use of dexamethasone-sodium-phosphate (DEX)-chitosan nanoparticles (CSNPs) coated with hyaluronic acid (HA) as a controlled release ocular delivery vehicle for the treatment of endotoxin-induced-uveitis (EIU) in a rabbit model [3]. The CSNPs were stable at 25 °C for 3 months and in vitro studies showed a similar DEX release in a range of 74–77% for uncoated and HA-coated nanoparticles. Drug-loaded CSNPs were safe for ocular applications and showed a noTable 10-fold increase in transcorneal flux and permeability of DEX in the case of HA-CSNPs vs. DEX-aqueous solution (DEX-AqS). The findings suggest improved delivery properties and promising anti-inflammatory effects of DEX-CSNPs in EIU rabbits with ocular bioavailability, with the half-life and ocular MRT0-inf of DEX being significantly higher than DEX-AqS.

Another study focused on extracellular nanovesicles (EVs) that have great potential as drug delivery systems for precision therapy but are limited due to technical challenges to purify and characterize the EVs. To address this issue, Nguyen et al. developed a 3D inner filter-based technique for the simple extraction of apoplastic fluid from blueberries, enabling EV purification [4]. The high drug loading capability and properties to modulate the release of proinflammatory cytokine IL-8 and total glutathione have enabled blueberry-derived EVs (BENVs) to be a promising edible multifunctional nano-bio-platform for future immunomodulatory therapies.

Vaccination is the most effective way to prevent infectious diseases but suffers from fading immunity requiring frequent boosters to maintain the immune response. In a novel approach, Kooji et al. demonstrated the effectiveness of a single injection with sustained-release microspheres as an alternative to the conventional multiple injection (prime-boost) immunization schedule of bovine serum albumin in terms of eliciting the same levels of IgG antibody response in mice [5]. The microspheres were designed based on two novel biodegradable multi-block copolymers with an opportunity to tailor the release profile in a range of 4 to 9 weeks by varying the polymer ratios.

Adjuvants are ingredients used in many vaccines to elicit a stronger immune response. In a recent study, Liang et al. demonstrated the use of formulated phospholipid 1,2-dimyristoyl-sn-glycero-3-phosphocholine (DMPC), a component of oil-in-water vaccine adjuvant emulsion (known as a stable emulsion or SE), as non-canonical agonists for murine and human TLR4 [6]. The effects of DMPC on human cells were proven but were less pronounced than the composition of emulsion oil and were dependent on the saturation, size, and headgroup of the phospholipid.

The next article is focused on drug loaded-microneedles, which are minimally invasive systems capable of painless delivery and offer dose-sparing benefits with a potential to replace hypodermal needles and oral routes of delivery. In this study, Faizi et al. developed a deferasirox-nanosuspension (DFS-NS) loaded with dissolving microneedles (DMN) for intradermal delivery for effective treatment of iron overload [7]. DFS-NSs were formulated by the wet media milling procedure using PVA and showed a 3-fold higher dissolution rate vs. pure DFS. The skin deposition studies showed significantly higher drug deposition from DFS-NSs loaded with polymeric dissolving microneedles (NS-DMN) as compared to DFS-NS transdermal patches without needles (DFS-NS-TP) or pure DFS-DMNs. Hence, the authors showed that loading DFS-NSs into novel DMN devices can be effectively used for transdermal delivery of sparingly soluble drugs, i.e., DFS in aqueous systems.

In another study, Peng et al. demonstrated the development of amphotericin B (AMB)- and levofloxacin (LVX)-loaded chitosan films for potential use in antimicrobial wound dressings [8]. An HPLC method developed by the authors measured 100% and 60% release of LVX and AMB, respectively, from the chitosan film after a week. An ex vivo deposition study showed that 20.96 ± 13.54 and 0.35 ± 0.04 of LVX and AMB, respectively, were deposited in porcine skin 24 h after application. Further, the films were able to inhibit the growth of *Candida albicans* and *Staphylococcus aureus*, demonstrating their antimicrobial applications.

Wang et al. in their recent review discussed the translational challenges and prospective solutions for implementing biomimetic delivery systems (BDSs) for therapeutic delivery [9]. BDSs are based on complex designs of biological structures and have emerged as a powerful tool for drug and vaccine delivery. This review provides recent advances in the development of BDSs, discusses the challenges faced in the translation of BDs from research to clinical applications, and presents emerging solutions, emphasized by real-world case studies.

Luo et al. provide insights into the development of organs-on-chips (OCs) and their impact on precision medicine and advanced system simulation [10]. OCs are devices with micro-physiological systems containing small tissues grown inside microfluidic chips with controlled cell microenvironments to study the pathophysiology and effect of drugs on the human body. OCs represent a faster, economical, and precise approach to study drug safety, efficacy, disease modelling and treatments with a potential to complement/replace traditional preclinical cell cultures, animal studies, and even human clinical trials.

Ingle and Fang in their recent review present an overview of the stability and delivery challenges of commercial nucleic acid (NA)-based therapeutics, including DNA, RNA, oligonucleotides, siRNA, miRNA, mRNA, small activating RNA, and gene therapies [11]. The review highlights NA-based therapeutics approved by the European Medicines Agency (EMA) and US Food and Drug Administration (US FDA) with a focus on the current progress in improving the stability, delivery, cost, and regulatory acceptance of these therapeutics.

There is significant interest in developing approaches to overcome the blood–brain barrier (BBB) for treatment of central nervous system (CNS) diseases. Meyer et al. in their recent review described novel developments to enable the treatment of CNS diseases with targeted drug delivery [12]. The review focuses on unfolding the full potential of novel therapeutic entities, i.e., gene therapy and degradomers, using innovative delivery systems for possible application in the treatment of CNS diseases.

In conclusion, this Special Issue converses through the translation of therapeutic delivery from discovery to large-scale production for pharmaceutical and biotechnology applications. The discussed strategies, including the use of polymeric nanoparticles, extracellular nanovesicles, sustained release microspheres, microneedles, polymeric biofilms, biomimetic delivery systems, new adjuvants, and organ-on-chips, possess great potential in addressing the limitations of drug and vaccine delivery. The editors express their gratitude for the interest and cooperation of the contributors and believe this Special Issue of Pharmaceutics would be an interesting addition to the scientific community engaged in drug delivery research.

Funding: This research received no external funding.

Conflicts of Interest: The authors declare no conflict of interest.

References

1. Vargason, A.M.; Anselmo, A.C.; Mitragotri, S. The Evolution of Commercial Drug Delivery Technologies. *Nat. Biomed. Eng.* **2021**, *5*, 951–967. [CrossRef] [PubMed]
2. Agrahari, V.; Kumar, P. Novel Approaches for Overcoming Biological Barriers. *Pharmaceutics* **2022**, *14*, 1851. [CrossRef]
3. Alkholief, M.; Kalam, M.A.; Raish, M.; Ansari, M.A.; Alsaleh, N.B.; Almomen, A.; Ali, R.; Alshamsan, A. Topical Sustained-Release Dexamethasone-Loaded Chitosan Nanoparticles: Assessment of Drug Delivery Efficiency in a Rabbit Model of Endotoxin-Induced Uveitis. *Pharmaceutics* **2023**, *15*, 2273. [CrossRef] [PubMed]
4. Nguyen, T.N.; Pham, C.V.; Chowdhury, R.; Patel, S.; Jaysawal, S.K.; Hou, Y.; Xu, H.; Jia, L.; Duan, A.; Tran, P.H.; et al. Development of Blueberry-Derived Extracellular Nanovesicles for Immunomodulatory Therapy. *Pharmaceutics* **2023**, *15*, 2115. [CrossRef] [PubMed]
5. van der Kooij, R.S.; Beukema, M.; Huckriede, A.L.W.; Zuidema, J.; Steendam, R.; Frijlink, H.W.; Hinrichs, W.L.J. A Single Injection with Sustained-Release Microspheres and a Prime-Boost Injection of Bovine Serum Albumin Elicit the Same Igg Antibody Response in Mice. *Pharmaceutics* **2023**, *15*, 676. [CrossRef] [PubMed]
6. Liang, H.; Lykins, W.R.; Seydoux, E.; Guderian, J.A.; Phan, T.; Fox, C.B.; Orr, M.T. Formulated Phospholipids as Non-Canonical Tlr4 Agonists. *Pharmaceutics* **2022**, *14*, 2557. [CrossRef] [PubMed]
7. Faizi, H.S.; Vora, L.K.; Nasiri, M.I.; Wu, Y.; Mishra, D.; Anjani, Q.K.; Paredes, A.J.; Thakur, R.R.S.; Minhas, M.U.; Donnelly, R.F. Deferasirox Nanosuspension Loaded Dissolving Microneedles for Intradermal Delivery. *Pharmaceutics* **2022**, *14*, 2817. [CrossRef] [PubMed]
8. Peng, K.; Li, M.; Himawan, A.; Dominguez-Robles, J.; Vora, L.K.; Duncan, R.; Dai, X.; Zhang, C.; Zhao, L.; Li, L.; et al. Amphotericin B- and Levofloxacin-Loaded Chitosan Films for Potential Use in Antimicrobial Wound Dressings: Analytical Method Development and Its Application. *Pharmaceutics* **2022**, *14*, 2497. [CrossRef] [PubMed]
9. Wang, Z.; Wang, X.; Xu, W.; Li, Y.; Lai, R.; Qiu, X.; Chen, X.; Chen, Z.; Mi, B.; Wu, M.; et al. Translational Challenges and Prospective Solutions in the Implementation of Biomimetic Delivery Systems. *Pharmaceutics* **2023**, *15*, 2623. [CrossRef] [PubMed]
10. Luo, Y.; Li, X.; Zhao, Y.; Zhong, W.; Xing, M.; Lyu, G. Development of Organs-on-Chips and Their Impact on Precision Medicine and Advanced System Simulation. *Pharmaceutics* **2023**, *15*, 2094. [CrossRef] [PubMed]
11. Ingle, R.G.; Fang, W.J. An Overview of the Stability and Delivery Challenges of Commercial Nucleic Acid Therapeutics. *Pharmaceutics* **2023**, *15*, 1158. [CrossRef] [PubMed]
12. Meyer, A.H.; Feldsien, T.M.; Mezler, M.; Untucht, C.; Venugopalan, R.; Lefebvre, D.R. Novel Developments to Enable Treatment of Cns Diseases with Targeted Drug Delivery. *Pharmaceutics* **2023**, *15*, 1100. [CrossRef] [PubMed]

Disclaimer/Publisher's Note: The statements, opinions and data contained in all publications are solely those of the individual author(s) and contributor(s) and not of MDPI and/or the editor(s). MDPI and/or the editor(s) disclaim responsibility for any injury to people or property resulting from any ideas, methods, instructions or products referred to in the content.

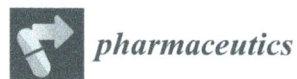

Review

Translational Challenges and Prospective Solutions in the Implementation of Biomimetic Delivery Systems

Zhe Wang [1], Xinpei Wang [2], Wanting Xu [2], Yongxiao Li [2], Ruizhi Lai [1], Xiaohui Qiu [2], Xu Chen [2], Zhidong Chen [2], Bobin Mi [3,4], Meiying Wu [2,*] and Junqing Wang [2,*]

1. Department of Pathology, The Eighth Affiliated Hospital, Sun Yat-sen University, Shenzhen 518033, China; wangzh379@mail.sysu.edu.cn (Z.W.); lairzh3@mail2.sysu.edu.cn (R.L.)
2. School of Pharmaceutical Sciences, Shenzhen Campus of Sun Yat-sen University, Shenzhen 518107, China; wangxp39@mail2.sysu.edu.cn (X.W.); xuwt27@mail2.sysu.edu.cn (W.X.); liyx356@mail2.sysu.edu.cn (Y.L.); qiuxh27@mail2.sysu.edu.cn (X.Q.); chenx589@mail2.sysu.edu.cn (X.C.); chenzhd9@mail2.sysu.edu.cn (Z.C.)
3. Department of Orthopaedics, Union Hospital, Tongji Medical College, Huazhong University of Science and Technology, Wuhan 430022, China; mibobin@hust.edu.cn
4. Hubei Province Key Laboratory of Oral and Maxillofacial Development and Regeneration, Wuhan 430022, China
* Correspondence: wumy53@mail.sysu.edu.cn (M.W.); wangjunqing@mail.sysu.edu.cn (J.W.)

Abstract: Biomimetic delivery systems (BDSs), inspired by the intricate designs of biological systems, have emerged as a groundbreaking paradigm in nanomedicine, offering unparalleled advantages in therapeutic delivery. These systems, encompassing platforms such as liposomes, protein-based nanoparticles, extracellular vesicles, and polysaccharides, are lauded for their targeted delivery, minimized side effects, and enhanced therapeutic outcomes. However, the translation of BDSs from research settings to clinical applications is fraught with challenges, including reproducibility concerns, physiological stability, and rigorous efficacy and safety evaluations. Furthermore, the innovative nature of BDSs demands the reevaluation and evolution of existing regulatory and ethical frameworks. This review provides an overview of BDSs and delves into the multifaceted translational challenges and present emerging solutions, underscored by real-world case studies. Emphasizing the potential of BDSs to redefine healthcare, we advocate for sustained interdisciplinary collaboration and research. As our understanding of biological systems deepens, the future of BDSs in clinical translation appears promising, with a focus on personalized medicine and refined patient-specific delivery systems.

Keywords: biomimetic; bioinspired; nanodiscs; liposomes; virus-like particles; albumin; ferritin; polysaccharides; extracellular vesicles

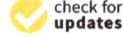

Citation: Wang, Z.; Wang, X.; Xu, W.; Li, Y.; Lai, R.; Qiu, X.; Chen, X.; Chen, Z.; Mi, B.; Wu, M.; et al. Translational Challenges and Prospective Solutions in the Implementation of Biomimetic Delivery Systems. *Pharmaceutics* **2023**, *15*, 2623. https://doi.org/10.3390/pharmaceutics15112623

Academic Editors: Anna Angela Barba and Juan José Torrado

Received: 25 September 2023
Revised: 3 November 2023
Accepted: 9 November 2023
Published: 14 November 2023

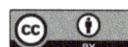

Copyright: © 2023 by the authors. Licensee MDPI, Basel, Switzerland. This article is an open access article distributed under the terms and conditions of the Creative Commons Attribution (CC BY) license (https:// creativecommons.org/licenses/by/ 4.0/).

1. Introduction

Biomimetic delivery systems (BDSs), defined by their ability to mimic biological systems, hold significant promise in the realm of biomedicine and nanomedicine. They leverage the principles of nature, emulating the structural or functional attributes of biological systems to enhance drug delivery capabilities [1–3]. BDSs often involve the use of naturally derived materials (Figure 1), the structural mimicry of biological entities, or the replication of biological processes, with the aim of improving drug delivery outcomes such as targeting ability, controlled release, and biocompatibility [4–6]. Recent advancements in biomimicry have resulted in the creation of innovative drug delivery systems [7–9] spanning various paradigms, such as liposomal carriers [10], virus-like nanoparticles (VLPs) for gene delivery [11–13], and hydrogel structures [14–16]. Additionally, new classes of delivery vehicles have emerged, including extracellular vesicles (EVs) [17,18], red blood cell (RBC)-based carriers [19,20], and nanodiscs (NDs), each presenting unique therapeutic prospects. EVs, naturally occurring cellular delivery systems, comprised of microvesicles and exosomes [21,22], hold promise due to their bio-compatibility and targeted delivery capability [23,24], stimulating interest in their use for delivering RNA-based therapeutics [21,25]. RBCs, with their advantageous properties such as a long circulatory half-life and immune evasion, are under investigation as potential drug carriers, with methods involving their engineering and manipulation into biomimetic nanoparticles [26–28]. NDs, mimicking high-density lipoproteins (HDL) [29,30], are versatile delivery platforms due to their ability to solubilize and present various drug molecules; additionally, they have potential benefits for targeted cancer therapy due to their preferential uptake by cancer cells [31,32].

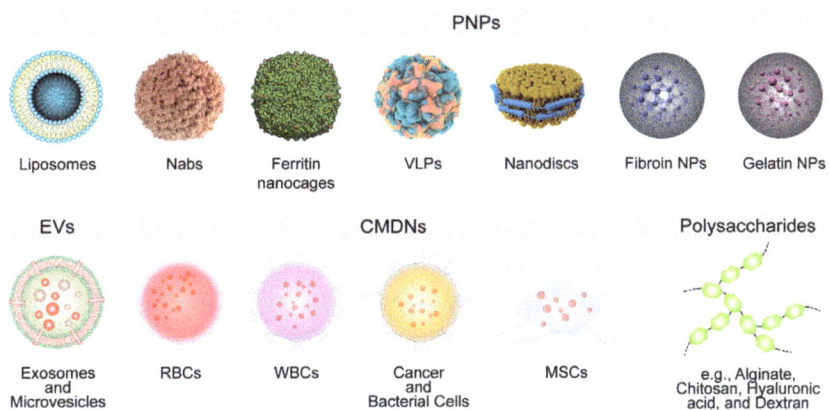

Figure 1. The general illustration of biomimetic delivery systems (BDSs). BDSs are designed to emulate natural structures, thereby augmenting therapeutic efficacy. Notable examples encompass liposomes, protein-based nanoparticles (PNPs), extracellular vesicles (EVs), cell membrane-derived nanocarriers (CMDNs), nanodiscs, and polysaccharides.

The theoretical bedrock of biomimetic delivery systems (BDSs) is fundamentally rooted in the principles of self-assembly, molecular recognition, and biocompatibility [1–3]. Self-assembly refers to the process by which molecules spontaneously organize into ordered structures [33,34]. This characteristic, borrowed from nature, is widely harnessed to construct nanoscale delivery vehicles [35]. Molecular recognition refers to the ability of molecules to interact specifically with others, typically resulting in a biological function or response. This principle allows for the precise targeting of therapeutic agents to disease sites, minimizing off-target effects. Lastly, the nano-bio interface effect and biocompatibility are critical attributes of any biomimetic nanosystem intended for clinical use, ensuring that the system does not elicit adverse immune responses or toxic effects [36,37]. The paradigm of drug delivery has seen revolutionary advancement with the burgeoning interest in BDSs, which intimately mimic biological structures to enhance therapeutic efficacy [38–40].

These advancements have catalyzed previously unattainable therapeutic opportunities, including targeted cancer therapies [41], gene editing [42], and regenerative medicine [43]. The diversity and adaptability of these BDSs underscore the significant potential of leveraging nature's design in the development of next-generation therapeutic interventions. However, the path from the bench to bedside translation is fraught with complexity. Despite the theoretical advantages of BDSs, their translation into clinical applications has been slower than expected, hindered by various technical, biological, and regulatory challenges. For instance, issues such as scalability of production, immunogenicity, stability of the systems under physiological conditions, and navigating regulatory approvals pose significant hurdles. The urgency for such a discourse is evident. The promise of biomimicry in healthcare can only be realized when these delivery systems transition from being experimental novelties to tools readily available in the clinician's arsenal.

This review elucidates the translational challenges prevalent in the field, focusing on their intricate aspects and contemplating potential resolutions (Figure 2). Given the broad scope of this review, emphasis is placed on general themes rather than meticulous analyses of individual cases. We initially provide an overview of the strengths and weaknesses of various BDSs, then we examine challenges segmented into technical, biological, and regulatory categories before presenting emerging solutions and strategies, highlighted by instances of successful translation. Conclusively, we offer insights into the future challenges in the BDS field, emphasizing the revolutionary impact of these technologies on healthcare and advocating for sustained research and collaboration in this realm.

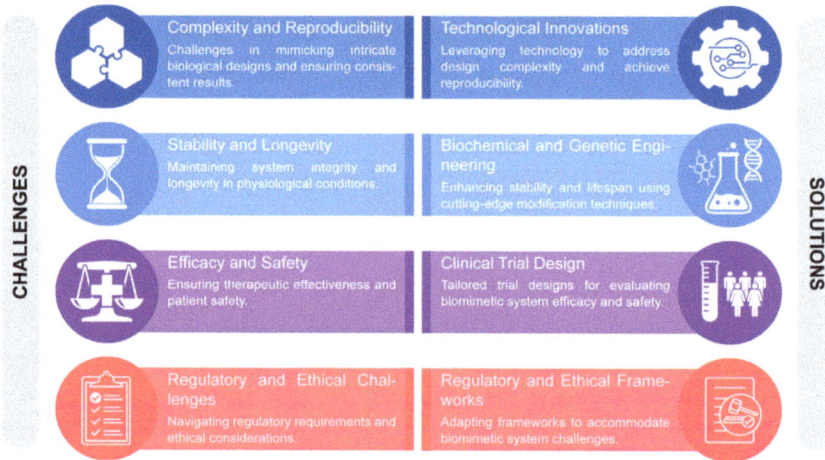

Figure 2. A schematic overview of the clinical translational hurdles and prospective solutions in BDS.

2. An Overview of the Strengths and Weaknesses of BDSs

In the rapidly evolving landscape of drug delivery, BDSs stand out as a beacon of innovation, drawing inspiration from biological structures and processes to optimize therapeutic delivery. By mimicking nature, BDSs aim to overcome the myriad challenges associated with traditional drug delivery, ranging from off-target effects to limited bioavailability [5]. BDSs span a broad spectrum, from liposomal structures to protein-based nanoparticles and CMDNs [1,8,42,44]. While the promise of BDSs is undeniable, it's imperative to evaluate their strengths and weaknesses in comparison with each other (Table 1).

Liposomes are spherical vesicles composed of phospholipid bilayers that can encapsulate a wide variety of therapeutic agents. Their biocompatibility arises from their resemblance to biological membranes, making them a preferred choice for drug delivery [45]. Despite their adaptability in drug loading, liposomes are not without limitations [46]. A critical issue pertains to their stability, which can be compromised during storage, necessitating the development of sophisticated stabilization strategies to ensure the longevity and efficacy of the liposomal formulation [47–50]. In vivo, liposomes may exhibit rapid clearance from the bloodstream, primarily due to opsonization and subsequent phagocytosis by the cells of the mononuclear phagocyte system [51,52]. This necessitates careful consideration of liposome size, surface charge, and surface modification with polymers such as polyethylene glycol (PEG) to extend their circulatory half-life [51,53].

Table 1. An overview of strengths, weaknesses, and therapeutic applications of BDSs.

BDS	Strengths	Weaknesses	Therapeutic Applications
Liposomes	Biocompatible, versatile in drug loading	Limited stability, potential for rapid clearance	Anticancer and antifungal therapy
Protein-based NPs			
Albumin NPs	Natural origin, good safety profile	Variable drug loading efficiency	Anticancer drug delivery
Protein-based nanocages	Defined structure, biodegradable	Complex production	Enzyme replacement therapy, vaccine delivery
VLPs	High immunogenicity, targeted delivery	Production challenges	Vaccines, cancer immunotherapy
NDs	Membrane protein stabilization, defined size	Limited drug loading	Drug and vaccines delivery, drug discovery
Silk Fibroin	Biocompatible, high mechanical strength, thermal stability	Potential immunogenicity, variable degradation rates, processing challenges	Bone tissue engineering, wound healing, anticancer drug delivery
Gelatin	Biodegradability, ease of modification	Potential risk of disease transmission, temperature sensitivity.	Drug delivery, tissue engineering
EVs	Natural origin, low immunogenicity	Isolation purity challenges	Regenerative medicine, anticancer therapy
CMDNs	Mimics natural cells, targeted delivery	Complex production	Targeted drug delivery, immunotherapy
Polysaccharides			
Alginate	Biocompatible, gel-forming	Rapid degradation in vivo	Wound healing, drug delivery
Chitosan	Biocompatible, mucoadhesive	Limited solubility in neutral and alkaline pH	Wound healing, vaccine delivery
Hyaluronic acid	Biocompatible, natural targeting to CD44 receptors	Rapid degradation in vivo	Osteoarthritis treatment, drug delivery
Dextran	Soluble, biocompatible	Potential for hypersensitivity reactions	Iron-deficiency treatment, drug delivery

Protein-based NPs, encompassing albumin NPs, protein-based nanocages, VLPs, and NDs, offer a versatile toolkit for enhancing drug delivery, each with distinct advantages and shared challenges. Albumin NPs utilize human serum albumin, which has a natural propensity to bind to various substances, thereby facilitating the transport of a wide range of molecules [54]. The biodegradability and lack of immunogenicity of albumin contribute to its appeal as a drug carrier. Notably, albumin has a unique ability to accumulate in tumor tissues due to the enhanced permeability and retention (EPR) effect, making it particularly useful for oncological applications [55,56]. However, the drug loading efficiency of albumin NPs can be unpredictable, and their interaction with the biological environment may sometimes lead to rapid clearance from the circulatory system. Despite this, the clinical success of albumin NPs is exemplified by the FDA-approved drug Abraxane, which is an albumin-bound form of paclitaxel used for the treatment of various cancers [57]. Protein-based nanocages are a novel form of protein NPs that offer a highly structured and uniform platform for drug delivery [58]. They are engineered by utilizing the self-assembling properties of certain proteins to form cage-like structures that can encapsulate therapeutic agents within their hollow interior [59]. This allows for precise control over the dosage and protection of the cargo from enzymatic degradation. However, the complexity of synthesizing these nanocages poses a significant challenge, potentially limiting their rapid deployment in clinical settings [60]. VLPs are multiprotein structures that mimic the organization and conformation of viruses but are devoid of viral genetic material, which mitigates safety concerns associated with live viral vectors. The repetitive, high-density display of antigens on their surface makes VLPs particularly effective as vaccine platforms, eliciting strong immune responses [11,61,62]. However, the production of VLPs is technically demanding, often requiring cell culture systems, and the scale-up for mass production can be challenging [63–65]. Nanodiscs are synthetic nanoscale particles that incorporate membrane proteins within a phospholipid bilayer stabilized by scaffold proteins. NDs provide a unique milieu for the study of membrane proteins in their near-native state, which is invaluable for drug discovery and development [66]. While they offer a controlled environment for membrane proteins, their therapeutic application as drug delivery vehicles is still nascent [30,67,68], with issues related to production scalability and drug loading capacity yet to be fully addressed. In a comparative context, while albumin NPs have achieved clinical use, protein-based nanocages and VLPs are still primarily in the research or early clinical trial stages. NDs, being relatively recent developments, and have not yet been extensively explored for therapeutic delivery but hold potential due to their unique ability to present membrane proteins and delivery of lipophilic drugs. Each of these protein-based NPs has its advantages in terms of specificity, biocompatibility, and targeting ability; however, they also face common challenges such as production complexity, stability, and potential immunogenicity.

Silk fibroin (SF) and gelatin (GA) epitomize the contrasting paradigms within BDSs, each with inherent strengths and challenges. SF is distinguished by its robust mechanical properties and sustained release potential, making it a quintessential candidate for structurally demanding applications such as in bone tissue engineering and targeted cancer therapies [69–71]. Nevertheless, its utility is occasionally circumscribed by intricate processing requirements and immunogenic concerns. Conversely, GA is celebrated for its facile chemical modifiability and hydrogel formation aptitude, characteristics that are pivotal for localized therapeutic delivery and tissue engineering scaffolds [72,73]. Yet, its application is sometimes compromised by inferior mechanical integrity, thermal instability, and the latent risk of pathogenic transmission [74]. The selection between SF and GA for DDSs is thus dictated by a nuanced balance between the therapeutic context and the material's physicochemical congruity, with each material offering distinctive contributions to the diversifying landscape of biomimetic therapeutic delivery.

EVs and CMDNs represent two innovative approaches in the realm of biomimetic drug delivery, each leveraging the innate properties of cellular components. EVs, owing to their natural origin, can transport a wide variety of biomolecules and have the ability to cross biological barriers with a low risk of immune response, positioning them as promising vectors for regenerative medicine and targeted cancer therapies [18,75,76]. Nevertheless, isolating EVs with high purity remains a significant technical challenge [77–79]. CMDNs, on the other hand, utilize the unique attributes of cell membranes to cloak nanoparticles, enabling them to evade the immune system and increase delivery specificity [27,80,81]. This strategy has shown considerable promise in targeted drug delivery and immunotherapy, capitalizing on the natural homing abilities of cells. Both EVs and CMDNs still face substantial production complexities (EVs in terms of isolation and CMDNs with membrane extraction and nanoparticle integration).

Polysaccharides, a diverse group of biopolymers, including alginate, chitosan, hyaluronic acid, and dextran, play a pivotal role in the landscape of therapeutic delivery due to their inherent biocompatibility and tailored biodegradability [82,83]. Alginate, renowned for its gel-forming capabilities, is widely used in wound healing applications and as a matrix for cell encapsulation, benefiting from its gentle gelation conditions that preserve cell viability [84,85]. Chitosan, with its distinctive mucoadhesive properties and ability to open tight junctions [86], is exploited for enhanced mucosal delivery of drugs, offering improved bioavailability and prolonged retention at the site of administration. Hyaluronic acid, by virtue of its specific interaction with CD44 receptors [87], which are overexpressed in many cancer cells, has emerged as a targeted delivery vehicle, especially in the treatment of osteoarthritis, where it can provide both viscosupplementation and targeted relief [88]. Dextran, due to its excellent solubility and minimal toxicity, is employed in various drug delivery systems and as a plasma volume expander, with its iron-conjugated forms used to treat iron-deficiency anemia [89,90].

Despite these advantages, the application of polysaccharides is not devoid of challenges; their susceptibility to rapid degradation in vivo may limit their utility, and potential immunogenicity cannot be entirely discounted. Moreover, the batch-to-batch variability and the complexity of producing highly purified, well-characterized polysaccharides can impact the reproducibility and scalability of pharmaceutical products. Hence, while polysaccharides offer considerable benefits for drug delivery, their clinical application requires meticulous optimization to ensure efficacy, safety, and manufacturability.

3. Challenges and Approaches in Clinical Translation of BDSs
3.1. Complexity and Reproducibility

In the realm of biomimetic delivery systems, different biomimetic materials and structures have been explored for their potential advantages in the delivery of therapeutic agents. Each of these systems brings unique complexities and challenges in terms of their production and ensuring their reproducibility (Table 2), which is vital for their successful translation into clinical applications.

Liposomes, vesicular structures composed of lipid bilayers, are valuable carriers for various drugs, improving their pharmacokinetics, biodistribution, and therapeutic index, exemplified by clinically approved liposomal drugs such as Doxil®/Caelyx® and AmBisome® [91]. However, challenges in clinical translation include the heterogeneous nature of liposomes affecting consistency between batches, impacting drug delivery efficacy and therapeutic outcomes [92]. Size and lipid composition variations, stability concerns related to environmental factors, and deviations in morphology and drug release under inappropriate storage temperatures or extreme pH levels are notable issues [47,51,93–95]. To mitigate these, real-time monitoring, process analytical technologies (PAT), and techniques such as nuclear magnetic resonance (NMR) spectroscopy and liquid chromatography–mass spectrometry (LC–MS) are crucial to ensure formulation consistency and rectify deviations immediately [96–98]. For instance, PAT provides real-time data that enables the monitoring and control of the manufacturing process, ensuring quality and consistency in the production of BDSs. LC-MS, on the other hand, is indispensable for the precise analysis of complex biodistributions and pharmacokinetics in BDSs, which is critical for the optimization of therapeutic delivery. Challenges in liposomal drug manufacturing include the need for meticulous control over storage and handling, stringent quality control, and managing the transition from the laboratory to the industrial scale, all contributing to increased costs and complexity [48]. However, continuous manufacturing processes and advanced technologies, such as high-throughput screening and microfluidic systems, can enhance consistency and uniformity, ensuring precise formulation control for therapeutic outcomes [99]. In silico methods aid in designing stable liposomal systems [100,101]. While it's improbable to eradicate all challenges in liposomal drug delivery systems (LDDS), integrating advanced technologies can alleviate them, ensuring efficient and consistent production of clinically effective LDDS. The integration of these technologies into formulation and production processes is crucial in addressing the challenges comprehensively.

Table 2. A summary of the complexities, reproducibility challenges, and prospective solutions related to various BDSs.

BDS	Complexity and Reproducibility	Prospective Solutions
Liposomes	Diverse lipids induce variability. Sustained stability is challenging. Surface alterations cause variability. Scaling up adds variability.	Advanced lipid-mixing technologies. Freeze–thaw increases reproducibility. Advanced ligand conjugation methods. Automated production control.
Protein-based NPs		
Albumin NPs	Influenced by albumin source. Uniform size and shape are difficult to attain. Altered surface for specific targeting. Efficient drug encapsulation control.	High-pressure homogenization. Improved purification techniques. High-throughput screening. Microfluidics and computational modeling.
Protein-based nanocages	Ensuring consistent protein folding. Reproducible encapsulation. Stable surface chemistry. Efficient drug encapsulation control. Consistent drug release profiles.	Advanced bioengineering methods. Monitoring protein folding in real-time. New modification methods for stability. Innovative drug-loading for consistency. Smart release systems for specific triggers.
VLPs	Complexity in VLP assembly. Attaining purity and reproducibility. Heterogeneous surface modifications. Inconsistent therapeutic encapsulation in VLPs.	Advanced purification such as SEC. Genomic engineering for optimized production. Developed specific bioconjugation techniques. High-throughput techniques for optimal encapsulation.
NDs	Component multiplicity causes variability. Consistent size and shape. Adding functional groups increases complexity. Batch-to-batch variability	Synthesis and purification for uniformity. Advanced assembly techniques. Site-specific functionalization and modular design. Standardized protocols, real-time QC, and advanced characterization.
Silk Fibroin and Gelatin	Source variability affecting properties. Controlling degradation profile. Ensuring efficient encapsulation. Batch-to-batch variability due to natural sourcing. Sensitivity to processing conditions leading to variability.	Implement strict source control and purification processes. Crosslinking and site-specific functionalization. Develop recombinant alternatives. Standardizing protocols. Quality assurance measures. Process analytical technology (PAT).
EVs	Heterogeneity of EV populations. Differentiating EV subtypes is challenging. Possible contamination with proteins. Ensuring efficient encapsulation. Controlling release kinetics. Maintaining EV properties post-modification. Ensuring targeting specificity. EV source depends on donor cells.	Advanced centrifugation. High-resolution imaging and flow cytometry. Improved purification processes. Sonication or electroporation. Covalent and non-covalent linking. Bio-orthogonal chemistry. Molecular imprinting techniques. Standardized cell lines/biofactories.

Table 2. Cont.

BDS	Complexity and Reproducibility	Prospective Solutions
CMDNs	Potential heterogeneity due to cell sources. Unpredictable biological interactions. Batch-to-batch differences. Enhanced nanocarrier functionality/specificity.	Improved cell culture techniques. Predictive molecular modeling and simulation. Controlled nanocarrier production via microfluidics. Surface engineering, genetic modifications, molecular tethering strategies.
Polysaccharides		
Alginate	Variability in alginate source/purity. Gelation process control. Encapsulation efficiency variability.	Advanced chromatography for purification. Microfluidics for consistent gel bead formation. Advanced sonication/emulsification.
Chitosan	Molecular weight influences properties. Degree of deacetylation influences properties. Replicating desired structures is challenging. Crosslinking variability affects stability. Uniform surface properties are challenging.	Advanced chromatographic techniques to standardize molecular weight. Spectroscopy for precise deacetylation. High-resolution microscopy and automated synthesis. Advanced controlled crosslinking techniques. Advanced surface characterization.
Hyaluronic acid	Variability in sources. Consistent molecular weight is crucial.	Microbial synthesis of HA for consistency. Real-time molecular weight monitoring.
Dextran	Variability in molecular weight distribution. Branching variation affects behavior. Functional group variation. Achieving consistent size/morphology is challenging.	Controlled polymerization methods. Detailed structure analysis via spectroscopy. Controlled enzymatic/chemical modifications. Microfluidics for controlled and reproducible nanosystem generation.

The exploration of endogenous proteins such as albumin in drug delivery is growing due to their biocompatibility and enhanced pharmacokinetics. However, the translation of albumin-based carriers is intricate due to challenges in modification and resultant variability [102]. The complexity arises from albumin's tendency to undergo conformational changes and the presence of a single free thiol group that is reactive under physiological conditions, complicating the controlled modification. Additionally, albumin's multiple drug-binding sites pose a challenge for achieving specific drug-to-protein ratios [103–105]. Methods such as covalent linkage and encapsulation are used for drug attachment to albumin [106], requiring precision to maintain albumin's integrity, and inconsistencies in these processes can lead to variations in drug loading and reproducibility [107]. While albumin is naturally benign, modifications can potentially induce immune reactions, impacting its biocompatibility, binding affinities, biodistribution, and pharmacokinetics, thereby posing a risk of undermining its inherent benefits [104,108]. Such modifications and variability in drug release kinetics can influence drug efficacy, plasma levels, and safety [109,110]. Utilizing high-resolution techniques and computational modeling can provide structural insights and predict interaction behaviors in biological settings, helping in refining drug loading and streamlining the design process [111–114]. Scaling from the lab to the industrial level can impact product quality and characteristics in albumin-based systems, and the complexity of albumin modification challenges the reproducibility [102,115]. Implementing microfluidic devices [116,117], utilizing standardized albumin sources such as rHSA [118], and employing automated synthesis platforms can enhance reproducibility by ensuring consistent reactions and minimizing variability and contamination [119]. The incorporation of sensors and analytical tools for real-time feedback and continuous monitoring of synthesis parameters further ensures product consistency [120–122]. The complexity and need for precise reproducibility in albumin-based delivery systems pose significant challenges, but technological advancements, from high-resolution analyses to automation, combined with strategic design, address these challenges [54,123], paving the way for broader clinical adoption.

Ferritin-based PNPs show promise for personalized medicine due to their encapsulation abilities but face translation challenges stemming from the complexity and reproducibility of assembly [124–126]. Notably, ferritin assembly is governed by both pH and ionic strength, which exert their influence through the modulation of amino acid ionization states and subunit interactivity, respectively [125,127–129]. Variations in pH alter the protonation state of amino acids at the subunit interfaces, consequently affecting their charge and dictating the electrostatic landscape critical for subunit alignment and stabilization. Ionic strength contributes to this regulation by screening these electrostatic charges; elevated ionic strength can shield repulsive interactions, thereby promoting assembly, whereas diminished ionic strength may not provide adequate shielding, potentially leading to disassembly [125,130]. This delicate balance of physicochemical conditions is essential for the proper biological functioning of ferritin, as it dictates both the structural integrity and iron-storage capacity of the complex. Therefore, precise control of pH and ionic strength is critical due to ferritin's conformational plasticity, and deviations can lead to irregular nanoparticles affecting drug delivery and therapeutic outcomes [129]. Standard assembly/disassembly methods and advanced spectroscopic techniques are pivotal for maintaining conditions and understanding ferritin conformational transitions [131,132]. Modifications to optimize encapsulation can disrupt self-assembly and affect size, thus impacting pharmacokinetics and pharmacodynamics [59,133,134]. Standardized modification protocols, including directed evolution and genetic fusion, are crucial for maintaining consistency [135]. The inherent size variability of ferritin nanoparticles poses further challenges [136], necessitating advanced separation methods and size-exclusion techniques to ensure uniform therapeutic outcomes [137]. Real-time monitoring and advanced characterization techniques such as cryo-electron microscopy provide insights into structures, aiding in addressing polydispersity [138]. Integration of technology advancements such as molecular dynamics simulations offers perspectives on ferritin assembly behavior, aiding in addressing the polydispersity [128,139] for informed design. A comprehensive approach focusing on control and standardization can help overcome challenges and realize ferritin's clinical potential in personalized medicine.

Virus-like particles (VLPs) use the infectious properties of viruses for therapeutic delivery, relying on complex recombinant DNA technology [13], and face inherent production variability. Advanced bioinformatics tools can refine the integration of foreign DNA [140,141], reducing genetic risks and enabling exact cellular condition control, assisted by modern bioreactors and real-time monitoring [65]. These innovations, along with high-throughput screening and synthetic biology, can mitigate biological system variability and genetic instability, promoting consistent VLP manufacturing [141–143]. However, purifying VLPs is complex due to their similarity to host proteins and size variation. Variations in purification methods can affect VLP yield and characteristics [144], possibly causing inconsistent therapeutic results. Nanotechnology and advanced filtration [145,146], coupled with real-time monitoring and cutting-edge spectroscopy [147–149], address these challenges by distinguishing VLPs from impurities and ensuring structural integrity. A deeper understanding of fundamental biological processes and targeted interventions, backed by advancements in technology and knowledge, are crucial for developing more efficient and reliable production strategies for VLP delivery systems.

Nanodiscs (NDs), stabilized by membrane scaffold proteins (MSPs), are discoidal structures apt for studying membrane proteins and delivering bioactive agents due to their biomimetic nature [29,30]. However, their clinical application is hindered by challenges in the complex, multi-step assembly process and reproducibility. The assembly involves the self-assembly of phospholipids and MSPs, and the correct protein-to-lipid ratio is crucial for ND integrity and function [150]. Factors such as lipid type, MSP variant, and assembly conditions necessitate optimization and significantly impact the assembly complexity and reproducibility [150,151], which are essential for complying with strict pharmaceutical regulations. Minor variations could alter ND properties, affecting their in vivo behavior and therapeutic efficacy, leading to batch variability and translational challenges. Microfluidic automation [152], real-time monitoring [153], and design strategies, such as molecular dynamics simulations [154–156] can address assembly complexity and enhance understanding of ND behavior. The scalability of ND production is pivotal, with continuous flow synthesis being a potential solution to maintain quality and meet regulatory demands for manufacturing consistency, as traditional batch processes introduce variability and are challenging to scale [157,158]. Efficient detergent-removal strategies and the exploration of biocompatible, biodegradable detergents are vital to mitigate toxicity concerns and simplify post-assembly purification [159–161]. In conclusion, overcoming the challenges in assembly complexity, reproducibility, and scalability is crucial to harness the full potential of NDs in innovative therapeutic delivery systems.

Silk fibroin (SF) and gelatin (GA) have been extensively researched for their potential in biomimetic delivery systems, owing to their biocompatibility and adjustable degradation rates, essential for in vivo nanoparticle application, especially in drug delivery [72–74,162]. However, translational challenges arise from their inherent complexity and the associated reproducibility issues in nanoparticle fabrication. For SF, clinical application is hindered by product heterogeneity arising from variability in silk sources and fibroin properties [163]. Advanced genetic engineering tools, such as CRISPR/Cas systems, and standardized fibroin extraction methods can help overcome such variability, ensuring consistent quality and properties essential for drug delivery [164–166]. Similarly, GA faces variability and reproducibility challenges due to differences in source animals and extraction methods [167–169]. High-throughput screening techniques and process standardization [170–172], including controlled crosslinking conditions and microfluidic platforms [171–174], are crucial for maintaining consistency in nanoparticle production. These enhancements, along with computational models predicting interactions between SF or GA and encapsulated drugs, contribute to achieving optimal and consistent biological performance [175–177]. Thus, standardized sourcing, purification, and fabrication procedures coupled with a comprehensive understanding of their impacts are imperative for the successful clinical translation of these biomimetic systems.

Extracellular vesicles (EVs) are notable for their potential in targeted therapeutic delivery and have gained prominence in biomedical research due to their capacity to transfer cellular information. However, their clinical transition is impeded by challenges related to their production, heterogeneity, scalability, and stability [178,179]. EVs, originating from cell cultures, play roles in cellular communication and waste management but exhibit considerable variability in size, content, and origin, complicating manufacturing and impacting therapeutic predictability and reproducibility [180]. Controlling this variability is crucial and can be achieved using single-vesicle analysis techniques, such as nanoscale flow cytometry, and potentially through synthetic biology approaches to ensure uniform EV production [178,181–183]. Scalability remains a significant challenge, with existing methods such as ultracentrifugation being inefficient and inducing structural alterations in vesicles [184]. The introduction of novel technologies such as bioreactors and microfluidic platforms has revolutionized EV production by optimizing cell conditions and enhancing yield and process efficiency [185–188]. The stability of EVs is paramount, with external factors impacting their functionality and safety. Advanced lyophilization, nano-encapsulation, and cryoprotectants have been employed to enhance EV shelf life, protect vesicle integrity, and prevent aggregation [189–191]. The application of artificial intelligence and machine learning can expedite and standardize EV analysis for quality control [192]. Despite their immense therapeutic potential, the realization of EVs necessitates advancements in their biology, production optimization, and rigorous quality control to address the prevailing challenges.

Cell membrane-derived nanocarriers (CMDNs), particularly from erythrocytes, present a promising frontier in targeted therapeutic delivery due to their biological stealth characteristics [20,26,27]. Nonetheless, the complexities in isolation, modification, and loading processes, coupled with the need for rigorous quality control and reproducibility, impede their clinical translation [193]. The isolation of CMDNs is intricate, involving donor cell selection, cell lysis, and the removal of cellular components, and each stage introduces potential variability, affecting product consistency [194]. Donor cell selection, influenced by age, health, and genetics, affects nanocarrier characteristics and performance. Implementations of microfluidic technologies, automation, and the utilization of 'cell banks' with optimal donor cells can standardize processes and diminish variability [152,195]. Additionally, post-isolation engineering of CMDNs for enhanced stability, circulation, and targeted delivery introduces further complexity. Controlled conditions and precision are requisite for consistent modifications across batches, facilitated by techniques such as atomic layer deposition and bio-orthogonal chemistries [196,197], with real-time monitoring ensuring uniformity [198,199]. Rigorous validation is vital for confirming drug loading and release profiles, crucial for therapeutic efficacy. The need for stringent quality control amid varied CMDN properties necessitates comprehensive quality control approaches. Techniques such as nanoparticle tracking analysis and dynamic light scattering are fundamental for characterizing CMDN parameters [200]. However, inherent biological variability and multifaceted production processes exacerbate the challenges in capturing CMDN diversity. Feedback-controlled systems, such as process analytical technology (PAT) [201], and computational models leveraging molecular dynamics and machine learning provide predictive insights into nanocarrier behavior and aid in optimizing production parameters [202,203]. Overcoming the production complexities, variability, and quality control challenges is pivotal for the clinical realization of CMDNs.

Polysaccharides such as alginate, chitosan, hyaluronic acid (HA), and dextran are prominent in nanoparticle synthesis due to their biocompatibility and safety [204]. However, their natural origins introduce variability in source, purification, and modification, yielding heterogeneity in nanoparticle properties which can impact the stability and reproducibility of delivery systems. The diverse sources, with variations in biological, chemical, and physical properties, influence polysaccharide properties, such as molecular weight and degree of deacetylation, thereby affecting nanoparticle attributes such as size, charge, stability, and, ultimately, therapeutic efficacy [205–207]. Modern extraction techniques and purification processes can mitigate batch variability, while sensor-based technologies and process adjustments aim to enhance consistency [208–211]. However, residual contaminants and modifications to polysaccharides amplify heterogeneity issues, impacting solubility, degradation, and drug loading. The employment of machine learning and artificial intelligence optimizes modification parameters, ensuring consistent processes and reduced product variability. The inherent variability in polysaccharide-based nanoparticles alters biological interactions and poses challenges in clinical translation, affecting pharmacokinetics, biodistribution, and therapeutic efficacy [212]. Advanced characterization methods and real-time monitoring technologies, such as PAT and digital twins of the production process, are crucial to control heterogeneity and enhance reproducibility [201,213]. The inherent complexity and reproducibility challenges of polysaccharides necessitate the development of standardized methods for extraction, purification, and modification, as well as advanced characterization techniques. Integrating technological advancements and innovative design strategies is pivotal for developing consistent and effective polysaccharide-based delivery systems, essential for bridging the gap from laboratory to clinical application.

3.2. Stability and Longevity

The quest for the stability and longevity of BDSs in physiological conditions is a complex journey marked by numerous challenges (Table 3). These systems, while crafted to mimic the natural biological environment, still encounter substantial difficulties in withstanding rapid clearance or degradation within the human body. This factor reduces their therapeutic window, undermining their effectiveness in achieving the desired clinical outcomes.

Table 3. An overview of the stability, longevity challenges, and prospective solutions related to various biomimetic delivery systems.

BDS	Stability and Longevity Challenges	Prospective Solutions
Liposomes	Sensitivity to oxidation and hydrolysis. Fusion/aggregation in serum. Rapid clearance from circulation.	Liposome coating (e.g., PEGylation). Incorporation of cholesterol. Antioxidant inclusion.
Protein-Based NPs		
Albumin nanoparticles	Instability in harsh environments (e.g., acidic pH). Enzymatic degradation.	Cross-linking of albumin molecules. Encapsulation with protective polymers. Surface modifications.
Protein-based nanocages	Structural disintegration at non-optimal conditions. Immune recognition and clearance.	Chemical surface modifications. Incorporation of stability enhancing ligands. Fusion with other stable proteins.
VLPs	Potential immunogenicity. Stability issues due to dynamic protein structures.	Genetic modifications. Encapsulation within protective matrices. Surface modifications to reduce immunogenicity.
NDs	Sensitivity to physiologic conditions, leading to structural alteration. Potential immune recognition.	Use of stable lipids. Protective protein inclusion. Surface modification.
Fibroin and Gelatin	Sensitivity to temperature and pH. Enzymatic degradation in vivo.	Chemical cross-linking. Incorporation into composite materials. Coating with protective polymers.
EVs	Susceptibility to clearance mechanisms. Sensitivity to physiologic conditions leading to vesicle disruption.	Surface modifications. PEGylation. Encapsulation within biomaterials. Cryopreservation techniques.
CMDNs	Potential immunogenicity. Sensitivity to in vivo degradation mechanisms.	Immune camouflage techniques. Genetic modifications for enhanced stability. Surface modifications.
Polysaccharides		
Alginate	Rapid degradation in vivo. Instability in the presence of divalent cations.	Cross-linking with divalent cations. Incorporation into composite materials. Layer-by-layer assembly.
Chitosan	Solubility issues in neutral and basic pH. Rapid degradation in vivo.	Chemical modifications for solubility. Cross-linking. Layer-by-layer assembly.
Hyaluronic acid	Rapid enzymatic degradation in vivo. Instability under harsh conditions.	Derivatization and cross-linking. Hydrogel formulations. Composite materials incorporation.
Dextran	Sensitivity to oxidative conditions. Enzymatic degradation.	Cross-linking. Encapsulation within protective matrices. Blend with other stable polymers.

Liposomes are inherently unstable due to the susceptibility of phospholipids to oxidation and hydrolysis, affecting their structural integrity and function [214,215]. Oxidation leads to the formation of cytotoxic peroxidation by-products, posing substantial challenges to clinical applications [52]. Antioxidants such as vitamin E and ferulic acid can neutralize oxidative damage, and their uniform distribution is facilitated by advanced techniques such as high-pressure homogenization [49,216,217]. The incorporation of stable phospholipids such as sphingomyelin and cholesterol can further enhance membrane stability [218]. Conversely, hydrolysis disrupts liposomal structure and compromises the stability and the encapsulated agents' efficacy in physiological environments [219–222]. Encapsulation with lipid-polymer conjugates such as PEG-PE and emerging techniques such as electrospinning can mitigate hydrolytic degradation [223,224]. Utilizing hydrolytically stable phospholipid analogs and designing liposomes with interdigitated lipid phases or incorporating ceramides can also bolster resistance to hydrolytic degradation [225]. Therefore, a profound understanding of phospholipid oxidation and hydrolysis is essential for developing stabilization strategies, which are crucial for liposomes' successful clinical translation.

Albumin-based BDSs, revered for their biocompatibility and molecule-binding potential, encounter numerous challenges in clinical transition due to their interactions with various bodily substances, leading to aggregation and premature therapeutic release [109,110,226]. Such interactions risk sub-optimal outcomes and affect pharmacokinetics and efficacy as they are quickly cleared by the immune system. Furthermore, enzymatic actions in the body can jeopardize their structural integrity and result in variable drug levels and adverse events [102]. Storage and transport also present challenges, including denaturation, oxidation, and aggregation [111,227–229]. Generally, protein-based BDS are highly sensitive to environmental conditions such as temperature fluctuations and light exposure, which can significantly compromise their structural integrity and stability [228,230]. Elevated temperatures may cause denaturation and aggregation of the biomimetic components while exposure to light, particularly UV light, can initiate oxidative reactions and photoinduced damage that further destabilize the protein structure. These changes not only lead to altered pharmacokinetics and reduced drug-binding efficacy, but also raise safety concerns due to the potential for increased immunogenicity. Thus, maintaining controlled storage and transport conditions is critical to preserve the functionality of protein-based BDSs. Several strategies have been developed to mitigate these challenges, including nanoencapsulation and PEGylation to prevent premature interactions and extend circulation half-life [231–233]. Modifying nanoparticle size and shape, utilizing enzyme-inhibiting coatings, and employing cryopreservation and lyophilization address issues related to immune evasion, enzymatic degradation, and structural integrity [234,235]. Implementations of antioxidants, hydrogel encapsulation, and optimized buffer solutions offer protection against various stresses and maintain albumin structure [236,237]. Molecular imprinting and stimuli-responsive elements have also been utilized for improved drug loading and controlled delivery [238–241]. Hence, integrating these methodologies is pivotal in addressing the complications associated with albumin-based BDSs, enabling enhanced therapeutic delivery.

Protein-based nanocages, led by ferritin, are a breakthrough in theranostic devices. They promise innovative drug delivery systems based on biomimetic principles. However, the journey to clinical use presents challenges, including structural disruption in varying in vivo environments, which might trigger unintended drug release [129]. These nanocages also risk denaturation, aggregation, or deactivation under certain conditions, necessitating specialized storage solutions. While ferritin's capability to traverse biological barriers is notable, controlling sustained drug release remains complex [127,242], with modifications for targeted delivery potentially introducing immunogenicity [243,244]. Ensuring uniformity in properties and drug potency during clinical manufacturing is imperative. Addressing these challenges demands a multidisciplinary approach, employing advancements in material science, innovative storage technologies, molecular engineering for precise drug release, advanced bioconjugation, computational simulations, high-resolution analytics, and machine learning for real-time monitoring [245,246]. This integrated methodology, combining the expertise of nanotechnologists, biologists, and pharmacologists, is crucial for unleashing the full potential of ferritin-based systems in targeted oncology.

VLPs are renowned for their precise control, defined structures, and adjustable immunogenicity, marking them as ideal candidates for targeted delivery platforms. However, their stability is compromised in demanding physiological environments due to factors such as pH fluctuations and the presence of proteases, causing potential premature therapeutic release and impacting targeting capabilities [140,247–249]. The inherent immunogenicity of VLPs, while advantageous for vaccines, poses a significant challenge for drug delivery, as it can provoke immune responses leading to rapid clearance and possible side effects [12]. Addressing these issues involves incorporating pH-responsive modifications and protease-resistant motifs to enhance stability [250–253], leveraging nanotechnology and surface modifications to augment targeting precision [254–256], and developing innovative strategies including "stealth" VLPs and biomimetic coatings to balance immunogenicity [257,258]. Such developments are pivotal in evolving VLPs into efficient, stable therapeutic delivery systems poised to yield enhanced clinical outcomes.

NDs serve as versatile drug delivery platforms but are hampered by challenges stemming from their amphiphilic lipid nature, causing instability in size, shape, and functional efficacy. Factors including temperature, pH, and ionic strength can induce lipid phase transitions and nanodisc aggregation, potentially causing premature drug release and reducing therapeutic efficacy [259,260]. The vulnerability of NDs to oxidation and enzymatic degradation poses significant concerns regarding their longevity, and interaction with serum proteins can further induce instability [261]. Additionally, the formation of a protein corona can lead to swift immune clearance and can elicit immune responses, thereby raising safety concerns [262]. Strategies to enhance ND stability include reinforcing the lipid layer, incorporating antioxidants, PEGylation, and developing stimuli-responsive NDs, all of which are crucial to maintaining ND biocompatibility and therapeutic potency [29,40,263,264]. The advancement in these strategies holds the potential to revolutionize ND-based drug delivery systems.

Fibroin and gelatin, due to their biocompatibility and biodegradability, are widely used in biomimetic delivery systems but face challenges related to stability and longevity under physiological conditions [265,266]. These proteins are susceptible to enzymatic degradation and pH variations, which affect their structural integrity and could lead to premature therapeutic release. Additionally, traditional sterilization methods can compromise their structural effectiveness for drug delivery. Several strategies are being developed to overcome these challenges. Chemical crosslinking and blending with synthetic polymers enhance resistance to degradation and improve mechanical properties [267–270]. Integration of bioinert nanoparticles and lyophilization offers stability and controlled drug release [271,272]. Innovations such as pH-responsive coatings [273,274], coacervation- and electrospinning-optimized encapsulation technologies [275–278], and novel fabrication and sterilization methods, including supercritical carbon dioxide-based NP formation methodologies and cold plasma sterilization [71,279], are being explored to maintain material integrity and safety. These advancements reinforce the significance of fibroin and gelatin in evolving biomedical applications.

EVs exhibit promising capabilities for targeted therapies due to their unique biological functionality but face substantial challenges in maintaining stability and longevity [190,280–282]. Physiological factors, along with difficulties in isolation, purification, and modification, can alter EV structure and hinder therapeutic delivery capabilities [77–79,282,283]. The unstable nature of EVs necessitates advancements in methodology to preserve functionality during storage, transport, and therapeutic loading, with issues such as sensitivity to freeze–thaw cycles and long-term storage further complicating their utilization [191,284]. Strategies such as encapsulation technologies [285,286], surface modifications [287], and advanced isolation methods are being developed to address these challenges [187,188,288]. Additionally, innovations in cryoprotectants, packaging, and transport solutions are being explored to enhance EV stability and integrity [235,289]. The advancement of these strategies, coupled with interdisciplinary collaboration, is pivotal for harnessing the therapeutic potential of EVs in modern medicine.

In biomimetic delivery, CMDNs, particularly those derived from red blood cells (RBCs), display significant stability and longevity challenges and can trigger immune responses leading to premature clearance due to alterations during the extraction and modification processes [290]. The mononuclear phagocyte system (MPS) recognizes altered RBC-derived nanocarriers, reducing their bloodstream longevity [291]. Solutions including surface camouflage (immune evasion through surface engineering with biocompatible polymers such as polyethylene glycol (PEG) or proteins that mimic the natural RBC surface), synthetic RBC mimetics, and the controlled release (response to pH, temperature, or particular biomolecules) of immunosuppressive agents are being explored to mitigate these challenges and prolong circulation [292,293]. Furthermore, preserving structural integrity and maintaining optimal stability and efficacy during storage and transport is crucial, with enhancements via nanoengineering, refined cryopreservation, lyophilization methods, and innovative preservatives being pivotal [294–296]. The development of CMDNs necessitates a multidisciplinary approach, combining biotechnology, material science, and pharmacology, to optimize the stability, longevity, and controlled-release kinetics of RBC-derived nanocarriers, heralding advancements in therapeutic delivery systems.

Polysaccharide-based carriers such as alginate, chitosan, hyaluronic acid, and dextran exhibit unique stability issues. Alginate and chitosan are notable for their biocompatibility and biodegradability but are susceptible to instability due to their hydrophilic nature, resulting in vulnerability to environmental factors such as pH and ionic strength [297,298]. Chemical modifications and protective coatings can address these vulnerabilities, improving their resilience. Hyaluronic acid faces stability issues due to susceptibility to enzymatic degradation by hyaluronidases, affecting its longevity and therapeutic effect [299]. The introduction of enzyme inhibitors or structural modifications can improve its resistance. Dextran, while soluble and biocompatible, is sensitive to microbial contamination, affecting its long-term stability [299]. Enhanced sterilization, incorporation of antimicrobial agents, and encapsulation techniques can mitigate this susceptibility. The formulation of these polysaccharides into nanoparticles or microspheres offers improved stability and controlled therapeutic release, symbolizing a promising development in creating robust delivery platforms [204,211,300]. Furthermore, the profound potential of polysaccharide-based BDSs is notably challenged by inherent stability issues. The integration of technological advancements, innovative design, chemical modifications, and protective strategies is crucial for realizing their full therapeutic capabilities, promoting the development of more resilient and efficient delivery platforms. Despite the revolutionary prospects of these delivery systems in drug delivery, stability and longevity challenges in physiological conditions, storage, and transport require continuous research, development, and optimization of fabrication and handling processes. This emphasizes the need for stabilizing agents and optimized procedures to enhance the clinical translatability of these promising systems.

3.3. Efficacy and Safety

The efficacy and safety of therapeutic agents, especially BDSs that emulate natural biological entities, are fundamental to their clinical utility. These BDSs are anticipated to provide efficacy comparable or superior to existing treatments with a satisfactory safety profile, but their clinical translation encounters substantial challenges such as unpredictable in vivo behavior, potential off-target effects, and unexpected immune responses [301]. Comprehensive evaluation, including preclinical and clinical studies of pharmacokinetics, pharmacodynamics, and immunogenicity, is pivotal to establish therapeutic validity.

Liposome-based BDSs, noted for their ability to encapsulate diverse agents, promise enhanced drug solubility and targeted delivery [91]. However, intrinsic challenges exist, impacting therapeutic efficacy and safety [302]. Variations in entrapment efficiency can result in sub-optimal drug concentrations, affecting therapeutic outcomes. Challenges with drug release kinetics, premature or delayed, can compromise drug effectiveness [303]. Rapid clearance and degradation in biological fluids and interactions with serum proteins, enzymes, or immune cells diminish drug bioavailability [301]. Inaccurate targeting and off-target interactions can necessitate higher doses, inducing potential side effects. Liposomal formulations, especially those modified with targeting ligands, may elicit immune responses, ranging from allergies to severe anaphylaxis [304,305], and certain liposomal components can exhibit toxicity. The variability in the enhanced permeability and retention (EPR) effect introduces an additional complexity [306]. Rapid drug release due to destabilization presents overdose risks [307]. Despite the potential of liposomal systems, these multifaceted concerns necessitate meticulous consideration and ongoing refinement.

The clinical translation of liposomal technologies, exemplified by pioneering formulations such as Doxil® and AmBisome®, highlights the innovation in therapeutic delivery. Doxil®, a paradigmatic FDA-approved nanodrug, utilized adaptive trial designs for dynamic dose adjustments, balancing efficacy with safety and showcasing the importance of real-time data-based refinements [308]. AmBisome® distinguished itself with a meticulous comparative approach in clinical trials, revealing its superior therapeutic index in antifungal treatments [309,310]. The imperative theme is the necessity of adaptable and flexible trial designs; MAMS, or multi-arm multi-stage designs are a novel approach in clinical trial methodology, allowing for multiple treatments to be tested simultaneously against a common control group [311,312]. This design provides flexibility to add or drop treatment arms based on interim results. Therefore, MAMS designs are efficient by allowing simultaneous evaluations of various formulations, accelerating development and optimizing resource allocation. In the post-approval phase, the integration of real-world evidence (RWE) and stringent post-marketing surveillance are crucial, providing insights into long-term safety, rare side effects, adherence patterns, and therapeutic outcomes in diverse populations [313,314]. This approach, drawing from the foundational successes of Doxil® and AmBisome®, informs and refines subsequent clinical trials and therapeutic guidelines. The clinical success of liposomal technologies underscores the essential role of innovative trial designs, adaptability, and ongoing evaluation in advancing liposomal therapeutics from experimental to established clinical treatments.

PNPs, encompassing a diverse set of biomaterials such as Albumin nanoparticles, protein-based nanocages (exemplified by ferritin), VLPs, NDs, fibroin, and gelatin, are advancing to the forefront of drug delivery research due to their inherent biocompatibility, biodegradability, and potential for precision-targeted therapeutic delivery. For Albumin nanoparticles, despite being synthesized from endogenous proteins, the inherent risk lies in the potential elicitation of immunogenic reactions, stemming from slight alterations or impurities during the nanoparticle formation process [315]; moreover, their inherent stability is also a concern, as degradation can substantially affect drug release kinetics, leading to suboptimal therapeutic effects [102,229]. Turning to protein-based nanocages, specifically ferritin, they display the dual challenges of potentially inconsistent drug loading efficiencies, which directly impact the therapeutic dosing [127,316], and a heightened sensitivity to environmental factors such as pH or temperature; this sensitivity might result in unintended, premature drug release [127,129]. Additionally, their natural role in iron storage poses concerns over inadvertently disrupting iron homeostasis in the body [317]. VLPs, while ingeniously designed to lack viral genetic material, are not without concerns, primarily rooted in the potential of evoking systemic immune reactions. Their complex synthesis pathway also introduces the risk of production inconsistencies and, albeit rarely, a shadow of concern regarding potential mutations, raising the specter of inadvertently reintroducing pathogenic properties [12,318]. NDs, in their design, carry lipid-based structures, which render them susceptible to oxidation or hydrolysis, challenges further exacerbated by potential size inconsistencies that can lead to variable biodistribution, affecting their therapeutic reach and efficacy [150]. Finally, the naturally-derived PNPs, fibroin and gelatin, introduce their own set of challenges: their natural sourcing can lead to variability in nanoparticle properties between batches, potential toxicity stemming from the use of chemical crosslinkers, and the concern of rapid degradation in physiological settings, which can obstruct the controlled, sustained release of therapeutic agents [162,167,173,319]. In summation, while the promise of PNPs in revolutionizing therapeutic delivery is undeniable, their path is fraught with multifaceted scientific challenges that mandate rigorous research and optimization before clinical fruition.

EVs and CMDNs, including exosomes, microvesicles, and apoptotic bodies, are prominent for their therapeutic delivery potential due to their biocompatibility and capability for targeted delivery, offering advantages over synthetic carriers. Nevertheless, integrating them into clinical paradigms requires rigorous evaluation of therapeutic efficacy and safety [320,321]. Achieving site-specific delivery is challenging, potentially leading to off-target effects [322]. Stability during storage is vital, with factors such as temperature fluctuations compromising therapeutic potential [190]. Immunogenicity is a significant concern; while autologous sources mitigate risks, large-scale production from allogenic or xenogenic sources amplifies associated risks [323]. Batch-to-batch variability and contamination risks during isolation compound safety concerns [324]. The potential for horizontal gene transfer by exosomes could inadvertently transfer detrimental genes. As the biomedical field progresses with the rise of EVs and CMDNs, there's an escalating need for reconfigured clinical trial frameworks to address the unique challenges associated with these therapies, particularly due to variable cargo loading efficiencies influenced by variations in vesicular dimensions, intricate lipidomic architectures, and membrane biomechanics [325,326]. Adaptive clinical trial designs become indispensable, allowing for modifiable responses based on interim findings and leveraging real-time pharmacokinetic feedback to optimize dosages [327,328]. The MAMS designs are noteworthy, enabling concurrent evaluations to optimize therapeutic precision [329]. Integration of real-world data is crucial to understand the longitudinal stability and efficacy in real clinical settings, balancing trial controls with patient variability. Safety evaluations should consider the diverse origins of EVs, employing basket and umbrella trial structures to assess immunogenicity risks across different patient cohorts [330]. Sequential multiple assignment randomized trial (SMART) designs, renowned for flexibility, are pivotal to counter variability and contamination threats, allowing treatment recalibrations based on evolving responses or risks [331,332]. The latent risk in exosomes mediating detrimental horizontal gene transfers demands meticulous dynamic surveillance mechanisms supported by Bayesian analytical paradigms. In conclusion, to realize the potential of EVs and cell membrane-based nanocarriers without compromising safety, clinical trial methodologies must evolve, incorporating innovative, adaptive, and rigorous designs.

Polysaccharide-based BDSs are renowned for their biocompatibility, biodegradability, and functional modification capacities, making them prominent in drug delivery research [83,204,211,300]. However, alginate exhibits challenges including burst release patterns and syneresis, impacting optimal drug concentrations and release kinetics and posing potential overdose concerns [333,334]. Contaminants in alginate can also provoke inflammatory responses. Chitosan's solubility is pH-dependent, affecting its efficacy in diverse bodily microenvironments, and variations in its molecular weight distribution can lead to discrepancies in drug loading and release profiles [298]. Its biodegradation kinetics can leave residual fragments in vivo, raising safety concerns including rare allergic reactions. HA's propensity for rapid enzymatic degradation limits its suitability for sustained drug delivery, and its purity is crucial if derived from animal sources to avoid immune responses or pathogen transmission [299]. Dextran, though versatile, presents challenges, with variable molecular weights affecting delivery profiles, and has rare instances of induced anaphylactic reactions associated with higher molecular weights [205,335].

A holistic assessment of polysaccharide-based BDSs necessitates a transition from traditional to more innovative, flexible clinical trial designs, with adaptive designs becoming pivotal for modifications including dose titrations based on interim analyses, addressing biomimetics' unpredictability [308,327,328]. The efficient MAMS design allows simultaneous evaluations of diverse formulations, swiftly sidelining suboptimal candidates, while platform trials provide a dynamic scaffold for continuous comparison of polysaccharide derivatives [312,328,329]. The specificity of umbrella and basket trials is invaluable for discerning patient subpopulations benefiting from particular formulations, enhancing precision medicine [330]. Integration of RWE is crucial, offering insights into broader clinical scenarios and assessing the real-world effectiveness of polysaccharide-based BDSs [314]. Incorporating patient feedback in patient-centric trials facilitates comprehensive assessments of biocompatibility and efficacy [336]. However, the employment of such innovative designs involves complexities; they require sophisticated statistical methodologies, continuous monitoring, and transparent, ethical decision-making. In summary, the clinical validation of polysaccharide-based BDS systems is intrinsically linked to the strategic employment of these innovative, nuanced trial designs in therapeutic applications.

In conclusion, while each biomimetic delivery system carries unique opportunities, they all share common challenges in terms of their in vivo behavior, safety, and efficacy profiles. To enable their clinical translation, a comprehensive understanding of these challenges and the development of strategies to address them is crucial. This should include extensive preclinical and clinical evaluation of their pharmacokinetics, pharmacodynamics, and potential for inducing immunogenicity. The successful resolution of these challenges will unlock the therapeutic potential of these biomimetic delivery systems, improving patient outcomes across a range of diseases and conditions.

3.4. Regulatory and Ethical Challenges

The clinical implementation journey of BDSs encompasses intricate regulatory necessities and significant ethical considerations, often aligning with advanced therapy medicinal products (ATMPs) or nanomedicines, requiring specialized regulatory pathways [337,338]. The diverse forms of BDSs, such as liposomes, albumin, CMDNs, and various polysaccharides, necessitate the formulation of innovative regulatory guidelines and consistent dialogue between researchers and regulatory entities to navigate the clinical translation pathway. Ethical considerations become paramount, especially with human-derived biomimetic materials such as EVs or RBCs [339], necessitating thorough informed consent processes, strict privacy protection measures, and equitable access considerations encompassing production cost, pricing, and healthcare infrastructure disparities. While addressing technical challenges is crucial, ethical concerns require equal emphasis, requiring a multidimensional approach to harmonize scientific innovation, regulatory compliance, and ethical responsibility in the clinical translation of biomimetic delivery systems.

Liposomes require intricate characterization due to their diverse properties, raising regulatory and informed consent complexities [46], and their predisposition to degradation necessitates stabilization efforts. PNPs such as albumin and ferritin pose risks of adverse immune reactions, batch variability, and contamination, particularly from animal-derived proteins, which elevate ethical concerns and can limit acceptability among certain demographics [340]. VLPs, although non-pathogenic, invoke apprehension about potential immunogenic responses and necessitate elevated consent standards due to uncertainties surrounding their long-term effects [64]. NDs, being relatively novel, face challenges in standardization and harbor unresolved ethical considerations. EVs present hurdles in achieving reproducible isolation and purification protocols and pose potential risks in transmitting undesired biomolecules, emphasizing the need for transparency [77–79,323]. CMDNs face challenges in preserving native membrane characteristics while balancing potential immunogenic reactions, especially when sourced from human tissues. Polysaccharides bring forth challenges related to consistency and contamination [211], with their derivation methods potentially conflicting with the preferences or beliefs of certain patient groups, thus intensifying ethical dilemmas.

The emerging BDSs epitomize the integration of nature's complex designs with human technological developments and have brought to the forefront an urgent necessity for advanced regulatory and ethical frameworks tailored to their nuances (Table 4). Historically, the edifice of regulatory standards has been anchored on principles of safety, efficacy, and quality, further buttressed by ethical cornerstones such as informed consent, equitability, and transparency. These tried-and-true paradigms, though effective for conventional therapeutics, grapple with the multifaceted challenges inherent to BDS. A hallmark feature of these systems is their biological variability and complexity, which, while promising targeted precision, complicates the path to achieving consistent reproducibility, i.e., a gold standard in therapeutic evaluations. This variability is compounded by BDSs' novel and potentially multifactorial mechanisms of action, which can diverge significantly from traditional therapeutics and demand a deeper level of scrutiny. Further, owing to their intimate mimicry of biological systems, BDSs introduce the possibility of unprecedented interactions with native biological entities, necessitating rigorous preemptive assessment and monitoring. On the ethical front, the material source variability of BDSs introduces intricate layers of concerns, spanning from informed consent and potential exploitation to uncharted territories of long-term biocompatibility and unforeseen systemic effects. The sophistication and innovation underlying BDSs, while promising groundbreaking therapeutic solutions, might also inadvertently escalate production and distribution costs, thus catalyzing debates on equitable accessibility, especially in socioeconomically diverse settings. As the biomedical community stands at this crossroads, a forward-thinking regulatory strategy is of paramount importance. This strategy should champion adaptive oversight mechanisms, foster interdisciplinary dialogues, and advocate for harmonized global standards, ensuring that BDS innovations are not siloed but shared collaboratively. Concurrently, ethical protocols require a renaissance, one that broadens the boundaries of informed consent, deepens stakeholder participation, and relentlessly pursues transparency, ensuring that the transformative potential of BDSs is harmoniously balanced with societal, moral, and patient-centric imperatives. The dawn of biomimetic delivery systems demands a rethinking of our regulatory and ethical scaffolds. While the challenges are intricate, they present an opportunity: to shape a future where innovation flourishes within robust societal safeguards, ensuring that advancements in drug delivery truly serve humanity's best interests.

Table 4. Overall insights into regulatory and ethical challenges for BDS.

Categories	Insights
Regulatory Challenges	<ul><li>Biological variability and complexity</li><li>Achieving consistent reproducibility</li><li>Potential unprecedented interactions with biological entities</li></ul>
Regulatory Frameworks	<ul><li>Adaptive oversight mechanisms</li><li>Interdisciplinary dialogues</li><li>Harmonized global standards</li></ul>
Ethical Challenges	<ul><li>Sourcing material from sentient entities (humans/animals)</li><li>Informed consent and potential exploitation</li><li>Equitable accessibility in diverse settings</li></ul>
Ethical Frameworks	<ul><li>Broadened boundaries of informed consent</li><li>Stakeholder participation</li><li>Pursuit of transparency</li></ul>

4. Conclusions

BDSs have emerged as a transformative frontier in nanomedicine, promising unparalleled advantages in drug delivery and therapeutic modalities. These systems, rooted in the principles of self-assembly, molecular recognition, and biocompatibility, encompass a variety of platforms such as liposomes [91], PNPs [30,74,162,242,341,342], extracellular vesicles [17], and polysaccharides [300]. Their clinical applications have been praised for achievements in targeted delivery, reduced side effects, and improved therapeutic outcomes. However, the journey of these innovative delivery systems from the lab bench to the bedside is not without its hurdles. The inherent complexity of biomimetic designs poses challenges in ensuring reproducibility, a crucial factor in clinical applications. The physiological environment presents issues related to the stability and longevity of these delivery systems. Moreover, the efficacy and safety of these novel therapies, although promising, need rigorous evaluation. Beyond the technical challenges lie intricate regulatory mazes and ethical considerations that must be navigated to achieve successful clinical translation. To overcome these challenges, the scientific community has turned to various strategies. Technological innovations have been at the forefront, addressing issues of complexity and reproducibility. The exploration and integration of advanced biomaterials aim to bolster the stability and lifespan of biomimetic systems in physiological settings. Recognizing the unique properties and challenges of biomimetic delivery, there has been a push for innovative clinical trial designs that can more aptly evaluate their efficacy and safety. Furthermore, it's evident that the traditional regulatory and ethical frameworks might fall short, necessitating the evolution of these frameworks in alignment with the innovative nature of biomimetic delivery systems. Real-world case studies provide tangible evidence of these challenges and, more importantly, shed light on successful strategies and interventions that have paved the way for clinical translation. These instances not only offer insights, but also inspire confidence in the potential of biomimetic delivery systems to revolutionize healthcare.

The future holds substantial promise for the clinical translation of BDSs as advancements in understanding biological systems continue to refine the design and capabilities of BDSs. Anticipated innovations, emerging from interdisciplinary collaborations among biologists, chemists, engineers, and clinicians, will likely be more refined, efficient, and personalized, aligning with individual patient profiles for optimized outcomes. The evolving familiarity of global regulatory bodies with BDSs anticipates the establishment of more streamlined guidelines, expediting clinical translation. Initial challenges and learnings in clinical translation will be instrumental in refining subsequent iterations of BDSs for enhanced clinical application. In essence, BDSs, merging nature's design with human ingenuity, have immense potential in revolutionizing drug delivery, and despite existing challenges, the commitment of the scientific community and ongoing technological and regulatory advancements underline a future replete with potential.

Author Contributions: Conceptualization, J.W. and Z.W.; resources acquisition and analysis, W.X., W.X., Y.L., X.Q., X.C., R.L. and Z.C.; writing—original draft preparation, Z.W. and J.W.; writing—review and revision, Z.W., J.W., X.W., M.W. and B.M.; visualization, J.W.; supervision, J.W. and M.W.; project administration, J.W.; funding acquisition, Z.W. and J.W. All authors have read and agreed to the published version of the manuscript.

Funding: This research was funded by the National Natural Science Foundation of China (grant No. 82001887), Shenzhen Science and Technology Program (grant No. JCYJ20210324115003009, 202206193000001; JCYJ20220530144401004), Futian Healthcare Research Project (grant No. FTWS2022018), and the Program of 'Transverse' Research Project at Sun Yat-sen University (grant No. K2175110-007).

Institutional Review Board Statement: Not applicable.

Informed Consent Statement: Not applicable.

Data Availability Statement: Data sharing is not applicable.

Conflicts of Interest: The authors declare no conflict of interest.

References

1. Sheikhpour, M.; Barani, L.; Kasaeian, A. Biomimetics in drug delivery systems: A critical review. *J. Control. Release* **2017**, *253*, 97–109. [CrossRef]
2. Vincent, J.F.V. Biomimetics—A review. *Proc. Inst. Mech. Eng. Part H J. Eng. Med.* **2009**, *223*, 919–939. [CrossRef] [PubMed]
3. Vincent, J.F.V.; Bogatyreva, O.A.; Bogatyrev, N.R.; Bowyer, A.; Pahl, A.-K. Biomimetics: Its practice and theory. *J. R. Soc. Interface* **2006**, *3*, 471–482. [CrossRef]
4. Venkatesh, S.; Byrne, M.E.; Peppas, N.A.; Hilt, J.Z. Applications of biomimetic systems in drug delivery. *Expert Opin. Drug Deliv.* **2005**, *2*, 1085–1096. [CrossRef] [PubMed]
5. Fukuta, T.; Kogure, K. Biomimetic Nanoparticle Drug Delivery Systems to Overcome Biological Barriers for Therapeutic Applications. *Chem. Pharm. Bull.* **2022**, *70*, 334–340. [CrossRef]
6. Chen, Y.-X.; Wei, C.-X.; Lyu, Y.-Q.; Chen, H.-Z.; Jiang, G.; Gao, X.-L. Biomimetic drug-delivery systems for the management of brain diseases. *Biomater. Sci.* **2020**, *8*, 1073–1088. [CrossRef] [PubMed]

7. Chen, L.; Hong, W.; Ren, W.; Xu, T.; Qian, Z.; He, Z. Recent progress in targeted delivery vectors based on biomimetic nanoparticles. *Signal Transduct. Target. Ther.* **2021**, *6*, 225. [CrossRef]
8. Rasheed, T.; Nabeel, F.; Raza, A.; Bilal, M.; Iqbal, H.M.N. Biomimetic nanostructures/cues as drug delivery systems: A review. *Mater. Today Chem.* **2019**, *13*, 147–157. [CrossRef]
9. Zhang, M.; Du, Y.; Wang, S.; Chen, B. A Review of Biomimetic Nanoparticle Drug Delivery Systems Based on Cell Membranes. *Drug Des. Dev. Ther.* **2020**, *14*, 5495–5503. [CrossRef]
10. Chandrawati, R.; Caruso, F. Biomimetic Liposome- and Polymersome-Based Multicompartmentalized Assemblies. *Langmuir* **2012**, *28*, 13798–13807. [CrossRef]
11. Tariq, H.; Batool, S.; Asif, S.; Ali, M.; Abbasi, B.H. Virus-Like Particles: Revolutionary Platforms for Developing Vaccines Against Emerging Infectious Diseases. *Front. Microbiol.* **2022**, *12*, 790121. [CrossRef]
12. Nooraei, S.; Bahrulolum, H.; Hoseini, Z.S.; Katalani, C.; Hajizade, A.; Easton, A.J.; Ahmadian, G. Virus-like particles: Preparation, immunogenicity and their roles as nanovaccines and drug nanocarriers. *J. Nanobiotechnol.* **2021**, *19*, 59. [CrossRef] [PubMed]
13. Banskota, S.; Raguram, A.; Suh, S.; Du, S.W.; Davis, J.R.; Choi, E.H.; Wang, X.; Nielsen, S.C.; Newby, G.A.; Randolph, P.B.; et al. Engineered virus-like particles for efficient in vivo delivery of therapeutic proteins. *Cell* **2022**, *185*, 250–265.e216. [CrossRef] [PubMed]
14. Geckil, H.; Xu, F.; Zhang, X.; Moon, S.; Demirci, U. Engineering hydrogels as extracellular matrix mimics. *Nanomedicine* **2010**, *5*, 469–484. [CrossRef] [PubMed]
15. Zhang, Y.; Xu, Y.; Gao, J. The engineering and application of extracellular matrix hydrogels: A review. *Biomater. Sci.* **2023**, *11*, 3784–3799. [CrossRef] [PubMed]
16. González-Díaz, E.C.; Varghese, S. Hydrogels as Extracellular Matrix Analogs. *Gels* **2016**, *2*, 20. [CrossRef]
17. Vader, P.; Mol, E.A.; Pasterkamp, G.; Schiffelers, R.M. Extracellular vesicles for drug delivery. *Adv. Drug Deliv. Rev.* **2016**, *106*, 148–156. [CrossRef]
18. Herrmann, I.K.; Wood, M.J.A.; Fuhrmann, G. Extracellular vesicles as a next-generation drug delivery platform. *Nat. Nanotechnol.* **2021**, *16*, 748–759. [CrossRef]
19. Muzykantov, V.R. Drug delivery by red blood cells: Vascular carriers designed by mother nature. *Expert Opin. Drug Deliv.* **2010**, *7*, 403–427. [CrossRef]
20. Villa, C.H.; Anselmo, A.C.; Mitragotri, S.; Muzykantov, V. Red blood cells: Supercarriers for drugs, biologicals, and nanoparticles and inspiration for advanced delivery systems. *Adv. Drug Deliv. Rev.* **2016**, *106*, 88–103. [CrossRef]
21. Kalluri, R.; LeBleu, V.S. The biology, function, and biomedical applications of exosomes. *Science* **2020**, *367*, eaau6977. [CrossRef] [PubMed]
22. Raposo, G.; Stoorvogel, W. Extracellular vesicles: Exosomes, microvesicles, and friends. *J. Cell Biol.* **2013**, *200*, 373–383. [CrossRef] [PubMed]
23. Muralidharan-Chari, V.; Clancy, J.W.; Sedgwick, A.; D'Souza-Schorey, C. Microvesicles: Mediators of extracellular communication during cancer progression. *J. Cell Sci.* **2010**, *123*, 1603–1611. [CrossRef]
24. Théry, C.; Zitvogel, L.; Amigorena, S. Exosomes: Composition, biogenesis and function. *Nat. Rev. Immunol.* **2002**, *2*, 569–579. [CrossRef]
25. O'Brien, K.; Breyne, K.; Ughetto, S.; Laurent, L.C.; Breakefield, X.O. RNA delivery by extracellular vesicles in mammalian cells and its applications. *Nat. Rev. Mol. Cell Biol.* **2020**, *21*, 585–606. [CrossRef]
26. Villa, C.H.; Cines, D.B.; Siegel, D.L.; Muzykantov, V. Erythrocytes as Carriers for Drug Delivery in Blood Transfusion and Beyond. *Transfus. Med. Rev.* **2017**, *31*, 26–35. [CrossRef] [PubMed]
27. Xia, Q.; Zhang, Y.; Li, Z.; Hou, X.; Feng, N. Red blood cell membrane-camouflaged nanoparticles: A novel drug delivery system for antitumor application. *Acta Pharm. Sin. B* **2019**, *9*, 675–689. [CrossRef]
28. Glassman, P.M.; Villa, C.H.; Ukidve, A.; Zhao, Z.; Smith, P.; Mitragotri, S.; Russell, A.J.; Brenner, J.S.; Muzykantov, V.R. Vascular Drug Delivery Using Carrier Red Blood Cells: Focus on RBC Surface Loading and Pharmacokinetics. *Pharmaceutics* **2020**, *12*, 440. [CrossRef]
29. Murakami, T. Phospholipid nanodisc engineering for drug delivery systems. *Biotechnol. J.* **2012**, *7*, 762–767. [CrossRef]
30. Bariwal, J.; Ma, H.; Altenberg, G.A.; Liang, H. Nanodiscs: A versatile nanocarrier platform for cancer diagnosis and treatment. *Chem. Soc. Rev.* **2022**, *51*, 1702–1728. [CrossRef]
31. Traughber, C.A.; Opoku, E.; Brubaker, G.; Major, J.; Lu, H.; Lorkowski, S.W.; Neumann, C.; Hardaway, A.; Chung, Y.M.; Gulshan, K.; et al. Uptake of high-density lipoprotein by scavenger receptor class B type 1 is associated with prostate cancer proliferation and tumor progression in mice. *J. Biol. Chem.* **2020**, *295*, 8252–8261. [CrossRef] [PubMed]
32. Baranova, I.N.; Kurlander, R.; Bocharov, A.V.; Vishnyakova, T.G.; Chen, Z.; Remaley, A.T.; Csako, G.; Patterson, A.P.; Eggerman, T.L. Role of human CD36 in bacterial recognition, phagocytosis, and pathogen-induced JNK-mediated signaling. *J. Immunol.* **2008**, *181*, 7147–7156. [CrossRef] [PubMed]
33. Lei, Z.; Wang, J.; Lv, P.; Liu, G. Biomimetic synthesis of nanovesicles for targeted drug delivery. *Sci. Bull.* **2018**, *63*, 663–665. [CrossRef] [PubMed]
34. Tu, R.S.; Tirrell, M. Bottom-up design of biomimetic assemblies. *Adv. Drug Deliv. Rev.* **2004**, *56*, 1537–1563. [CrossRef]
35. Chen, Z.; Chen, X.; Huang, J.; Wang, J.; Wang, Z. Harnessing Protein Corona for Biomimetic Nanomedicine Design. *Biomimetics* **2022**, *7*, 126. [CrossRef]

36. Tang, Z.; Xiao, Y.; Kong, N.; Liu, C.; Chen, W.; Huang, X.; Xu, D.; Ouyang, J.; Feng, C.; Wang, C.; et al. Nano-bio interfaces effect of two-dimensional nanomaterials and their applications in cancer immunotherapy. *Acta Pharm. Sin. B* **2021**, *11*, 3447–3464. [CrossRef]
37. Liu, Y.; Wang, J.; Xiong, Q.; Hornburg, D.; Tao, W.; Farokhzad, O.C. Nano–Bio Interactions in Cancer: From Therapeutics Delivery to Early Detection. *Accounts Chem. Res.* **2021**, *54*, 291–301. [CrossRef]
38. Chen, Z.; Chen, X.; Liu, G.; Han, K.; Chen, J.; Wang, J. Editorial: The Application of Nanoengineering in Advanced Drug Delivery and Translational Research. *Front. Bioeng. Biotechnol.* **2022**, *10*, 886109. [CrossRef]
39. Li, L.; Wang, J.; Kong, H.; Zeng, Y.; Liu, G. Functional biomimetic nanoparticles for drug delivery and theranostic applications in cancer treatment. *Sci. Technol. Adv. Mater.* **2018**, *19*, 771–790. [CrossRef]
40. Wang, J.; Wang, A.Z.; Lv, P.; Tao, W.; Liu, G. Advancing the Pharmaceutical Potential of Bioinorganic Hybrid Lipid-Based Assemblies. *Adv. Sci.* **2018**, *5*, 1800564. [CrossRef]
41. Guido, C.; Maiorano, G.; Cortese, B.; D'Amone, S.; Palamà, I.E. Biomimetic Nanocarriers for Cancer Target Therapy. *Bioengineering* **2020**, *7*, 111. [CrossRef] [PubMed]
42. Sabu, C.; Rejo, C.; Kotta, S.; Pramod, K. Bioinspired and biomimetic systems for advanced drug and gene delivery. *J. Control. Release* **2018**, *287*, 142–155. [CrossRef] [PubMed]
43. Liu, S.; Yu, J.-M.; Gan, Y.-C.; Qiu, X.-Z.; Gao, Z.-C.; Wang, H.; Chen, S.-X.; Xiong, Y.; Liu, G.-H.; Lin, S.-E.; et al. Biomimetic natural biomaterials for tissue engineering and regenerative medicine: New biosynthesis methods, recent advances, and emerging applications. *Mil. Med. Res.* **2023**, *10*, 16. [CrossRef]
44. Soprano, E.; Polo, E.; Pelaz, B.; del Pino, P. Biomimetic cell-derived nanocarriers in cancer research. *J. Nanobiotechnol.* **2022**, *20*, 538. [CrossRef] [PubMed]
45. Nsairat, H.; Khater, D.; Sayed, U.; Odeh, F.; Al Bawab, A.; Alshaer, W. Liposomes: Structure, composition, types, and clinical applications. *Heliyon* **2022**, *8*, e09394. [CrossRef]
46. Belfiore, L.; Saunders, D.N.; Ranson, M.; Thurecht, K.J.; Storm, G.; Vine, K.L. Towards clinical translation of ligand-functionalized liposomes in targeted cancer therapy: Challenges and opportunities. *J. Control. Release* **2018**, *277*, 1–13. [CrossRef]
47. Sułkowski, W.W.; Pentak, D.; Nowak, K.; Sułkowska, A. The influence of temperature, cholesterol content and pH on liposome stability. *J. Mol. Struct.* **2005**, *744–747*, 737–747. [CrossRef]
48. Wagner, A.; Vorauer-Uhl, K. Liposome Technology for Industrial Purposes. *J. Drug Deliv.* **2011**, *2011*, 591325. [CrossRef]
49. Sainaga Jyothi, V.G.S.; Bulusu, R.; Venkata Krishna Rao, B.; Pranothi, M.; Banda, S.; Kumar Bolla, P.; Kommineni, N. Stability characterization for pharmaceutical liposome product development with focus on regulatory considerations: An update. *Int. J. Pharm.* **2022**, *624*, 122022. [CrossRef]
50. Frøkjaer, S.; Hjorth, E.L.; Wørts, O. Stability testing of liposomes during storage. In *Liposome Technology*; CRC Press: Boca Raton, FL, USA, 2019; pp. 235–245.
51. Senior, J.H. Fate and behavior of liposomes in vivo: A review of controlling factors. *Crit. Rev. Ther. Drug Carr. Syst.* **1987**, *3*, 123–193.
52. Inglut, C.T.; Sorrin, A.J.; Kuruppu, T.; Vig, S.; Cicalo, J.; Ahmad, H.; Huang, H.-C. Immunological and Toxicological Considerations for the Design of Liposomes. *Nanomaterials* **2020**, *10*, 190. [CrossRef] [PubMed]
53. Mare, R.; Paolino, D.; Celia, C.; Molinaro, R.; Fresta, M.; Cosco, D. Post-insertion parameters of PEG-derivatives in phosphocholine-liposomes. *Int. J. Pharm.* **2018**, *552*, 414–421. [CrossRef] [PubMed]
54. Spada, A.; Emami, J.; Tuszynski, J.A.; Lavasanifar, A. The Uniqueness of Albumin as a Carrier in Nanodrug Delivery. *Mol. Pharm.* **2021**, *18*, 1862–1894. [CrossRef] [PubMed]
55. Elsadek, B.; Kratz, F. Impact of albumin on drug delivery—New applications on the horizon. *J. Control. Release* **2012**, *157*, 4–28. [CrossRef] [PubMed]
56. Elzoghby, A.O.; Samy, W.M.; Elgindy, N.A. Albumin-based nanoparticles as potential controlled release drug delivery systems. *J. Control. Release* **2012**, *157*, 168–182. [CrossRef] [PubMed]
57. Miele, E.; Spinelli, G.P.; Miele, E.; Tomao, F.; Tomao, S. Albumin-bound formulation of paclitaxel (Abraxane® ABI-007) in the treatment of breast cancer. *Int. J. Nanomed.* **2009**, *4*, 99–105. [CrossRef]
58. Todd, T.J.; Zhen, Z.; Xie, J. Ferritin nanocages: Great potential as clinically translatable drug delivery vehicles? *Nanomedicine* **2013**, *8*, 1555–1557. [CrossRef]
59. Zhang, B.; Tang, G.; He, J.; Yan, X.; Fan, K. Ferritin nanocage: A promising and designable multi-module platform for constructing dynamic nanoassembly-based drug nanocarrier. *Adv. Drug Deliv. Rev.* **2021**, *176*, 113892. [CrossRef]
60. Bhaskar, S.; Lim, S. Engineering protein nanocages as carriers for biomedical applications. *NPG Asia Mater.* **2017**, *9*, e371. [CrossRef]
61. Tissot, A.C.; Renhofa, R.; Schmitz, N.; Cielens, I.; Meijerink, E.; Ose, V.; Jennings, G.T.; Saudan, P.; Pumpens, P.; Bachmann, M.F. Versatile Virus-Like Particle Carrier for Epitope Based Vaccines. *PLoS ONE* **2010**, *5*, e9809. [CrossRef]
62. Noad, R.; Roy, P. Virus-like particles as immunogens. *Trends Microbiol.* **2003**, *11*, 438–444. [CrossRef]
63. Zeltins, A. Construction and Characterization of Virus-Like Particles: A Review. *Mol. Biotechnol.* **2013**, *53*, 92–107. [CrossRef]
64. Mittal, M.; Banerjee, M.; Lua, L.H.; Rathore, A.S. Current status and future challenges in transitioning to continuous bioprocessing of virus-like particles. *J. Chem. Technol. Biotechnol.* **2022**, *97*, 2376–2385. [CrossRef]
65. Fuenmayor, J.; Gòdia, F.; Cervera, L. Production of virus-like particles for vaccines. *New Biotechnol.* **2017**, *39*, 174–180. [CrossRef]

66. Tsujita, M.; Wolska, A.; Gutmann, D.A.P.; Remaley, A.T. Reconstituted Discoidal High-Density Lipoproteins: Bioinspired Nanodiscs with Many Unexpected Applications. *Curr. Atheroscler. Rep.* **2018**, *20*, 59. [CrossRef]
67. Kuai, R.; Ochyl, L.J.; Bahjat, K.S.; Schwendeman, A.; Moon, J.J. Designer vaccine nanodiscs for personalized cancer immunotherapy. *Nat. Mater.* **2017**, *16*, 489–496. [CrossRef]
68. Chen, L.; Yu, C.; Xu, W.; Xiong, Y.; Cheng, P.; Lin, Z.; Zhang, Z.; Knoedler, L.; Panayi, A.C.; Knoedler, S.; et al. Dual-Targeted Nanodiscs Revealing the Cross-Talk between Osteogenic Differentiation of Mesenchymal Stem Cells and Macrophages. *ACS Nano* **2023**, *17*, 3153–3167. [CrossRef]
69. Melke, J.; Midha, S.; Ghosh, S.; Ito, K.; Hofmann, S. Silk fibroin as biomaterial for bone tissue engineering. *Acta Biomater.* **2016**, *31*, 1–16. [CrossRef]
70. Xu, H.-L.; ZhuGe, D.-L.; Chen, P.-P.; Tong, M.-Q.; Lin, M.-T.; Jiang, X.; Zheng, Y.-W.; Chen, B.; Li, X.-K.; Zhao, Y.-Z. Silk fibroin nanoparticles dyeing indocyanine green for imaging-guided photo-thermal therapy of glioblastoma. *Drug Deliv.* **2018**, *25*, 364–375. [CrossRef]
71. Xie, M.; Fan, D.; Li, Y.; He, X.; Chen, X.; Chen, Y.; Zhu, J.; Xu, G.; Wu, X.; Lan, P. Supercritical carbon dioxide-developed silk fibroin nanoplatform for smart colon cancer therapy. *Int. J. Nanomed.* **2017**, *12*, 7751–7761. [CrossRef]
72. Yasmin, R.; Shah, M.; Khan, S.A.; Ali, R. Gelatin nanoparticles: A potential candidate for medical applications. *Nanotechnol. Rev.* **2017**, *6*, 191–207. [CrossRef]
73. Foox, M.; Zilberman, M. Drug delivery from gelatin-based systems. *Expert Opin. Drug Deliv.* **2015**, *12*, 1547–1563. [CrossRef] [PubMed]
74. Elzoghby, A.O. Gelatin-based nanoparticles as drug and gene delivery systems: Reviewing three decades of research. *J. Control. Release* **2013**, *172*, 1075–1091. [CrossRef] [PubMed]
75. Wiklander, O.P.B.; Brennan, M.Á.; Lötvall, J.; Breakefield, X.O.; EL Andaloussi, S. Advances in therapeutic applications of extracellular vesicles. *Sci. Transl. Med.* **2019**, *11*, eaav8521. [CrossRef] [PubMed]
76. De Jong, O.G.; Van Balkom, B.W.M.; Schiffelers, R.M.; Bouten, C.V.C.; Verhaar, M.C. Extracellular Vesicles: Potential Roles in Regenerative Medicine. *Front. Immunol.* **2014**, *5*, 608. [CrossRef]
77. Melling, G.E.; Carollo, E.; Conlon, R.; Simpson, J.C.; Carter, D.R.F. The Challenges and Possibilities of Extracellular Vesicles as Therapeutic Vehicles. *Eur. J. Pharm. Biopharm.* **2019**, *144*, 50–56. [CrossRef]
78. Clemmens, H.; Lambert, D.W. Extracellular vesicles: Translational challenges and opportunities. *Biochem. Soc. Trans.* **2018**, *46*, 1073–1082. [CrossRef]
79. Ramirez, M.I.; Amorim, M.G.; Gadelha, C.; Milic, I.; Welsh, J.A.; Freitas, V.M.; Nawaz, M.; Akbar, N.; Couch, Y.; Makin, L. Technical challenges of working with extracellular vesicles. *Nanoscale* **2018**, *10*, 881–906. [CrossRef]
80. Dash, P.; Piras, A.M.; Dash, M. Cell membrane coated nanocarriers—An efficient biomimetic platform for targeted therapy. *J. Control. Release* **2020**, *327*, 546–570. [CrossRef]
81. Miao, Y.; Yang, Y.; Guo, L.; Chen, M.; Zhou, X.; Zhao, Y.; Nie, D.; Gan, Y.; Zhang, X. Cell Membrane-Camouflaged Nanocarriers with Biomimetic Deformability of Erythrocytes for Ultralong Circulation and Enhanced Cancer Therapy. *ACS Nano* **2022**, *16*, 6527–6540. [CrossRef]
82. Sun, Y.; Jing, X.; Ma, X.; Feng, Y.; Hu, H. Versatile Types of Polysaccharide-Based Drug Delivery Systems: From Strategic Design to Cancer Therapy. *Int. J. Mol. Sci.* **2020**, *21*, 9159. [CrossRef] [PubMed]
83. Miao, T.; Wang, J.; Zeng, Y.; Liu, G.; Chen, X. Polysaccharide-Based Controlled Release Systems for Therapeutics Delivery and Tissue Engineering: From Bench to Bedside. *Adv. Sci.* **2018**, *5*, 1700513. [CrossRef]
84. Barbu, A.; Neamtu, B.; Zăhan, M.; Iancu, G.M.; Bacila, C.; Mireșan, V. Current Trends in Advanced Alginate-Based Wound Dressings for Chronic Wounds. *J. Pers. Med.* **2021**, *11*, 890. [CrossRef] [PubMed]
85. Ashimova, A.; Yegorov, S.; Negmetzhanov, B.; Hortelano, G. Cell Encapsulation Within Alginate Microcapsules: Immunological Challenges and Outlook. *Front. Bioeng. Biotechnol.* **2019**, *7*, 380. [CrossRef] [PubMed]
86. Sonaje, K.; Chuang, E.-Y.; Lin, K.-J.; Yen, T.-C.; Su, F.-Y.; Tseng, M.T.; Sung, H.-W. Opening of Epithelial Tight Junctions and Enhancement of Paracellular Permeation by Chitosan: Microscopic, Ultrastructural, and Computed-Tomographic Observations. *Mol. Pharm.* **2012**, *9*, 1271–1279. [CrossRef] [PubMed]
87. Mattheolabakis, G.; Milane, L.; Singh, A.; Amiji, M.M. Hyaluronic acid targeting of CD44 for cancer therapy: From receptor biology to nanomedicine. *J. Drug Target.* **2015**, *23*, 605–618. [CrossRef]
88. Mao, L.; Wu, W.; Wang, M.; Guo, J.; Li, H.; Zhang, S.; Xu, J.; Zou, J. Targeted treatment for osteoarthritis: Drugs and delivery system. *Drug Deliv.* **2021**, *28*, 1861–1876. [CrossRef]
89. Huang, G.; Huang, H. Application of dextran as nanoscale drug carriers. *Nanomedicine* **2018**, *13*, 3149–3158. [CrossRef]
90. Varshosaz, J. Dextran conjugates in drug delivery. *Expert Opin. Drug Deliv.* **2012**, *9*, 509–523. [CrossRef]
91. Liu, P.; Chen, G.; Zhang, J. A Review of Liposomes as a Drug Delivery System: Current Status of Approved Products, Regulatory Environments, and Future Perspectives. *Molecules* **2022**, *27*, 1372. [CrossRef]
92. Agmo Hernández, V.; Karlsson, G.; Edwards, K. Intrinsic Heterogeneity in Liposome Suspensions Caused by the Dynamic Spontaneous Formation of Hydrophobic Active Sites in Lipid Membranes. *Langmuir* **2011**, *27*, 4873–4883. [CrossRef] [PubMed]
93. Maritim, S.; Boulas, P.; Lin, Y. Comprehensive analysis of liposome formulation parameters and their influence on encapsulation, stability and drug release in glibenclamide liposomes. *Int. J. Pharm.* **2021**, *592*, 120051. [CrossRef] [PubMed]

94. Mayer, L.D.; Tai, L.C.L.; Ko, D.S.C.; Masin, D.; Ginsberg, R.S.; Cullis, P.R.; Bally, M.B. Influence of Vesicle Size, Lipid Composition, and Drug-to-Lipid Ratio on the Biological Activity of Liposomal Doxorubicin in Mice1. *Cancer Res.* **1989**, *49*, 5922–5930.
95. Crowe, J.H.; Crowe, L.M. Factors affecting the stability of dry liposomes. *Biochim. Biophys. Acta (BBA)-Biomembr.* **1988**, *939*, 327–334. [CrossRef]
96. Hupfeld, S.; Holsæter, A.M.; Skar, M.; Frantzen, C.B.; Brandl, M. Liposome Size Analysis by Dynamic/Static Light Scattering upon Size Exclusion-/Field Flow-Fractionation. *J. Nanosci. Nanotechnol.* **2006**, *6*, 3025–3031. [CrossRef] [PubMed]
97. Doyen, C.; Larquet, E.; Coureux, P.-D.; Frances, O.; Herman, F.; Sablé, S.; Burnouf, J.-P.; Sizun, C.; Lescop, E. Nuclear Magnetic Resonance Spectroscopy: A Multifaceted Toolbox to Probe Structure, Dynamics, Interactions, and Real-Time In Situ Release Kinetics in Peptide-Liposome Formulations. *Mol. Pharm.* **2021**, *18*, 2521–2539. [CrossRef]
98. Siriwardane, D.A.; Wang, C.; Jiang, W.; Mudalige, T. Quantification of phospholipid degradation products in liposomal pharmaceutical formulations by ultra performance liquid chromatography-mass spectrometry (UPLC-MS). *Int. J. Pharm.* **2020**, *578*, 119077. [CrossRef]
99. Carugo, D.; Bottaro, E.; Owen, J.; Stride, E.; Nastruzzi, C. Liposome production by microfluidics: Potential and limiting factors. *Sci. Rep.* **2016**, *6*, 25876. [CrossRef]
100. Parchekani, J.; Allahverdi, A.; Taghdir, M.; Naderi-Manesh, H. Design and simulation of the liposomal model by using a coarse-grained molecular dynamics approach towards drug delivery goals. *Sci. Rep.* **2022**, *12*, 2371. [CrossRef]
101. Jämbeck, J.P.M.; Eriksson, E.S.E.; Laaksonen, A.; Lyubartsev, A.P.; Eriksson, L.A. Molecular Dynamics Studies of Liposomes as Carriers for Photosensitizing Drugs: Development, Validation, and Simulations with a Coarse-Grained Model. *J. Chem. Theory Comput.* **2014**, *10*, 5–13. [CrossRef]
102. Langer, K.; Anhorn, M.G.; Steinhauser, I.; Dreis, S.; Celebi, D.; Schrickel, N.; Faust, S.; Vogel, V. Human serum albumin (HSA) nanoparticles: Reproducibility of preparation process and kinetics of enzymatic degradation. *Int. J. Pharm.* **2008**, *347*, 109–117. [CrossRef]
103. Fanciullino, R.; Ciccolini, J.; Milano, G. Challenges, expectations and limits for nanoparticles-based therapeutics in cancer: A focus on nano-albumin-bound drugs. *Crit. Rev. Oncol. Hematol.* **2013**, *88*, 504–513. [CrossRef]
104. Hornok, V. Serum Albumin Nanoparticles: Problems and Prospects. *Polymers* **2021**, *13*, 3759. [CrossRef]
105. Yan, S.; Zhang, H.; Piao, J.; Chen, Y.; Gao, S.; Lu, C.; Niu, L.; Xia, Y.; Hu, Y.; Ji, R.; et al. Studies on the Preparation, Characterization and Intracellular Kinetics of JD27-loaded Human Serum Albumin Nanoparticles. *Procedia Eng.* **2015**, *102*, 590–601. [CrossRef]
106. Bertucci, C.; Domenici, E. Reversible and covalent binding of drugs to human serum albumin: Methodological approaches and physiological relevance. *Curr. Med. Chem.* **2002**, *9*, 1463–1481. [CrossRef]
107. Galisteo-González, F.; Molina-Bolívar, J.A. Systematic study on the preparation of BSA nanoparticles. *Colloids Surf. B Biointerfaces* **2014**, *123*, 286–292. [CrossRef]
108. Maciążek-Jurczyk, M.; Szkudlarek, A.; Chudzik, M.; Pożycka, J.; Sułkowska, A. Alteration of human serum albumin binding properties induced by modifications: A review. *Spectrochim. Acta Part A Mol. Biomol. Spectrosc.* **2018**, *188*, 675–683. [CrossRef]
109. Das, S.; Jagan, L.; Isiah, R.; Rajesh, B.; Backianathan, S.; Subhashini, J. Nanotechnology in oncology: Characterization and in vitro release kinetics of cisplatin-loaded albumin nanoparticles: Implications in anticancer drug delivery. *Indian J. Pharmacol.* **2011**, *43*, 409. [CrossRef]
110. Kulig, K.; Ziąbka, M.; Pilarczyk, K.; Owczarzy, A.; Rogóż, W.; Maciążek-Jurczyk, M. Physicochemical Study of Albumin Nanoparticles with Chlorambucil. *Processes* **2022**, *10*, 1170. [CrossRef]
111. Baler, K.; Martin, O.A.; Carignano, M.A.; Ameer, G.A.; Vila, J.A.; Szleifer, I. Electrostatic Unfolding and Interactions of Albumin Driven by pH Changes: A Molecular Dynamics Study. *J. Phys. Chem. B* **2014**, *118*, 921–930. [CrossRef]
112. Narwal, M.; Kumar, D.; Mukherjee, T.K.; Bhattacharyya, R.; Banerjee, D. Molecular dynamics simulation as a tool for assessment of drug binding property of human serum albumin. *Mol. Biol. Rep.* **2018**, *45*, 1647–1652. [CrossRef] [PubMed]
113. Kaboli, S.F.; Mehrnejad, F.; Nematollahzadeh, A. Molecular modeling prediction of albumin-based nanoparticles and experimental preparation, characterization, and in-vitro release kinetics of prednisolone from the nanoparticles. *J. Drug Deliv. Sci. Technol.* **2021**, *64*, 102588. [CrossRef]
114. Amirinasab, M.; Dehestani, M. Theoretical aspects of interaction of the anticancer drug cytarabine with human serum albumin. *Struct. Chem.* **2023**, 1–9. [CrossRef] [PubMed]
115. Muthu, M.S.; Wilson, B. Challenges posed by the scale-up of nanomedicines. *Nanomedicine* **2012**, *7*, 307–309. [CrossRef] [PubMed]
116. Shrimal, P.; Jadeja, G.; Patel, S. A review on novel methodologies for drug nanoparticle preparation: Microfluidic approach. *Chem. Eng. Res. Des.* **2020**, *153*, 728–756. [CrossRef]
117. Hakala, T.A.; Davies, S.; Toprakcioglu, Z.; Bernardim, B.; Bernardes, G.J.L.; Knowles, T.P.J. A Microfluidic Co-Flow Route for Human Serum Albumin-Drug-Nanoparticle Assembly. *Chem. -A Eur. J.* **2020**, *26*, 5965–5969. [CrossRef] [PubMed]
118. Tuan Giam Chuang, V.; Kragh-Hansen, U.; Otagiri, M. Pharmaceutical Strategies Utilizing Recombinant Human Serum Albumin. *Pharm. Res.* **2002**, *19*, 569–577. [CrossRef]
119. Liu, X.; Mohanty, R.P.; Maier, E.Y.; Peng, X.; Wulfe, S.; Looney, A.P.; Aung, K.L.; Ghosh, D. Controlled loading of albumin-drug conjugates ex vivo for enhanced drug delivery and antitumor efficacy. *J. Control. Release* **2020**, *328*, 1–12. [CrossRef]
120. Ghadami, S.A.; Ahmadi, Z.; Moosavi-Nejad, Z. The albumin-based nanoparticle formation in relation to protein aggregation. *Spectrochim. Acta Part A Mol. Biomol. Spectrosc.* **2021**, *252*, 119489. [CrossRef]

121. Dawoud, M.H.S.; Abdel-Daim, A.; Nour, M.S.; Sweed, N.M. A Quality by Design Paradigm for Albumin-Based Nanoparticles: Formulation Optimization and Enhancement of the Antitumor Activity. *J. Pharm. Innov.* **2023**. [CrossRef]
122. Sønderby, P.; Bukrinski, J.T.; Hebditch, M.; Peters, G.H.J.; Curtis, R.A.; Harris, P. Self-Interaction of Human Serum Albumin: A Formulation Perspective. *ACS Omega* **2018**, *3*, 16105–16117. [CrossRef] [PubMed]
123. Vogel, V.; Langer, K.; Balthasar, S.; Schuck, P.; Mächtle, W.; Haase, W.; van den Broek, J.A.; Tziatzios, C.; Schubert, D. *Characterization of Serum Albumin Nanoparticles by Sedimentation Velocity Analysis and Electron Microscopy*; Springer: Berlin/Heidelberg, Germany, 2002; pp. 31–36.
124. Tesarova, B.; Musilek, K.; Rex, S.; Heger, Z. Taking advantage of cellular uptake of ferritin nanocages for targeted drug delivery. *J. Control. Release* **2020**, *325*, 176–190. [CrossRef] [PubMed]
125. Zhang, Y.; Orner, B.P. Self-Assembly in the Ferritin Nano-Cage Protein Superfamily. *Int. J. Mol. Sci.* **2011**, *12*, 5406–5421. [CrossRef]
126. Honarmand Ebrahimi, K.; Hagedoorn, P.-L.; Hagen, W.R. Unity in the Biochemistry of the Iron-Storage Proteins Ferritin and Bacterioferritin. *Chem. Rev.* **2015**, *115*, 295–326. [CrossRef]
127. Yin, S.; Davey, K.; Dai, S.; Liu, Y.; Bi, J. A critical review of ferritin as a drug nanocarrier: Structure, properties, comparative advantages and challenges. *Particuology* **2022**, *64*, 65–84. [CrossRef]
128. Li, Z.; Maity, B.; Hishikawa, Y.; Ueno, T.; Lu, D. Importance of the Subunit–Subunit Interface in Ferritin Disassembly: A Molecular Dynamics Study. *Langmuir* **2022**, *38*, 1106–1113. [CrossRef] [PubMed]
129. Stühn, L.; Auernhammer, J.; Dietz, C. pH-depended protein shell dis- and reassembly of ferritin nanoparticles revealed by atomic force microscopy. *Sci. Rep.* **2019**, *9*, 17755. [CrossRef] [PubMed]
130. Mohanty, A.; K, M.; Jena, S.S.; Behera, R.K. Kinetics of Ferritin Self-Assembly by Laser Light Scattering: Impact of Subunit Concentration, pH, and Ionic Strength. *Biomacromolecules* **2021**, *22*, 1389–1398. [CrossRef]
131. Nakahara, Y.; Endo, Y.; Inoue, I. Construction Protocol of Drug-Protein Cage Complexes for Drug Delivery System. In *Protein Cages: Design, Structure, and Applications*; Ueno, T., Lim, S., Xia, K., Eds.; Springer: New York, NY, USA, 2023; pp. 335–347. [CrossRef]
132. Liu, Y.; Zhao, G. Reassembly Design of Ferritin Cages. In *Protein Cages: Design, Structure, and Applications*; Ueno, T., Lim, S., Xia, K., Eds.; Springer: New York, NY, USA, 2023; pp. 69–78. [CrossRef]
133. Wade, V.J.; Levi, S.; Arosio, P.; Treffry, A.; Harrison, P.M.; Mann, S. Influence of site-directed modifications on the formation of iron cores in ferritin. *J. Mol. Biol.* **1991**, *221*, 1443–1452. [CrossRef]
134. Yang, C.; Cao, C.; Cai, Y.; Zhang, T.; Pan, Y. The Surface Modification of Ferritin and Its Applications. *Prog. Chem.* **2016**, *28*, 91–102. [CrossRef]
135. Wang, C.; Zhang, C.; Li, Z.; Yin, S.; Wang, Q.; Guo, F.; Zhang, Y.; Yu, R.; Liu, Y.; Su, Z. Extending Half Life of H-Ferritin Nanoparticle by Fusing Albumin Binding Domain for Doxorubicin Encapsulation. *Biomacromolecules* **2018**, *19*, 773–781. [CrossRef] [PubMed]
136. Zhang, S.; Zang, J.; Chen, H.; Li, M.; Xu, C.; Zhao, G. The Size Flexibility of Ferritin Nanocage Opens a New Way to Prepare Nanomaterials. *Small* **2017**, *13*, 1701045. [CrossRef] [PubMed]
137. Giddings, J.C.; Yang, F.J.; Myers, M.N. Flow field-flow fractionation as a methodology for protein separation and characterization. *Anal. Biochem.* **1977**, *81*, 395–407. [CrossRef] [PubMed]
138. He, D.; Hughes, S.; Vanden-Hehir, S.; Georgiev, A.; Altenbach, K.; Tarrant, E.; Mackay, C.L.; Waldron, K.J.; Clarke, D.J.; Marles-Wright, J. Structural characterization of encapsulated ferritin provides insight into iron storage in bacterial nanocompartments. *eLife* **2016**, *5*, e18972. [CrossRef] [PubMed]
139. Anjum, F.; Shahwan, M.; Alhumaydhi, F.A.; Sharaf, S.E.; Al Abdulmonem, W.; Shafie, A.; Bilgrami, A.L.; Shamsi, A.; Md Ashraf, G. Mechanistic insight into the binding between Ferritin and Serotonin: Possible implications in neurodegenerative diseases. *J. Mol. Liq.* **2022**, *351*, 118618. [CrossRef]
140. Zhang, L.; Lua, L.H.L.; Middelberg, A.P.J.; Sun, Y.; Connors, N.K. Biomolecular engineering of virus-like particles aided by computational chemistry methods. *Chem. Soc. Rev.* **2015**, *44*, 8608–8618. [CrossRef]
141. Charlton Hume, H.K.; Vidigal, J.; Carrondo, M.J.T.; Middelberg, A.P.J.; Roldão, A.; Lua, L.H.L. Synthetic biology for bioengineering virus-like particle vaccines. *Biotechnol. Bioeng.* **2019**, *116*, 919–935. [CrossRef]
142. Santi, L.; Huang, Z.; Mason, H. Virus-like particles production in green plants. *Methods* **2006**, *40*, 66–76. [CrossRef]
143. Mohr, J.; Chuan, Y.P.; Wu, Y.; Lua, L.H.L.; Middelberg, A.P.J. Virus-like particle formulation optimization by miniaturized high-throughput screening. *Methods* **2013**, *60*, 248–256. [CrossRef]
144. Huhti, L.; Blazevic, V.; Nurminen, K.; Koho, T.; Hytönen, V.P.; Vesikari, T. A comparison of methods for purification and concentration of norovirus GII-4 capsid virus-like particles. *Arch. Virol.* **2010**, *155*, 1855–1858. [CrossRef]
145. Rocha, J.M. Aqueous two-phase systems and monolithic chromatography as alternative technological platforms for virus and virus-like particle purification. *J. Chem. Technol. Biotechnol.* **2021**, *96*, 309–317. [CrossRef]
146. Marchel, M.; Niewisiewicz, J.; Coroadinha, A.S.; Marrucho, I.M. Purification of virus-like particles using aqueous biphasic systems composed of natural deep eutectic solvents. *Sep. Purif. Technol.* **2020**, *252*, 117480. [CrossRef]
147. Ladd Effio, C.; Oelmeier, S.A.; Hubbuch, J. High-throughput characterization of virus-like particles by interlaced size-exclusion chromatography. *Vaccine* **2016**, *34*, 1259–1267. [CrossRef] [PubMed]

148. Pereira Aguilar, P.; González-Domínguez, I.; Schneider, T.A.; Gòdia, F.; Cervera, L.; Jungbauer, A. At-line multi-angle light scattering detector for faster process development in enveloped virus-like particle purification. *J. Sep. Sci.* **2019**, *42*, 2640–2649. [CrossRef] [PubMed]
149. Durous, L.; Rosa-Calatrava, M.; Petiot, E. Advances in influenza virus-like particles bioprocesses. *Expert Rev. Vaccines* **2019**, *18*, 1285–1300. [CrossRef]
150. Denisov, I.G.; Grinkova, Y.V.; Lazarides, A.A.; Sligar, S.G. Directed Self-Assembly of Monodisperse Phospholipid Bilayer Nanodiscs with Controlled Size. *J. Am. Chem. Soc.* **2004**, *126*, 3477–3487. [CrossRef]
151. Xu, D.; Chen, X.; Li, Y.; Chen, Z.; Xu, W.; Wang, X.; Lv, Y.; Wang, Z.; Wu, M.; Liu, G.; et al. Reconfigurable Peptide Analogs of Apolipoprotein A-I Reveal Tunable Features of Nanodisc Assembly. *Langmuir* **2023**, *39*, 1262–1276. [CrossRef]
152. Wade, J.H.; Jones, J.D.; Lenov, I.L.; Riordan, C.M.; Sligar, S.G.; Bailey, R.C. Microfluidic platform for efficient Nanodisc assembly, membrane protein incorporation, and purification. *Lab A Chip* **2017**, *17*, 2951–2959. [CrossRef]
153. Goluch, E.D.; Shaw, A.W.; Sligar, S.G.; Liu, C. Microfluidic patterning of nanodisc lipid bilayers and multiplexed analysis of protein interaction. *Lab A Chip* **2008**, *8*, 1723–1728. [CrossRef]
154. Xu, D.; Chen, X.; Chen, Z.; Lv, Y.; Li, Y.; Li, S.; Xu, W.; Mo, Y.; Wang, X.; Chen, Z.; et al. An in Silico Approach to Reveal the Nanodisc Formulation of Doxorubicin. *Front. Bioeng. Biotechnol.* **2022**, *10*, 859255. [CrossRef]
155. Bengtsen, T.; Holm, V.L.; Kjølbye, L.R.; Midtgaard, S.R.; Johansen, N.T.; Tesei, G.; Bottaro, S.; Schiøtt, B.; Arleth, L.; Lindorff-Larsen, K. Structure and dynamics of a nanodisc by integrating NMR, SAXS and SANS experiments with molecular dynamics simulations. *eLife* **2020**, *9*, e56518. [CrossRef] [PubMed]
156. Pourmousa, M.; Pastor, R.W. Molecular dynamics simulations of lipid nanodiscs. *Biochim. Biophys. Acta (BBA)-Biomembr.* **2018**, *1860*, 2094–2107. [CrossRef] [PubMed]
157. Yoshida, J.-I.; Nagaki, A.; Yamada, D. Continuous flow synthesis. *Drug Discov. Today: Technol.* **2013**, *10*, e53–e59. [CrossRef] [PubMed]
158. Julien, J.A.; Fernandez, M.G.; Brandmier, K.M.; Del Mundo, J.T.; Bator, C.M.; Loftus, L.A.; Gomez, E.W.; Gomez, E.D.; Glover, K.J. Rapid preparation of nanodiscs for biophysical studies. *Arch. Biochem. Biophys.* **2021**, *712*, 109051. [CrossRef]
159. Pedrazzani, R.; Ceretti, E.; Zerbini, I.; Casale, R.; Gozio, E.; Bertanza, G.; Gelatti, U.; Donato, F.; Feretti, D. Biodegradability, toxicity and mutagenicity of detergents: Integrated experimental evaluations. *Ecotoxicol. Environ. Saf.* **2012**, *84*, 274–281. [CrossRef] [PubMed]
160. Sobrino-Figueroa, A.S. Evaluation of oxidative stress and genetic damage caused by detergents in the zebrafish Danio rerio (Cyprinidae). *Comp. Biochem. Physiol. Part A Mol. Integr. Physiol.* **2013**, *165*, 528–532. [CrossRef]
161. Justesen, B.H.; Günther-Pomorski, T. Chromatographic and electrophoretic methods for nanodisc purification and analysis. *Rev. Anal. Chem.* **2014**, *33*, 165–172. [CrossRef]
162. Howard, F.H.; Gao, Z.; Mansor, H.B.; Yang, Z.; Muthana, M. Silk Fibroin Nanoparticles: A Biocompatible Multi-Functional Polymer for Drug Delivery. In *Biotechnology—Biosensors, Biomaterials and Tissue Engineering—Annual Volume 2022*; Intech Open: Rijeka, Croatia, 2023.
163. Nguyen, T.P.; Nguyen, Q.V.; Nguyen, V.-H.; Le, T.-H.; Huynh, V.Q.N.; Vo, D.-V.N.; Trinh, Q.T.; Kim, S.Y.; Le, Q.V. Silk Fibroin-Based Biomaterials for Biomedical Applications: A Review. *Polymers* **2019**, *11*, 1933. [CrossRef]
164. Baci, G.-M.; Cucu, A.-A.; Giurgiu, A.-I.; Muscă, A.-S.; Bagameri, L.; Moise, A.R.; Bobiș, O.; Rațiu, A.C.; Dezmirean, D.S. Advances in Editing Silkworms (Bombyx mori) Genome by Using the CRISPR-Cas System. *Insects* **2022**, *13*, 28. [CrossRef]
165. Aznar-Cervantes, S.D.; Vicente-Cervantes, D.; Meseguer-Olmo, L.; Cenis, J.L.; Lozano-Pérez, A.A. Influence of the protocol used for fibroin extraction on the mechanical properties and fiber sizes of electrospun silk mats. *Mater. Sci. Eng. C Mater. Biol. Appl.* **2013**, *33*, 1945–1950. [CrossRef]
166. DeBari, M.K.; King, C.I., III; Altgold, T.A.; Abbott, R.D. Silk Fibroin as a Green Material. *ACS Biomater. Sci. Eng.* **2021**, *7*, 3530–3544. [CrossRef] [PubMed]
167. Khan, S.A. Mini-Review: Opportunities and challenges in the techniques used for preparation of gelatin nanoparticles. *Pak. J. Pharm. Sci.* **2020**, *33*, 221–228.
168. Ahmed, M.A.; Al-Kahtani, H.A.; Jaswir, I.; AbuTarboush, H.; Ismail, E.A. Extraction and characterization of gelatin from camel skin (potential halal gelatin) and production of gelatin nanoparticles. *Saudi J. Biol. Sci.* **2020**, *27*, 1596–1601. [CrossRef] [PubMed]
169. Zhou, P.; Regenstein, J.M. Effects of Alkaline and Acid Pretreatments on Alaska Pollock Skin Gelatin Extraction. *J. Food Sci.* **2005**, *70*, c392–c396. [CrossRef]
170. Eggert, S.; Kahl, M.; Bock, N.; Meinert, C.; Friedrich, O.; Hutmacher, D.W. An open-source technology platform to increase reproducibility and enable high-throughput production of tailorable gelatin methacryloyl (GelMA)—Based hydrogels. *Mater. Des.* **2021**, *204*, 109619. [CrossRef]
171. Xia, Y.; Xu, R.; Ye, S.; Yan, J.; Kumar, P.; Zhang, P.; Zhao, X. Microfluidic Formulation of Curcumin-Loaded Multiresponsive Gelatin Nanoparticles for Anticancer Therapy. *ACS Biomater. Sci. Eng.* **2023**, *9*, 3402–3413. [CrossRef]
172. Solomun, J.I.; Totten, J.D.; Wongpinyochit, T.; Florence, A.J.; Seib, F.P. Manual Versus Microfluidic-Assisted Nanoparticle Manufacture: Impact of Silk Fibroin Stock on Nanoparticle Characteristics. *ACS Biomater. Sci. Eng.* **2020**, *6*, 2796–2804. [CrossRef]
173. Jahanshahi, M.; Sanati, M.H.; Hajizadeh, S.; Babaei, Z. Gelatin nanoparticle fabrication and optimization of the particle size. *Phys. Status Solidi (A)* **2008**, *205*, 2898–2902. [CrossRef]

174. Madkhali, O.; Mekhail, G.; Wettig, S.D. Modified gelatin nanoparticles for gene delivery. *Int. J. Pharm.* **2019**, *554*, 224–234. [CrossRef]
175. Gharehnazifam, Z.; Dolatabadi, R.; Baniassadi, M.; Shahsavari, H.; Kajbafzadeh, A.-M.; Abrinia, K.; Baghani, M. Computational analysis of vincristine loaded silk fibroin hydrogel for sustained drug delivery applications: Multiphysics modeling and experiments. *Int. J. Pharm.* **2021**, *609*, 121184. [CrossRef]
176. Hathout, R.M.; Metwally, A.A.; Woodman, T.J.; Hardy, J.G. Prediction of Drug Loading in the Gelatin Matrix Using Computational Methods. *ACS Omega* **2020**, *5*, 1549–1556. [CrossRef] [PubMed]
177. Carmelo-Luna, F.J.; Mendoza-Wilson, A.M.; Ramos-Clamont Montfort, G.; Lizardi-Mendoza, J.; Madera-Santana, T.; Lardizábal-Gutiérrez, D.; Quintana-Owen, P. Synthesis and experimental/computational characterization of sorghum procyanidins–gelatin nanoparticles. *Bioorganic Med. Chem.* **2021**, *42*, 116240. [CrossRef]
178. Bordanaba-Florit, G.; Royo, F.; Kruglik, S.G.; Falcón-Pérez, J.M. Using single-vesicle technologies to unravel the heterogeneity of extracellular vesicles. *Nat. Protoc.* **2021**, *16*, 3163–3185. [CrossRef] [PubMed]
179. Ingato, D.; Lee, J.U.; Sim, S.J.; Kwon, Y.J. Good things come in small packages: Overcoming challenges to harness extracellular vesicles for therapeutic delivery. *J. Control. Release* **2016**, *241*, 174–185. [CrossRef]
180. Tkach, M.; Théry, C. Communication by Extracellular Vesicles: Where We Are and Where We Need to Go. *Cell* **2016**, *164*, 1226–1232. [CrossRef]
181. Vogel, R.; Coumans, F.A.W.; Maltesen, R.G.; Böing, A.N.; Bonnington, K.E.; Broekman, M.L.; Broom, M.F.; Buzás, E.I.; Christiansen, G.; Hajji, N.; et al. A standardized method to determine the concentration of extracellular vesicles using tunable resistive pulse sensing. *J. Extracell. Vesicles* **2016**, *5*, 31242. [CrossRef]
182. Morales-Kastresana, A.; Telford, B.; Musich, T.A.; McKinnon, K.; Clayborne, C.; Braig, Z.; Rosner, A.; Demberg, T.; Watson, D.C.; Karpova, T.S.; et al. Labeling Extracellular Vesicles for Nanoscale Flow Cytometry. *Sci. Rep.* **2017**, *7*, 1878. [CrossRef] [PubMed]
183. Srivastava, A.; Amreddy, N.; Pareek, V.; Chinnappan, M.; Ahmed, R.; Mehta, M.; Razaq, M.; Munshi, A.; Ramesh, R. Progress in extracellular vesicle biology and their application in cancer medicine. *Wiley Interdiscip. Rev. Nanomed. Nanobiotechnol.* **2020**, *12*, e1621. [CrossRef]
184. Allelein, S.; Medina-Perez, P.; Lopes, A.L.H.; Rau, S.; Hause, G.; Kölsch, A.; Kuhlmeier, D. Potential and challenges of specifically isolating extracellular vesicles from heterogeneous populations. *Sci. Rep.* **2021**, *11*, 11585. [CrossRef]
185. Yan, I.K.; Shukla, N.; Borrelli, D.A.; Patel, T. Use of a Hollow Fiber Bioreactor to Collect Extracellular Vesicles from Cells in Culture. In *Extracellular RNA: Methods and Protocols*; Patel, T., Ed.; Springer: New York, NY, USA, 2018; pp. 35–41. [CrossRef]
186. Kang, H.; Bae, Y.-h.; Kwon, Y.; Kim, S.; Park, J. Extracellular Vesicles Generated Using Bioreactors and their Therapeutic Effect on the Acute Kidney Injury Model. *Adv. Healthc. Mater.* **2022**, *11*, 2101606. [CrossRef] [PubMed]
187. Davies, R.T.; Kim, J.; Jang, S.C.; Choi, E.-J.; Gho, Y.S.; Park, J. Microfluidic filtration system to isolate extracellular vesicles from blood. *Lab A Chip* **2012**, *12*, 5202–5210. [CrossRef] [PubMed]
188. Gholizadeh, S.; Shehata Draz, M.; Zarghooni, M.; Sanati-Nezhad, A.; Ghavami, S.; Shafiee, H.; Akbari, M. Microfluidic approaches for isolation, detection, and characterization of extracellular vesicles: Current status and future directions. *Biosens. Bioelectron.* **2017**, *91*, 588–605. [CrossRef] [PubMed]
189. Görgens, A.; Corso, G.; Hagey, D.W.; Jawad Wiklander, R.; Gustafsson, M.O.; Felldin, U.; Lee, Y.; Bostancioglu, R.B.; Sork, H.; Liang, X.; et al. Identification of storage conditions stabilizing extracellular vesicles preparations. *J. Extracell. Vesicles* **2022**, *11*, e12238. [CrossRef] [PubMed]
190. Zeng, Y.; Qiu, Y.; Jiang, W.; Shen, J.; Yao, X.; He, X.; Li, L.; Fu, B.; Liu, X. Biological Features of Extracellular Vesicles and Challenges. *Front. Cell Dev. Biol.* **2022**, *10*, 816698. [CrossRef]
191. Trenkenschuh, E.; Richter, M.; Heinrich, E.; Koch, M.; Fuhrmann, G.; Friess, W. Enhancing the Stabilization Potential of Lyophilization for Extracellular Vesicles. *Adv. Healthc. Mater.* **2022**, *11*, 2100538. [CrossRef]
192. Gómez-de-Mariscal, E.; Maška, M.; Kotrbová, A.; Pospíchalová, V.; Matula, P.; Muñoz-Barrutia, A. Deep-Learning-Based Segmentation of Small Extracellular Vesicles in Transmission Electron Microscopy Images. *Sci. Rep.* **2019**, *9*, 13211. [CrossRef]
193. Bourgeaux, V.; Lanao, J.M.; Bax, B.E.; Godfrin, Y. Drug-loaded erythrocytes: On the road toward marketing approval. *Drug Des. Dev. Ther.* **2016**, *10*, 665–676. [CrossRef] [PubMed]
194. Chugh, V.; Vijaya Krishna, K.; Pandit, A. Cell Membrane-Coated Mimics: A Methodological Approach for Fabrication, Characterization for Therapeutic Applications, and Challenges for Clinical Translation. *ACS Nano* **2021**, *15*, 17080–17123. [CrossRef]
195. Rao, L.; Cai, B.; Bu, L.-L.; Liao, Q.-Q.; Guo, S.-S.; Zhao, X.-Z.; Dong, W.-F.; Liu, W. Microfluidic Electroporation-Facilitated Synthesis of Erythrocyte Membrane-Coated Magnetic Nanoparticles for Enhanced Imaging-Guided Cancer Therapy. *ACS Nano* **2017**, *11*, 3496–3505. [CrossRef]
196. Yang, H.-C.; Waldman, R.Z.; Chen, Z.; Darling, S.B. Atomic layer deposition for membrane interface engineering. *Nanoscale* **2018**, *10*, 20505–20513. [CrossRef]
197. Huang, L.-L.; Nie, W.; Zhang, J.; Xie, H.-Y. Cell-Membrane-Based Biomimetic Systems with Bioorthogonal Functionalities. *Accounts Chem. Res.* **2020**, *53*, 276–287. [CrossRef] [PubMed]
198. Yousefi, N.; Tufenkji, N. Probing the Interaction between Nanoparticles and Lipid Membranes by Quartz Crystal Microbalance with Dissipation Monitoring. *Front. Chem.* **2016**, *4*, 46. [CrossRef] [PubMed]
199. McDonnell, J.M. Surface plasmon resonance: Towards an understanding of the mechanisms of biological molecular recognition. *Curr. Opin. Chem. Biol.* **2001**, *5*, 572–577. [CrossRef] [PubMed]

200. Fang, R.H.; Kroll, A.V.; Gao, W.; Zhang, L. Cell Membrane Coating Nanotechnology. *Adv. Mater.* **2018**, *30*, 1706759. [CrossRef]
201. Read, E.K.; Park, J.T.; Shah, R.B.; Riley, B.S.; Brorson, K.A.; Rathore, A.S. Process analytical technology (PAT) for biopharmaceutical products: Part I. concepts and applications. *Biotechnol. Bioeng.* **2010**, *105*, 276–284. [CrossRef]
202. Zhang, X.; Ma, G.; Wei, W. Simulation of nanoparticles interacting with a cell membrane: Probing the structural basis and potential biomedical application. *NPG Asia Mater.* **2021**, *13*, 52. [CrossRef]
203. Singh, A.V.; Maharjan, R.-S.; Kanase, A.; Siewert, K.; Rosenkranz, D.; Singh, R.; Laux, P.; Luch, A. Machine-Learning-Based Approach to Decode the Influence of Nanomaterial Properties on Their Interaction with Cells. *ACS Appl. Mater. Interfaces* **2021**, *13*, 1943–1955. [CrossRef]
204. Barclay, T.G.; Day, C.M.; Petrovsky, N.; Garg, S. Review of polysaccharide particle-based functional drug delivery. *Carbohydr. Polym.* **2019**, *221*, 94–112. [CrossRef]
205. Díaz-Montes, E. Dextran: Sources, Structures, and Properties. *Polysaccharides* **2021**, *2*, 554–565. [CrossRef]
206. Huang, M.; Khor, E.; Lim, L.-Y. Uptake and Cytotoxicity of Chitosan Molecules and Nanoparticles: Effects of Molecular Weight and Degree of Deacetylation. *Pharm. Res.* **2004**, *21*, 344–353. [CrossRef]
207. Bhattacharya, D.S.; Svechkarev, D.; Bapat, A.; Patil, P.; Hollingsworth, M.A.; Mohs, A.M. Sulfation Modulates the Targeting Properties of Hyaluronic Acid to P-Selectin and CD44. *ACS Biomater. Sci. Eng.* **2020**, *6*, 3585–3598. [CrossRef]
208. Mena-García, A.; Ruiz-Matute, A.I.; Soria, A.C.; Sanz, M.L. Green techniques for extraction of bioactive carbohydrates. *TrAC Trends Anal. Chem.* **2019**, *119*, 115612. [CrossRef]
209. Huang, G.; Chen, F.; Yang, W.; Huang, H. Preparation, deproteinization and comparison of bioactive polysaccharides. *Trends Food Sci. Technol.* **2021**, *109*, 564–568. [CrossRef]
210. Zheng, D.; Yang, K.; Nie, Z. Engineering heterogeneity of precision nanoparticles for biomedical delivery and therapy. *VIEW* **2021**, *2*, 20200067. [CrossRef]
211. Plucinski, A.; Lyu, Z.; Schmidt, B.V. Polysaccharide nanoparticles: From fabrication to applications. *J. Mater. Chem. B* **2021**, *9*, 7030–7062. [CrossRef]
212. Galmarini, S.; Hanusch, U.; Giraud, M.; Cayla, N.; Chiappe, D.; von Moos, N.; Hofmann, H.; Maurizi, L. Beyond Unpredictability: The Importance of Reproducibility in Understanding the Protein Corona of Nanoparticles. *Bioconjugate Chem.* **2018**, *29*, 3385–3393. [CrossRef]
213. Bastogne, T. Quality-by-design of nanopharmaceuticals—A state of the art. *Nanomedicine* **2017**, *13*, 2151–2157. [CrossRef] [PubMed]
214. Schnitzer, E.; Pinchuk, I.; Bor, A.; Leikin-Frenkel, A.; Lichtenberg, D. Oxidation of liposomal cholesterol and its effect on phospholipid peroxidation. *Chem. Phys. Lipids* **2007**, *146*, 43–53. [CrossRef] [PubMed]
215. Schnitzer, E.; Pinchuk, I.; Lichtenberg, D. Peroxidation of liposomal lipids. *Eur. Biophys. J.* **2007**, *36*, 499–515. [CrossRef] [PubMed]
216. Barnadas-Rodríguez, R.; Sabés, M. Factors involved in the production of liposomes with a high-pressure homogenizer. *Int. J. Pharm.* **2001**, *213*, 175–186. [CrossRef]
217. Karn, P.R.; Cho, W.; Park, H.-J.; Park, J.-S.; Hwang, S.-J. Characterization and stability studies of a novel liposomal cyclosporin A prepared using the supercritical fluid method: Comparison with the modified conventional Bangham method. *Int. J. Nanomed.* **2013**, *8*, 365–377. [CrossRef]
218. Webb, M.S.; Harasym, T.O.; Masin, D.; Bally, M.B.; Mayer, L.D. Sphingomyelin-cholesterol liposomes significantly enhance the pharmacokinetic and therapeutic properties of vincristine in murine and human tumour models. *Br. J. Cancer* **1995**, *72*, 896–904. [CrossRef]
219. Roy, B.; Guha, P.; Bhattarai, R.; Nahak, P.; Karmakar, G.; Chettri, P.; Panda, A.K. Influence of Lipid Composition, pH, and Temperature on Physicochemical Properties of Liposomes with Curcumin as Model Drug. *J. Oleo Sci.* **2016**, *65*, 399–411. [CrossRef]
220. Grit, M.; Crommelin, D.J.A. Chemical stability of liposomes: Implications for their physical stability. *Chem. Phys. Lipids* **1993**, *64*, 3–18. [CrossRef] [PubMed]
221. Arouri, A.; Hansen, A.H.; Rasmussen, T.E.; Mouritsen, O.G. Lipases, liposomes and lipid-prodrugs. *Curr. Opin. Colloid Interface Sci.* **2013**, *18*, 419–431. [CrossRef]
222. Flaten, G.E.; Chang, T.-T.; Phillips, W.T.; Brandl, M.; Bao, A.; Goins, B. Liposomal formulations of poorly soluble camptothecin: Drug retention and biodistribution. *J. Liposome Res.* **2013**, *23*, 70–81. [CrossRef] [PubMed]
223. Basáñez, G.; Goñi, F.M.; Alonso, A. Poly(ethylene glycol)-lipid conjugates inhibit phospholipase C-induced lipid hydrolysis, liposome aggregation and fusion through independent mechanisms. *FEBS Lett.* **1997**, *411*, 281–286. [CrossRef] [PubMed]
224. Mickova, A.; Buzgo, M.; Benada, O.; Rampichova, M.; Fisar, Z.; Filova, E.; Tesarova, M.; Lukas, D.; Amler, E. Core/Shell Nanofibers with Embedded Liposomes as a Drug Delivery System. *Biomacromolecules* **2012**, *13*, 952–962. [CrossRef] [PubMed]
225. Maurer, N.; Fenske, D.B.; Cullis, P.R. Developments in liposomal drug delivery systems. *Expert Opin. Biol. Ther.* **2001**, *1*, 923–947. [CrossRef] [PubMed]
226. Mishra, V.; Heath, R.J. Structural and Biochemical Features of Human Serum Albumin Essential for Eukaryotic Cell Culture. *Int. J. Mol. Sci.* **2021**, *22*, 8411. [CrossRef]
227. Lebedeva, N.S.; Yurina, E.S.; Gubarev, Y.A.; Koifman, O.I. Molecular mechanisms causing albumin aggregation. The main role of the porphyrins of the blood group. *Spectrochim. Acta Part A Mol. Biomol. Spectrosc.* **2021**, *246*, 118975. [CrossRef]

228. Wang, S.-L.; Lin, S.-Y.; Li, M.-J.; Wei, Y.-S.; Hsieh, T.-F. Temperature effect on the structural stability, similarity, and reversibility of human serum albumin in different states. *Biophys. Chem.* **2005**, *114*, 205–212. [CrossRef] [PubMed]
229. Oliva, A.; Santoveña, A.; Llabres, M.; Fariña, J.B. Stability Study of Human Serum Albumin Pharmaceutical Preparations. *J. Pharm. Pharmacol.* **2010**, *51*, 385–392. [CrossRef] [PubMed]
230. Ruzza, P.; Honisch, C.; Hussain, R.; Siligardi, G. Free Radicals and ROS Induce Protein Denaturation by UV Photostability Assay. *Int. J. Mol. Sci.* **2021**, *22*, 6512. [CrossRef] [PubMed]
231. Aljabali, A.A.A.; Bakshi, H.A.; Hakkim, F.L.; Haggag, Y.A.; Al-Batanyeh, K.M.; Al Zoubi, M.S.; Al-Trad, B.; Nasef, M.M.; Satija, S.; Mehta, M.; et al. Albumin Nano-Encapsulation of Piceatannol Enhances Its Anticancer Potential in Colon Cancer Via Downregulation of Nuclear p65 and HIF-1α. *Cancers* **2020**, *12*, 113. [CrossRef]
232. Narayana, S.; Gulzar Ahmed, M.; Nasrine, A. Effect of nano-encapsulation using human serum albumin on anti-angiogenesis activity of bevacizumab to target corneal neovascularization: Development, optimization and in vitro assessment. *Mater. Today: Proc.* **2022**, *68*, 93–104. [CrossRef]
233. Fahrländer, E.; Schelhaas, S.; Jacobs, A.H.; Langer, K. PEGylated human serum albumin (HSA) nanoparticles: Preparation, characterization and quantification of the PEGylation extent. *Nanotechnology* **2015**, *26*, 145103. [CrossRef]
234. Niknejad, H.; Mahmoudzadeh, R. Comparison of different crosslinking methods for preparation of docetaxel-loaded albumin nanoparticles. *Iran. J. Pharm. Res.* **2015**, *14*, 385.
235. Anhorn, M.G.; Mahler, H.-C.; Langer, K. Freeze drying of human serum albumin (HSA) nanoparticles with different excipients. *Int. J. Pharm.* **2008**, *363*, 162–169. [CrossRef]
236. Anraku, M.; Kouno, Y.; Kai, T.; Tsurusaki, Y.; Yamasaki, K.; Otagiri, M. The role of N-acetyl-methioninate as a new stabilizer for albumin products. *Int. J. Pharm.* **2007**, *329*, 19–24. [CrossRef]
237. Meng, R.; Zhu, H.; Deng, P.; Li, M.; Ji, Q.; He, H.; Jin, L.; Wang, B. Research progress on albumin-based hydrogels: Properties, preparation methods, types and its application for antitumor-drug delivery and tissue engineering. *Front. Bioeng. Biotechnol.* **2023**, *11*, 1137145. [CrossRef]
238. Zhao, M.; Li, Z.; Li, X.; Xie, H.; Zhao, Q.; Zhao, M. Molecular imprinting of doxorubicin by refolding thermally denatured bovine serum albumin and cross-linking with hydrogel network. *React. Funct. Polym.* **2021**, *168*, 105036. [CrossRef]
239. Zhang, J.; Hao, Y.; Tian, X.; Liang, Y.; He, X.; Gao, R.; Chen, L.; Zhang, Y. Multi-stimuli responsive molecularly imprinted nanoparticles with tailorable affinity for modulated specific recognition of human serum albumin. *J. Mater. Chem. B* **2022**, *10*, 6634–6643. [CrossRef]
240. Raja, S.T.K.; Thiruselvi, T.; Mandal, A.B.; Gnanamani, A. pH and redox sensitive albumin hydrogel: A self-derived biomaterial. *Sci. Rep.* **2015**, *5*, 15977. [CrossRef] [PubMed]
241. Zheng, C.; Wang, L.; Gao, C. pH-sensitive bovine serum albumin nanoparticles for paclitaxel delivery and controlled release to cervical cancer. *Appl. Nanosci.* **2022**, *12*, 4047–4057. [CrossRef]
242. Khoshnejad, M.; Parhiz, H.; Shuvaev, V.V.; Dmochowski, I.J.; Muzykantov, V.R. Ferritin-based drug delivery systems: Hybrid nanocarriers for vascular immunotargeting. *J. Control. Release* **2018**, *282*, 13–24. [CrossRef] [PubMed]
243. Houser, K.V.; Chen, G.L.; Carter, C.; Crank, M.C.; Nguyen, T.A.; Burgos Florez, M.C.; Berkowitz, N.M.; Mendoza, F.; Hendel, C.S.; Gordon, I.J.; et al. Safety and immunogenicity of a ferritin nanoparticle H2 influenza vaccine in healthy adults: A phase 1 trial. *Nat. Med.* **2022**, *28*, 383–391. [CrossRef]
244. Morikawa, K.; Oseko, F.; Morikawa, S. A Role for Ferritin in Hematopoiesis and the Immune System. *Leuk. Lymphoma* **1995**, *18*, 429–433. [CrossRef]
245. Sun, X.; Hong, Y.; Gong, Y.; Zheng, S.; Xie, D. Bioengineered Ferritin Nanocarriers for Cancer Therapy. *Int. J. Mol. Sci.* **2021**, *22*, 7023. [CrossRef]
246. Singh, A.; Singhal, B. Role of Machine Learning in Bioprocess Engineering: Current Perspectives and Future Directions. In *Design and Applications of Nature Inspired Optimization: Contribution of Women Leaders in the Field*; Singh, D., Garg, V., Deep, K., Eds.; Springer International Publishing: Cham, Switzerland, 2022; pp. 39–54. [CrossRef]
247. Gupta, R.; Arora, K.; Roy, S.S.; Joseph, A.; Rastogi, R.; Arora, N.M.; Kundu, P.K. Platforms, advances, and technical challenges in virus-like particles-based vaccines. *Front. Immunol.* **2023**, *14*, 1123805. [CrossRef]
248. Lv, P.; Liu, X.; Chen, X.; Liu, C.; Zhang, Y.; Chu, C.; Wang, J.; Wang, X.; Chen, X.; Liu, G. Genetically Engineered Cell Membrane Nanovesicles for Oncolytic Adenovirus Delivery: A Versatile Platform for Cancer Virotherapy. *Nano Lett.* **2019**, *19*, 2993–3001. [CrossRef] [PubMed]
249. Suffian, I.F.B.M.; Al-Jamal, K.T. Bioengineering of virus-like particles as dynamic nanocarriers for in vivo delivery and targeting to solid tumours. *Adv. Drug Deliv. Rev.* **2022**, *180*, 114030. [CrossRef] [PubMed]
250. Biabanikhankahdani, R.; Alitheen, N.B.M.; Ho, K.L.; Tan, W.S. pH-responsive Virus-like Nanoparticles with Enhanced Tumour-targeting Ligands for Cancer Drug Delivery. *Sci. Rep.* **2016**, *6*, 37891. [CrossRef]
251. Hu, H.; Steinmetz, N.F. Doxorubicin-Loaded Physalis Mottle Virus Particles Function as a pH-Responsive Prodrug Enabling Cancer Therapy. *Biotechnol. J.* **2020**, *15*, 2000077. [CrossRef] [PubMed]
252. Serradell, M.C.; Rupil, L.L.; Martino, R.A.; Prucca, C.G.; Carranza, P.G.; Saura, A.; Fernández, E.A.; Gargantini, P.R.; Tenaglia, A.H.; Petiti, J.P.; et al. Efficient oral vaccination by bioengineering virus-like particles with protozoan surface proteins. *Nat. Commun.* **2019**, *10*, 361. [CrossRef]

253. Ali, A.; Ganguillet, S.; Turgay, Y.; Keys, T.; Causa, E.; Fradique, R.; Lutz-Bueno, V.; Chesnov, S.; Lin, C.-w.; Lentsch, V.; et al. Surface crosslinking of virus-like particles increases resistance to proteases, low pH and mechanical stress for mucosal applications. *bioRxiv* **2023**. [CrossRef]
254. Shi, L.; Sanyal, G.; Ni, A.; Luo, Z.; Doshna, S.; Wang, B.; Graham, T.L.; Wang, N.; Volkin, D.B. Stabilization of human papillomavirus virus-like particles by non-ionic surfactants. *J. Pharm. Sci.* **2005**, *94*, 1538–1551. [CrossRef]
255. Schumacher, J.; Bacic, T.; Staritzbichler, R.; Daneschdar, M.; Klamp, T.; Arnold, P.; Jägle, S.; Türeci, Ö.; Markl, J.; Sahin, U. Enhanced stability of a chimeric hepatitis B core antigen virus-like-particle (HBcAg-VLP) by a C-terminal linker-hexahistidine-peptide. *J. Nanobiotechnol.* **2018**, *16*, 39. [CrossRef]
256. Gleiter, S.; Lilie, H. Coupling of antibodies via protein Z on modified polyoma virus-like particles. *Protein Sci.* **2001**, *10*, 434–444. [CrossRef]
257. Segel, M.; Lash, B.; Song, J.; Ladha, A.; Liu, C.C.; Jin, X.; Mekhedov, S.L.; Macrae, R.K.; Koonin, E.V.; Zhang, F. Mammalian retrovirus-like protein PEG10 packages its own mRNA and can be pseudotyped for mRNA delivery. *Science* **2021**, *373*, 882–889. [CrossRef]
258. Himbert, S.; Rheinstädter, M. Erythro-VLP: Erythrocyte Virus-Like-Particles. *Biophys. J.* **2021**, *120*, 196a. [CrossRef]
259. Grushin, K.; White, M.A.; Stoilova-McPhie, S. Reversible stacking of lipid nanodiscs for structural studies of clotting factors. *Nanotechnol. Rev.* **2017**, *6*, 139–148. [CrossRef]
260. Hoi, K.K.; Robinson, C.V.; Marty, M.T. Unraveling the Composition and Behavior of Heterogeneous Lipid Nanodiscs by Mass Spectrometry. *Anal. Chem.* **2016**, *88*, 6199–6204. [CrossRef] [PubMed]
261. Damiati, S.; Scheberl, A.; Zayni, S.; Damiati, S.A.; Schuster, B.; Kompella, U.B. Albumin-bound nanodiscs as delivery vehicle candidates: Development and characterization. *Biophys. Chem.* **2019**, *251*, 106178. [CrossRef]
262. Chen, T.; Pan, F.; Luo, G.; Jiang, K.; Wang, H.; Ding, T.; Li, W.; Zhan, C.; Wei, X. Morphology-driven protein corona manipulation for preferential delivery of lipid nanodiscs. *Nano Today* **2022**, *46*, 101609. [CrossRef]
263. Dane, E.L.; Belessiotis-Richards, A.; Backlund, C.; Wang, J.; Hidaka, K.; Milling, L.E.; Bhagchandani, S.; Melo, M.B.; Wu, S.; Li, N.; et al. STING agonist delivery by tumour-penetrating PEG-lipid nanodiscs primes robust anticancer immunity. *Nat. Mater.* **2022**, *21*, 710–720. [CrossRef]
264. Zhang, W.; Sun, J.; Liu, Y.; Tao, M.; Ai, X.; Su, X.; Cai, C.; Tang, Y.; Feng, Z.; Yan, X.; et al. PEG-Stabilized Bilayer Nanodisks As Carriers for Doxorubicin Delivery. *Mol. Pharm.* **2014**, *11*, 3279–3290. [CrossRef]
265. Li, Z.; Gu, L. Effects of Mass Ratio, pH, Temperature, and Reaction Time on Fabrication of Partially Purified Pomegranate Ellagitannin−Gelatin Nanoparticles. *J. Agric. Food Chem.* **2011**, *59*, 4225–4231. [CrossRef]
266. Lammel, A.S.; Hu, X.; Park, S.-H.; Kaplan, D.L.; Scheibel, T.R. Controlling silk fibroin particle features for drug delivery. *Biomaterials* **2010**, *31*, 4583–4591. [CrossRef]
267. Yan, H.-B.; Zhang, Y.-Q.; Ma, Y.-L.; Zhou, L.-X. Biosynthesis of insulin-silk fibroin nanoparticles conjugates and in vitro evaluation of a drug delivery system. *J. Nanoparticle Res.* **2009**, *11*, 1937–1946. [CrossRef]
268. Leo, E.; Angela Vandelli, M.; Cameroni, R.; Forni, F. Doxorubicin-loaded gelatin nanoparticles stabilized by glutaraldehyde: Involvement of the drug in the cross-linking process. *Int. J. Pharm.* **1997**, *155*, 75–82. [CrossRef]
269. Kaul, G.; Amiji, M. Long-Circulating Poly(Ethylene Glycol)-Modified Gelatin Nanoparticles for Intracellular Delivery. *Pharm. Res.* **2002**, *19*, 1061–1067. [CrossRef] [PubMed]
270. Totten, J.D.; Wongpinyochit, T.; Carrola, J.; Duarte, I.F.; Seib, F.P. PEGylation-Dependent Metabolic Rewiring of Macrophages with Silk Fibroin Nanoparticles. *ACS Appl. Mater. Interfaces* **2019**, *11*, 14515–14525. [CrossRef] [PubMed]
271. Gonçalves, A.S.C.; Rodrigues, C.F.; Fernandes, N.; de Melo-Diogo, D.; Ferreira, P.; Moreira, A.F.; Correia, I.J. IR780 loaded gelatin-PEG coated gold core silica shell nanorods for cancer-targeted photothermal/photodynamic therapy. *Biotechnol. Bioeng.* **2022**, *119*, 644–656. [CrossRef]
272. Jia, L.; Guo, L.; Zhu, J.; Ma, Y. Stability and cytocompatibility of silk fibroin-capped gold nanoparticles. *Mater. Sci. Eng. C Mater. Biol. Appl.* **2014**, *43*, 231–236. [CrossRef]
273. Curcio, M.; Altimari, I.; Spizzirri, U.G.; Cirillo, G.; Vittorio, O.; Puoci, F.; Picci, N.; Iemma, F. Biodegradable gelatin-based nanospheres as pH-responsive drug delivery systems. *J. Nanoparticle Res.* **2013**, *15*, 1581. [CrossRef]
274. Sun, N.; Lei, R.; Xu, J.; Kundu, S.C.; Cai, Y.; Yao, J.; Ni, Q. Fabricated porous silk fibroin particles for pH-responsive drug delivery and targeting of tumor cells. *J. Mater. Sci.* **2019**, *54*, 3319–3330. [CrossRef]
275. Deveci, S.S.; Basal, G. Preparation of PCM microcapsules by complex coacervation of silk fibroin and chitosan. *Colloid Polym. Sci.* **2009**, *287*, 1455–1467. [CrossRef]
276. Zhou, Y.; Yang, H.; Liu, X.; Mao, J.; Gu, S.; Xu, W. Electrospinning of carboxyethyl chitosan/poly(vinyl alcohol)/silk fibroin nanoparticles for wound dressings. *Int. J. Biol. Macromol.* **2013**, *53*, 88–92. [CrossRef]
277. Fathollahipour, S.; Abouei Mehrizi, A.; Ghaee, A.; Koosha, M. Electrospinning of PVA/chitosan nanocomposite nanofibers containing gelatin nanoparticles as a dual drug delivery system. *J. Biomed. Mater. Res. Part A* **2015**, *103*, 3852–3862. [CrossRef]
278. Patra, S.; Basak, P.; Tibarewala, D.N. Synthesis of gelatin nano/submicron particles by binary nonsolvent aided coacervation (BNAC) method. *Mater. Sci. Eng. C Mater. Biol. Appl.* **2016**, *59*, 310–318. [CrossRef]
279. Rnjak-Kovacina, J.; DesRochers, T.M.; Burke, K.A.; Kaplan, D.L. The Effect of Sterilization on Silk Fibroin Biomaterial Properties. *Macromol. Biosci.* **2015**, *15*, 861–874. [CrossRef]

280. Jeyaram, A.; Jay, S.M. Preservation and Storage Stability of Extracellular Vesicles for Therapeutic Applications. *AAPS J.* **2017**, *20*, 1. [CrossRef] [PubMed]
281. Yuan, F.; Li, Y.-M.; Wang, Z. Preserving extracellular vesicles for biomedical applications: Consideration of storage stability before and after isolation. *Drug Deliv.* **2021**, *28*, 1501–1509. [CrossRef] [PubMed]
282. Midekessa, G.; Godakumara, K.; Ord, J.; Viil, J.; Lättekivi, F.; Dissanayake, K.; Kopanchuk, S.; Rinken, A.; Andronowska, A.; Bhattacharjee, S.; et al. Zeta Potential of Extracellular Vesicles: Toward Understanding the Attributes that Determine Colloidal Stability. *ACS Omega* **2020**, *5*, 16701–16710. [CrossRef] [PubMed]
283. Schulz, E.; Karagianni, A.; Koch, M.; Fuhrmann, G. Hot EVs—How temperature affects extracellular vesicles. *Eur. J. Pharm. Biopharm.* **2020**, *146*, 55–63. [CrossRef]
284. Bahr, M.M.; Amer, M.S.; Abo-El-Sooud, K.; Abdallah, A.N.; El-Tookhy, O.S. Preservation techniques of stem cells extracellular vesicles: A gate for manufacturing of clinical grade therapeutic extracellular vesicles and long-term clinical trials. *Int. J. Vet. Sci. Med.* **2020**, *8*, 1–8. [CrossRef]
285. Lv, K.; Li, Q.; Zhang, L.; Wang, Y.; Zhong, Z.; Zhao, J.; Lin, X.; Wang, J.; Zhu, K.; Xiao, C.; et al. Incorporation of small extracellular vesicles in sodium alginate hydrogel as a novel therapeutic strategy for myocardial infarction. *Theranostics* **2019**, *9*, 7403–7416. [CrossRef]
286. Piffoux, M.; Silva, A.K.A.; Wilhelm, C.; Gazeau, F.; Tareste, D. Modification of Extracellular Vesicles by Fusion with Liposomes for the Design of Personalized Biogenic Drug Delivery Systems. *ACS Nano* **2018**, *12*, 6830–6842. [CrossRef]
287. Richter, M.; Vader, P.; Fuhrmann, G. Approaches to surface engineering of extracellular vesicles. *Adv. Drug Deliv. Rev.* **2021**, *173*, 416–426. [CrossRef]
288. Gardiner, C.; Vizio, D.D.; Sahoo, S.; Théry, C.; Witwer, K.W.; Wauben, M.; Hill, A.F. Techniques used for the isolation and characterization of extracellular vesicles: Results of a worldwide survey. *J. Extracell. Vesicles* **2016**, *5*, 32945. [CrossRef] [PubMed]
289. de Jong, O.G.; Kooijmans, S.A.A.; Murphy, D.E.; Jiang, L.; Evers, M.J.W.; Sluijter, J.P.G.; Vader, P.; Schiffelers, R.M. Drug Delivery with Extracellular Vesicles: From Imagination to Innovation. *Accounts Chem. Res.* **2019**, *52*, 1761–1770. [CrossRef]
290. Malhotra, S.; Dumoga, S.; Singh, N. Red blood cells membrane-derived nanoparticles: Applications and key challenges in their clinical translation. *Wiley Interdisc. Rev. Nanomed. Nanobiotechnol.* **2022**, *14*, e1776. [CrossRef] [PubMed]
291. Abbina, S.; Parambath, A. 14—PEGylation and its alternatives: A summary. In *Engineering of Biomaterials for Drug Delivery Systems*; Parambath, A., Ed.; Woodhead Publishing: Sawston, UK, 2018; pp. 363–376. [CrossRef]
292. Doshi, N.; Zahr, A.S.; Bhaskar, S.; Lahann, J.; Mitragotri, S. Red blood cell-mimicking synthetic biomaterial particles. *Proc. Natl. Acad. Sci. USA* **2009**, *106*, 21495–21499. [CrossRef] [PubMed]
293. Krishnan, N.; Fang, R.H.; Zhang, L. Engineering of stimuli-responsive self-assembled biomimetic nanoparticles. *Adv. Drug Deliv. Rev.* **2021**, *179*, 114006. [CrossRef] [PubMed]
294. Hu, C.-M.J.; Fang, R.H.; Zhang, L. Erythrocyte-Inspired Delivery Systems. *Adv. Heal. Mater.* **2012**, *1*, 537–547. [CrossRef]
295. Scott, K.L.; Lecak, J.; Acker, J.P. Biopreservation of Red Blood Cells: Past, Present, and Future. *Transfus. Med. Rev.* **2005**, *19*, 127–142. [CrossRef]
296. Han, Y.; Quan, G.B.; Liu, X.Z.; Ma, E.P.; Liu, A.; Jin, P.; Cao, W. Improved preservation of human red blood cells by lyophilization. *Cryobiology* **2005**, *51*, 152–164. [CrossRef]
297. Lee, K.Y.; Mooney, D.J. Alginate: Properties and biomedical applications. *Prog. Polym. Sci.* **2012**, *37*, 106–126. [CrossRef]
298. Kumar, M.N.V.R.; Muzzarelli, R.A.A.; Muzzarelli, C.; Sashiwa, H.; Domb, A.J. Chitosan Chemistry and Pharmaceutical Perspectives. *Chem. Rev.* **2004**, *104*, 6017–6084. [CrossRef]
299. Meyer, K. The Biological Significance of Hyaluronic Acid and Hyaluronidase. *Physiol. Rev.* **1947**, *27*, 335–359. [CrossRef]
300. Sirisha, V.; D'Souza, J.S. Polysaccharide-based nanoparticles as drug delivery systems. *Mar. OMICS* **2016**, *18*, 663–702.
301. Moosavian, S.A.; Bianconi, V.; Pirro, M.; Sahebkar, A. Challenges and pitfalls in the development of liposomal delivery systems for cancer therapy. *Semin. Cancer Biol.* **2021**, *69*, 337–348. [CrossRef]
302. Sercombe, L.; Veerati, T.; Moheimani, F.; Wu, S.Y.; Sood, A.K.; Hua, S. Advances and Challenges of Liposome Assisted Drug Delivery. *Front. Pharmacol.* **2015**, *6*, 286. [CrossRef] [PubMed]
303. Sawant, R.R.; Torchilin, V.P. Challenges in Development of Targeted Liposomal Therapeutics. *AAPS J.* **2012**, *14*, 303–315. [CrossRef] [PubMed]
304. Guan, J.; Shen, Q.; Zhang, Z.; Jiang, Z.; Yang, Y.; Lou, M.; Qian, J.; Lu, W.; Zhan, C. Enhanced immunocompatibility of ligand-targeted liposomes by attenuating natural IgM absorption. *Nat. Commun.* **2018**, *9*, 2982. [CrossRef] [PubMed]
305. Muro, S. Challenges in design and characterization of ligand-targeted drug delivery systems. *J. Control. Release* **2012**, *164*, 125–137. [CrossRef]
306. Maeda, H. Toward a full understanding of the EPR effect in primary and metastatic tumors as well as issues related to its heterogeneity. *Adv. Drug Deliv. Rev.* **2015**, *91*, 3–6. [CrossRef]
307. Deshpande, P.P.; Biswas, S.; Torchilin, V.P. Current trends in the use of liposomes for tumor targeting. *Nanomedicine* **2013**, *8*, 1509–1528. [CrossRef]
308. Pallmann, P.; Bedding, A.W.; Choodari-Oskooei, B.; Dimairo, M.; Flight, L.; Hampson, L.V.; Holmes, J.; Mander, A.P.; Odondi, L.o.; Sydes, M.R.; et al. Adaptive designs in clinical trials: Why use them, and how to run and report them. *BMC Med.* **2018**, *16*, 29. [CrossRef]

309. Meunier, F.; Prentice, H.G.; Ringdén, O. Liposomal amphotericin B (AmBisome): Safety data from a phase II/III clinical trial. *J. Antimicrob. Chemother.* **1991**, *28*, 83–91. [CrossRef] [PubMed]
310. Stone, N.R.H.; Bicanic, T.; Salim, R.; Hope, W. Liposomal Amphotericin B (AmBisome®): A Review of the Pharmacokinetics, Pharmacodynamics, Clinical Experience and Future Directions. *Drugs* **2016**, *76*, 485–500. [CrossRef] [PubMed]
311. Parmar, M.K.B.; Barthel, F.M.-S.; Sydes, M.; Langley, R.; Kaplan, R.; Eisenhauer, E.; Brady, M.; James, N.; Bookman, M.A.; Swart, A.-M.; et al. Speeding up the Evaluation of New Agents in Cancer. *J. Natl. Cancer Inst.* **2008**, *100*, 1204–1214. [CrossRef] [PubMed]
312. Wason, J.M.S.; Jaki, T. Optimal design of multi-arm multi-stage trials. *Stat. Med.* **2012**, *31*, 4269–4279. [CrossRef] [PubMed]
313. Burcu, M.; Manzano-Salgado, C.B.; Butler, A.M.; Christian, J.B. A Framework for Extension Studies Using Real-World Data to Examine Long-Term Safety and Effectiveness. *Ther. Innov. Regul. Sci.* **2022**, *56*, 15–22. [CrossRef]
314. Sherman, R.E.; Anderson, S.A.; Dal Pan, G.J.; Gray, G.W.; Gross, T.; Hunter, N.L.; LaVange, L.; Marinac-Dabic, D.; Marks, P.W.; Robb, M.A.; et al. Real-World Evidence—What Is It and What Can It Tell Us? *N. Engl. J. Med.* **2016**, *375*, 2293–2297. [CrossRef]
315. Kianfar, E. Protein nanoparticles in drug delivery: Animal protein, plant proteins and protein cages, albumin nanoparticles. *J. Nanobiotechnol.* **2021**, *19*, 159. [CrossRef]
316. Mollazadeh, S.; Yazdimamaghani, M.; Yazdian-Robati, R.; Pirhadi, S. New insight into the structural changes of apoferritin pores in the process of doxorubicin loading at an acidic pH: Molecular dynamics simulations. *Comput. Biol. Med.* **2022**, *141*, 105158. [CrossRef]
317. Arosio, P.; Levi, S. Ferritin, iron homeostasis, and oxidative damage 1, 2. *Free Radic. Biol. Med.* **2002**, *33*, 457–463. [CrossRef]
318. Harro, C.D.; Pang, Y.-Y.S.; Roden, R.B.S.; Hildesheim, A.; Wang, Z.; Reynolds, M.J.; Mast, T.C.; Robinson, R.; Murphy, B.R.; Karron, R.A.; et al. Safety and Immunogenicity Trial in Adult Volunteers of a Human Papillomavirus 16 L1 Virus-Like Particle Vaccine. *J. Natl. Cancer Inst.* **2001**, *93*, 284–292. [CrossRef]
319. Carissimi, G.; Montalbán, M.G.; Fuster, M.G.; Víllora, G. Silk Fibroin Nanoparticles: Synthesis and Applications as Drug Nanocarriers. In *21st Century Nanostructured Materials: Physics, Chemistry, Classification, and Emerging Applications in Industry, Biomedicine, and Agriculture*; Intech Open: Rijeka, Croatia, 2022; p. 205.
320. Meng, W.; He, C.; Hao, Y.; Wang, L.; Li, L.; Zhu, G. Prospects and challenges of extracellular vesicle-based drug delivery system: Considering cell source. *Drug Deliv.* **2020**, *27*, 585–598. [CrossRef] [PubMed]
321. Le, Q.-V.; Lee, J.; Lee, H.; Shim, G.; Oh, Y.-K. Cell membrane-derived vesicles for delivery of therapeutic agents. *Acta Pharm. Sin. B* **2021**, *11*, 2096–2113. [CrossRef]
322. Noren Hooten, N.; Yáñez-Mó, M.; DeRita, R.; Russell, A.; Quesenberry, P.; Ramratnam, B.; Robbins, P.D.; Di Vizio, D.; Wen, S.; Witwer, K.W.; et al. Hitting the Bullseye: Are extracellular vesicles on target? *J. Extracell. Vesicles* **2020**, *10*, e12032. [CrossRef] [PubMed]
323. Ortiz, A. Not all extracellular vesicles were created equal: Clinical implications. *Ann. Transl. Med.* **2017**, *5*, 111. [CrossRef] [PubMed]
324. Ghodsi, M.; Cloos, A.-S.; Mozaheb, N.; Van Der Smissen, P.; Henriet, P.; Pierreux, C.E.; Cellier, N.; Mingeot, M.-P.; Najdovski, T.; Tyteca, D. Variability of extracellular vesicle release during storage of red blood cell concentrates is associated with differential membrane alterations, including loss of cholesterol-enriched domains. *Front. Physiol.* **2023**, *14*, 1205493. [CrossRef] [PubMed]
325. Loch-Neckel, G.; Matos, A.T.; Vaz, A.R.; Brites, D. Challenges in the Development of Drug Delivery Systems Based on Small Extracellular Vesicles for Therapy of Brain Diseases. *Front. Pharmacol.* **2022**, *13*, 839790. [CrossRef]
326. Ravasco, J.M.J.M.; Paiva-Santos, A.C.; Conde, J. Technological challenges of biomembrane-coated top-down cancer nanotherapy. *Nat. Rev. Bioeng.* **2023**, *1*, 156–158. [CrossRef]
327. Saxena, A.; Rubens, M.; Ramamoorthy, V.; Zhang, Z.; Ahmed, M.A.; McGranaghan, P.; Das, S.; Veledar, E. A Brief Overview of Adaptive Designs for Phase I Cancer Trials. *Cancers* **2022**, *14*, 1566. [CrossRef]
328. Angus, D.C.; Alexander, B.M.; Berry, S.; Buxton, M.; Lewis, R.; Paoloni, M.; Webb, S.A.R.; Arnold, S.; Barker, A.; Berry, D.A.; et al. Adaptive platform trials: Definition, design, conduct and reporting considerations. *Nat. Rev. Drug Discov.* **2019**, *18*, 797–807. [CrossRef]
329. Ghosh, P.; Liu, L.; Senchaudhuri, P.; Gao, P.; Mehta, C. Design and monitoring of multi-arm multi-stage clinical trials. *Biometrics* **2017**, *73*, 1289–1299. [CrossRef]
330. Park, J.J.H.; Hsu, G.; Siden, E.G.; Thorlund, K.; Mills, E.J. An overview of precision oncology basket and umbrella trials for clinicians. *CA A Cancer J. Clin.* **2020**, *70*, 125–137. [CrossRef] [PubMed]
331. Kidwell, K.M.; Almirall, D. Sequential, Multiple Assignment, Randomized Trial Designs. *JAMA* **2023**, *329*, 336–337. [CrossRef] [PubMed]
332. Kim, H.M. Get SMART—Understanding Sequential Multiple Assignment Randomized Trials. *NEJM Evid.* **2023**, *2*, EVIDe2300031. [CrossRef]
333. Yasmin, F.; Chen, X.; Eames, B.F. Effect of Process Parameters on the Initial Burst Release of Protein-Loaded Alginate Nanospheres. *J. Funct. Biomater.* **2019**, *10*, 42. [CrossRef]
334. Hannon, G.; Prina-Mello, A. Endotoxin contamination of engineered nanomaterials: Overcoming the hurdles associated with endotoxin testing. *Wiley Interdiscip Rev. Nanomed. Nanobiotechnol.* **2021**, *13*, e1738. [CrossRef]
335. Paull, J. A Prospective Study of Dextran-induced Anaphylactoid Reactions in 5745 Patients. *Anaesth. Intensive Care* **1987**, *15*, 163–167. [CrossRef]

336. Stegemann, S.; Klingmann, V.; Reidemeister, S.; Breitkreutz, J. Patient-centric drug product development: Acceptability across patient populations—Science and evidence. *Eur. J. Pharm. Biopharm.* **2023**, *188*, 1–5. [CrossRef]
337. Wasti, S.; Lee, I.H.; Kim, S.; Lee, J.-H.; Kim, H. Ethical and legal challenges in nanomedical innovations: A scoping review. *Front. Genet.* **2023**, *14*, 1163392. [CrossRef]
338. Paradise, J. Regulating nanomedicine at the food and drug administration. *AMA J. Ethics* **2019**, *21*, 347–355.
339. Allon, I.; Ben-Yehudah, A.; Dekel, R.; Solbakk, J.-H.; Weltring, K.-M.; Siegal, G. Ethical issues in nanomedicine: Tempest in a teapot? *Med. Health Care Philos.* **2017**, *20*, 3–11. [CrossRef]
340. Clark, D.P.; Pazdernik, N.J. Chapter 21—Viral and Prion Infections. In *Biotechnology*, 2nd ed.; Clark, D.P., Pazdernik, N.J., Eds.; Academic Cell: Boston, MA, USA, 2016; pp. 663–685. [CrossRef]
341. Larsen, M.T.; Kuhlmann, M.; Hvam, M.L.; Howard, K.A. Albumin-based drug delivery: Harnessing nature to cure disease. *Mol. Cell. Ther.* **2016**, *4*, 3. [CrossRef] [PubMed]
342. Rohovie, M.J.; Nagasawa, M.; Swartz, J.R. Virus-like particles: Next-generation nanoparticles for targeted therapeutic delivery. *Bioeng. Transl. Med.* **2017**, *2*, 43–57. [CrossRef] [PubMed]

Disclaimer/Publisher's Note: The statements, opinions and data contained in all publications are solely those of the individual author(s) and contributor(s) and not of MDPI and/or the editor(s). MDPI and/or the editor(s) disclaim responsibility for any injury to people or property resulting from any ideas, methods, instructions or products referred to in the content.

Article

Topical Sustained-Release Dexamethasone-Loaded Chitosan Nanoparticles: Assessment of Drug Delivery Efficiency in a Rabbit Model of Endotoxin-Induced Uveitis

Musaed Alkholief [1,*,†], Mohd Abul Kalam [1,†], Mohammad Raish [1], Mushtaq Ahmad Ansari [2], Nasser B. Alsaleh [2], Aliyah Almomen [3], Raisuddin Ali [1] and Aws Alshamsan [1,*]

1. Department of Pharmaceutics, College of Pharmacy, King Saud University, P.O. Box 2457, Riyadh 11451, Saudi Arabia; makalam@ksu.edu.sa (M.A.K.); mraish@ksu.edu.sa (M.R.); ramohammad@ksu.edu.sa (R.A.)
2. Department of Pharmacology and Toxicology, College of Pharmacy, King Saud University, P.O. Box 2457, Riyadh 11451, Saudi Arabia; muansari@ksu.edu.sa (M.A.A.); nbalsaleh@ksu.edu.sa (N.B.A.)
3. Department of Pharmaceutical Chemistry, College of Pharmacy, King Saud University, P.O. Box 2457, Riyadh 11451, Saudi Arabia; alalmomen@ksu.edu.sa
* Correspondence: malkholief@ksu.edu.sa (M.A.); aalshamsan@ksu.edu.sa (A.A.)
† These authors contributed equally to this work.

Abstract: Uveitis is an ocular illness that if not treated properly can lead to a total loss of vision. In this study, we evaluated the utility of HA-coated Dexamethasone-sodium-phosphate (DEX)-chitosan nanoparticles (CSNPs) coated with hyaluronic acid (HA) as a sustained ocular delivery vehicle for the treatment of endotoxin-induced-uveitis (EIU) in rabbits. The CSNPs were characterized for particle size, zeta potential, polydispersity, surface morphology, and physicochemical properties. Drug encapsulation, in vitro drug release, and transcorneal permeation were also evaluated. Finally, eye irritation, ocular pharmacokinetics, and pharmacodynamics were in vivo. The CSNPs ranged from 310.4 nm and 379.3 nm pre-(uncoated) and post-lyophilization (with HA-coated), respectively. The zeta potentials were +32 mV (uncoated) and −5 mV (HA-uncoated), while polydispersity was 0.178–0.427. Drug encapsulation and loading in the CSNPs were 73.56% and 6.94% (uncoated) and 71.07% and 5.54% (HA-coated), respectively. The in vitro DEX release over 12 h was 77.1% from the HA-coated and 74.2% from the uncoated NPs. The physicochemical properties of the CSNPs were stable over a 3-month period when stored at 25 °C. Around a 10-fold increased transcorneal-flux and permeability of DEX was found with HA-CSNPs compared to the DEX-aqueous solution (DEX-AqS), and the eye-irritation experiment indicated its ocular safety. After the ocular application of the CSNPs, DEX was detected in the aqueous humor (AH) till 24 h. The area under the concentrations curve (AUC_{0-24h}) for DEX from the CSNPs was 1.87-fold (uncoated) and 2.36-fold (HA-coated) higher than DEX-AqS. The half-life ($t_{1/2}$) of DEX from the uncoated and HA-coated NPs was 2.49-and 3.36-fold higher, and the ocular MRT_{0-inf} was 2.47- and 3.15-fold greater, than that of DEX-AqS, respectively. The EIU rabbit model showed increased levels of MPO, TNF-α, and IL-6 in AH. Topical DEX-loaded CSNPs reduced MPO, TNF-α, and IL-6 levels as well as inhibited NF-κB expression. Our findings demonstrate that the DEX-CSNPs platform has improved the delivery properties and, hence, the promising anti-inflammatory effects on EIU in rabbits.

Keywords: dexamethasone; chitosan-nanoparticles; hyaluronic-acid; ocular-pharmacokinetics; endotoxin; uveitis; cytokines; histopathology

1. Introduction

Uveitis is a prevalent condition with a prevalence of 24.9 cases per 100,000 persons that affects either gender population significantly by geographic location and all ages of patients [1]. Among the different types of uveitis, the anterior uveitis is the most prevalent and the posterior uveitis is the least prevalent [2,3]. The rodent model for endotoxin-induced uveitis (EUI) is widely applied to evaluate anterior uveitis [4]. EIU is an acute inflammation of the anterior chamber of the eye that is induced by the intravitreal injection of endotoxins (also known as lipopolysaccharides; LPSs) [4]. Prostaglandin E_2 (PGE_2) and tumor necrosis factor-alpha (TNF-α) are the primary mediates associated with EIU [5,6], but other chemokines and cytokines have also been shown to play a role in EIU [6,7]. Thus, suppressing pro-inflammatory mediators is a key strategy in controlling and resolving EIU.

Previous studies have revealed that systemic glucocorticoids such as dexamethasone (DEX) (9α-fluoro-16α-methyl-11β,17α,21-trihydroxy-1,4-pregnadiene-3,20-dione) mitigate the production of inflammatory mediators in EIU animal models [5,8]. DEX is a long-acting synthetic glucocorticoid and, among other corticosteroids, DEX sodium phosphate has the highest potency and efficacy against ocular inflammatory conditions [9,10]. It acts by binding to corticosteroid receptors found in human trabecular meshwork cells and the iris as well as the ciliary bodies of rabbit eyes. DEX sodium phosphate reduces pain and swelling by inhibiting the phospholipase-A_2 pathway and the associated inflammatory eicosanoids, including prostaglandins and leukotrienes. Thus, it is often used to reduce injury-, surgery-, and infection-induced eye inflammation.

However, the prolonged use of DEX may cause some systemic adverse effects such as muscle weakness, osteoporosis, cataracts, glaucoma, ecchymosis, insomnia, and skin changes (bruising/fragility/hirsutism) [11–14]. Some general side effects such as hypertension, hyperglycemia, and cognitive alterations have also been reported [15]. Although topical application can avoid such effects, the self-protective barriers of the eye and the tight junctions of the corneal and conjunctival epithelia allow only a small percentage of topically administered drugs to penetrate through ocular tissues [16], rendering limited drug availability to the anterior/posterior segments as well as corneal stroma [17]. Developing novel formulations that efficiently transport conventional ocular preparations across the cornea represents a major challenge. New ocular drug delivery carriers, such as mucoadhesive polymer-based nanoparticles, are needed to achieve effective ophthalmic drug levels. Chitosan (CS) polymer-based nanoparticles are believed to adhere to the surface of the eye for prolonged periods without causing significant irritation [18]. Furthermore, they have been shown to reversibly loosen corneal epithelial tight junctions and thereby improve the transcorneal flux of the applied drug [19].

Our previous studies exhibited less ocular bioavailability in terms of transcorneal permeation and aqueous humor drug concentration as compared to the HA-coated DEX-CSNPs [18]. Remarkably, prior evidence has demonstrated that DEX-loaded nanocarriers improved the efficiency of drug delivery applied to the eyes [20], with a high concentration of DEX accumulating on the ocular surface [18,21]. This in turn triggers transcorneal flux and delivery of DEX to the anterior and posterior segments of the eyes [22]. In that manner, DEX-loaded nanocarriers achieve controlled and constant delivery of DEX to the target site, ultimately reducing ocular inflammation [23].

The inherent properties of chitosan (CS) and hyaluronic acid (HA), such as biodegradability, biocompatibility, and susceptibility to enzyme-based hydrolysis and ocular safety make this a promising drug delivery platform [18,24,25]. Furthermore, HA has been shown to improve the proliferation (and hence regeneration) of corneal and conjunctival epithelial cells through direct interaction with CD44 receptors, which are increasingly expressed during ocular inflammation [17,26,27]. Additionally, the surfaces of HA and chitosan nanoparticles (CSNPs) bind to form an interfacial HA-CS complex, which has been shown to improve cellular targeting [28] and uptake via receptor-facilitated endocytosis [18].

The purpose of this study was to examine the therapeutic effects of DEX-loaded CSNPs in rabbits with LPS-induced uveitis. We evaluated the utility of uncoated and HA-coated DEX-CSNPs as a sustained ocular delivery vehicle to deliver DEX. The HA-coated DEX-CSNPs have been reported by many researchers, but in the present study, we focused on their pharmacodynamic application in EIU in rabbits. Furthermore, the transcorneal penetration of DEX on the excised rabbit cornea as well as the eye-irritation potential of the CSNPs, including ocular pharmacokinetics, were also assessed.

2. Materials and Methods

2.1. Chemicals

Dexamethasone sodium phosphate ($C_{22}H_{28}FNa_2O_8P$; MW: 516.4 g/mol), hydrocortisone ($C_{21}H_{30}O_5$; MW: 362.5 g/mol), low-molecular-weight chitosan (75–85% deacetylated) with viscosity average molecular weight of 50–190 k, sodium tripolyphosphate (sodium-TPP), and sodium dihydrogen phosphate were purchased from Sigma Aldrich (St. Louis, MO, USA). Glacial acetic acid was purchased from BDH Ltd. (Poole, UK). Hyaluronic acid (200 kDa) was obtained from Medipol SA (Lausanne, Switzerland). A Spectra/Por regenerated cellulose (RC) dialysis membrane with 12–14 kDa molecular weight cut-off was procured from Spectrum Laboratories, Inc. (Rancho Dominguez, CA, USA). Mannitol was purchased from Qualikems Fine Chem. Pvt. Ltd. (Vadodara, India). Methanol and acetonitrile (HiPerSolv CHROMANORM® for HPLC) were purchased from BDH Prolabo® (Leuven, Belgium). Purified water was obtained using a Milli-Q® water purifier (Millipore, Molsheim, France). All other solvents were of HPLC grade, and the remaining chemicals were of analytical grade. LPS from *Escherichia coli* was purchased from ChemCruz (Santa Cruz Biotechnology, Inc. Dallas, TX, USA), and the ELISA kits were purchased from MyBiosource, Inc. (San Diego, CA, USA).

2.2. Preparation of CSNPs, Surface Coating, and Lyophilization of DEX-CSNPs

The chitosan nanoparticles (CSNPs) were prepared by the ionic-gelation method at physiologic pH range [29]. Self-aggregation of CS and Tripolyphosphate-Sodium (TPP-Na) resulted in ionic crosslinking, where TPP-Na acts as a cross-linker. The magnetic stirring (for 2–3 h at 700 rpm) at low w/w ratio of TPP and CS ratio produced stable NPs. The detailed method for the preparation of DEX-loaded CSNPs and their surface coating with HA was reported previously [24]. Briefly, CS was solubilized in 1% (v/v) acetic acid to obtain a concentration range of CS (0.2, 0.4, 0.6, and 1.0 mgmL^{-1}). The DEX (10 mg) was dissolved in CS solution. The TPP was solubilized in Milli-Q® water to get different concentrations (0.2, 0.4, 0.6, 0.8, and 1.0 mgmL^{-1}) and the pH was maintained to 7.2 with 0.1 M sodium dihydrogen phosphate (NaH_2PO_4) buffer. Subsequently, TPP solution (6 mL) was added in CS solution (12 mL) at 1.5 mLmin^{-1} of rate of addition. For HA coating, 20 mg of CSNPs was suspended in 0.1 M acetic acid (2 mL) at pH 5. The suspension was added drop wise to 2 mL of HA containing (0.5, 1, 2, 5, 10, and 20 mgmL^{-1}) 0.1 M acetic acid solution. The process was performed at magnetic stirring (1000 rpm for 30 min). Thereafter, the nanosuspension was ultra-filtered against purified water through the dialysis membrane [30,31]. The suspensions of DEX-CSNPs and HA-coated DEX-CSNPs were lyophilized with and without mannitol (2.5%, 5%, and 7.5% w/v) [32,33] and then stored at 25 °C for further characterization. The nanosuspensions of CSNPs were filtered through the Millipore® syringe filters (450 μ), frozen at −80 °C, and lyophilized by FreeZone-4.5 Freeze Dry System (Labconco Corporation, Kansas City, MO, USA). The lyophilization was performed with and without mannitol at varying concentrations (2.5%, 5%, and 7.5%, w/v) as lyoprotectant. The lyophilized products were stored as mentioned above.

2.3. Physical and Physicochemical Characterizations

The physical characterizations including the size, distribution, polydispersity-index (PDI), and zeta potentials (ZP) of the DEX-CSNPs (HA-coated and uncoated, with and without mannitol) were determined by dynamic light scattering (DLS) using Zetasizer Nano-ZS (Malvern Instruments Ltd., Worcestershire, UK).

The morphologies of HA-coated and uncoated DEX-CSNPs were characterized by transmission electron microscopy (TEM). Concisely, the nanosuspensions were sonicated for 5 min prior to grid preparation. A copper grid (300 meshes) with carbon type-B support film (manufactured by Ted-Pella Inc. Redding, CA, USA) was kept on butter paper.

One drop of the CSNPs suspensions (previously sonicated for 5 min) was put separately on the grid and left for 15 min to settle down the NPs. The grid was left overnight to dry. The dried grid was then mounted in the sample holder of the machine, and the shape of the NPs was investigated under JEM-1010, TEM (JEOL, Tokyo, Japan). The machine operated at 80 kV (accelerating voltage) and 60,000- to 150,000-times magnification power at room temperature [34].

Drug encapsulation efficiency (EE) and loading capacity (DL) were estimated indirectly by measuring the free drug concentration of DEX via an ultra-performance liquid chromatography coupled with the ultraviolet detection (UPLC-UV) method [24,35]. Briefly, the Waters Acquity H-Class UPLC system coupled with a Waters TUV Detector by Acquity (Waters, Milford, MA, USA) for the analysis of DEX was used. Elution of DEX was completed on a Acquity UPLC BEH^{TM} C_{18} Column (1.7 µm, 2.1 × 50 mm) that was maintained at ambient temperature. The mobile phase (60/40 acetonitrile and water, where the pH of water was adjusted to 3.2 with O-phosphoric acid) was isocratically pumped at 0.14 mL.min^{-1} flow rate, and the volume of injection was 10 µL. The EMPOWER software was used for data acquisition, processing, as well as to control the UPLC system.

The transparency of the prepared nanosuspensions (coated and uncoated) was determined by visual observation under light against a black and white background. The pH was checked using a pH-meter (MP-220; Mettler Toledo, Switzerland), and the refractive index was estimated by an Abbe Refractometer (model DR-A1, ATAGO, Inc., Bellevue, Washington, USA). The viscosity of nanosuspensions was measured using a cone and plate viscometer (Physica Rheolab, Austria) with an MK-22 spindle. The above parameters were evaluated initially and after three months storage at 25 ± 2 °C, as reported previously [36–38].

2.4. In Vitro Drug Release

The dialysis membrane method was employed for the in vitro drug release experiment [39]. After maintaining the isotonicity by mannitol, an equivalent amount of NPs and DEX-solution in triplicate, containing 0.1% (w/v) of drug (i.e., 1.0 mg/mL), were placed in dialysis bags (MWCO 10–12 kDa) and both ends were tightly closed. The filled bags were put in beakers containing 50 mL of simulated tear fluids (STF). The whole assembly was placed in a water bath (shaken at 50 rpm and maintained at 35 ± 0.5 °C just to mimic the ocular surface temperature). Samples were withdrawn at predetermined time points and the same amount of fresh STF (maintained at 35 ± 0.5 °C) was replaced after each sampling to maintain the sink conditions. The withdrawn samples were centrifuged for 10 min at 13,000 rpm and 4 °C, supernatants were collected (diluted with STF, whenever needed), and the concentration of released DEX was analyzed using UPLC-UV as described previously [24,35,40]. A calibration curve (y = 10984x − 639.32), $R^2 = 0.999$, was used to calculate the DEX concentration. The cumulative amounts of drug released (%DR) was calculated using Equation (1) and plotted against time (h).

$$\% \, DR = \frac{Conc. \, (\mu g m L^{-1}) \times Dilution \, factor \times Volume \, of \, STF \, (mL)}{Initial \, dose \, (\mu g)} \times 100 \qquad (1)$$

2.5. In Vivo Animal Study

Thirty male New Zealand Albino rabbits (2.0–3.0 kg) were acquired from the College of Pharmacy (Animal Care and Use Center, King Saud University, Riyadh, Saudi Arabia). The animal experiments were performed as per the Association for Research in Vision and Ophthalmology (ARVO) statement regarding the use of animals in ophthalmic and vision research, and they were approved by the Institutional Animal Care and Use Committee of King Saud University (SE-19-90). The drug-loaded CSNPs were subjected to in vivo ocular experiments based on the results of the physicochemical characteristics, in vitro drug release study, and permeation parameters.

2.5.1. Ocular Irritation Study

The drug-loaded CSNPs intended for topical ocular application were cryoprotected by mannitol (2.5%, w/v), freeze-dried, and sterilized by UV-radiation. The formulations were exposed to UV-light at 254 nm wavelength for 2 h [41,42]. The formulations were reconstituted in sterile water for injection before ocular administration. Six rabbits were divided in two groups (n = 3). The eye irritation test was performed as per Draize's protocol for rabbits [43]. We instilled the sterilized formulations into rabbit eyes three times/day for 10 days and visually observed them throughout the experiment. The level of eye irritation was judged by observing the animals' uneasiness and assessing signs/symptoms in the cornea, conjunctiva, and eyelids according to previously reported scoring systems [44].

2.5.2. Transcorneal Permeation

After a washout period of three weeks, five rabbits (previously utilized for ocular irritation experiments) were sacrificed to excise ten corneas. Among these, nine corneas were used for transcorneal permeation study by the double-jacketed automated transdermal diffusion cell-equipped sampling system (SFDC-6; Logan, NJ, USA). The detailed methodology was as previously reported [18]. The cross-section of the cornea measured 0.636 cm^2. Phosphate buffered saline (PBS; 6.9 mL, pH = 7.4) was used as the release medium, and the initial drug concentration was 500 µg·mL^{-1}. The study was performed in triplicate for 6 h and the amount of permeated DEX was analyzed by UPLC-UV [35]. Permeation parameters such as steady-state flux (J, µgcm^{-2}s^{-1}) and apparent permeability (Papp, cms^{-1}) were determined by Equations (2) and (3).

$$J\ (\mu gcm^{-2}s^{-1}) = dQ/dt \qquad (2)$$

$$Papp\ (cms^{-1}) = J/C_0 \qquad (3)$$

where Q is the quantity of DEX that passes through the cornea, t is the exposure time, and C_0 is the initial DEX concentration (µg·mL^{-1}) in the donor compartment of the Franz diffusion cell.

2.5.3. Ocular Pharmacokinetics

Nine animals were divided into 3 groups (n = 3). As per the directive of the Association for Research in Vision and Ophthalmology (ARVO) for animal use in ophthalmic and vision research only one eye (either right or left) should be used for the experimental purpose. Therefore, only the left eye of all rabbits was treated. The concentration of DEX in AH was determined after the instillation of sterilized formulations such as DEX-CSNPs (group-A), HA-coated DEX-CSNPs (Group-B), and DEX-aqueous solution (DEX-AqS; Group-C). In addition, AH was collected at different time intervals, and its DEX concentration was analyzed by UPLC-UV as previously reported [18]. A non-compartmental approach was used for determining pharmacokinetic parameters. The area under the curve to the last measurable concentration (AUC$_{0-t}$), area under the curve to infinity (AUC$_{0-inf}$), maximum concentration (C$_{max}$), time to C$_{max}$ (t$_{max}$), and half-life (t$_{1/2}$) were computed using PK-Solver software (Nanjing, China) in Microsoft Excel 2013 [18,45]. The paired t-test (GraphPad Software, Inc., San Diego, CA, USA) was utilized to compare the obtained pharmacokinetic parameters; p-value < 0.05 was considered statistically significant.

2.5.4. Effect of DEX-CSNPs on LPS-Induced Ocular Inflammation

Study Design and Animal Model of Experimental Uveitis

Fifteen rabbits were divided in 5 groups (n = 3). Rabbits in Group-1 (normal control group) received 5% mannitol (vehicle). Group-2 was injected with LPS. Group-3 received DEX-AqS. Group-4 was treated with DEX-CSNPs and Group-5 was treated with HA-coated DEX-CSNPs. All groups except Group-1 received intravitreal injections of LPS (20 µL; 100 ng) in both eyes to induce uveitis [46,47]. Topical anesthesia was applied by administering one drop of 0.5% Proparacaine Hydrochloride. After retracting the upper lid, 100 ng (20 µL, dissolved in water for injection) of the endotoxin was injected intravitreally with a 29-gauge needle. After the induction of uveitis, the sterilized formulations were instilled topically into the animals' left eye 3 times a day for 3 days. Seventy-two hours after the induction of uveitis, AH was sampled for cell count, protein, interleukin-6 (IL6), myeloperoxidase (MPO), nuclear factor kappa B (NF-κB)-DNA binding activity, and estimated TNF-α [20]. Rabbits were re-examined for clinical signs of uveitis and then sacrificed. Animals' eyes were enucleated for histopathologic examination [48].

Grading System for Ocular Inflammation

The clinical signs of ocular inflammation were graded on a scale of 0 to 4 according to a previously reported scoring system [49] as follows: no inflammatory reaction (= 0), discrete inflammatory reaction (= 1), moderate dilation of the iris and conjunctival vessels (= 2), intense iridial hyperemia with flaring in the anterior chamber (= 3), intense iridial hyperemia with intense flaring in the anterior chamber and the presence of fibrinoid exudates in the papillary area (= 4). Grading was performed 24 and 72 h post intravitreal injection of LPS [47,48].

Aqueous Humor (AH) Sampling

A combination of Ketamine Hydrochloride (20–40 mg·kg^{-1} b. wt.) and Xylazine (1–2 mg·kg^{-1} of body weight) was intravenously injected into the rabbits' marginal ear veins to induce anesthesia. The Proparacaine Hydrochloride (0.5%, w/v) was instilled in the eyes to facilitate general anesthesia. A 29-gauge needle was used to remove approximately 50–100 µL of AH from the anterior chamber of the eyes while taking care not to injure the iris, lens, and other areas of the eyes.

Total Cell Count

Approximately 50 µL of AH was suspended in 50 µL of Turk's stain solution. Cells were counted using a hemocytometer with the aid of a light microscope. Afterward, the number of cells per milliliter of AH was calculated [50,51]. Cell counting was performed on the day of AH sampling.

Estimation of Total Protein and Inflammatory Cytokines (TNF-α and IL6)

The Estimation of total protein in AH samples was performed according to Lowry's method [52]. Briefly, AH (10 µL) samples were diluted with 990 µL of 1 N NaOH and reacted with 4 mL of copper reagent. After 10 min, 500 µL of Folin's reagent was added to each sample and the solutions were vortexed. Then, the samples were stored for 30 min in the dark. Absorbance was recorded with a spectrophotometer at 620 nm. Bovine serum albumin (BSA) was used as the standard for calculating the protein content of the samples. All estimations were performed in triplicate. Protein estimation was performed on the day of AH sampling. The levels of TNF-α and IL6 in AH were determined by using a commercially available ELISA kit per the manufacturer's instructions [53].

Western Blot Assay

Frozen eye tissues were homogenized in a 0.5% (w/v) hexadecyltrimethylammonium bromide solution, solubilized in 0.01 M potassium phosphate buffer (pH = 7), and centrifuged at 6000 rpm for 30 min at 4 °C. The concentration of protein in tissues was measured by Lowry's method [52]. Tissue lysates (25 µg/well) were loaded in 10% Mini-Protean TGX Gels (Bio-rad, Hercules, CA, USA), underwent electrophoresis, and were transferred to a PVDF membrane (Bio-rad, Hercules, CA, USA). The membrane was then blocked, and, with 5% (w/v) skimmed milk, prepared in Tris-buffered saline and Tween 20 (TBS-T). The membrane was then incubated with primary antibodies prepared based on the manufacturer's recommendation overnight at 4 °C. Membranes were then washed and incubated with the suitable secondary antibody, horseradish peroxidase-coupled anti-rabbit or anti-mouse antibody. Bands were visualized using the Western Bright ECL Kit for 5000 cm^2 Membrane and Blue Basic Autoradiography Film (Bioexpress, Kaysville, CA, USA) [54].

Histopathological Evaluation

The eyes of sacrificed rabbits were enucleated 72 h post intravitreal injection of LPS and stored in 10% (v/v) formaldehyde solution. Sections (approximately 4 to 5 μm thick) were cut and stained with Hematoxylin and Eosin stains (H&E) and evaluated using light microscopy.

2.6. Statistical Analysis

All results were expressed as mean of three measurements with standard deviation (Mean ± SD). The statistical analysis was performed using GraphPad Prism V 5.0 (Graph-Pad Software Inc., San Diego, CA, USA). All parameters were compared using one-way ANOVA. The paired t-test (GraphPad Software Inc., San Diego, CA, USA) was employed to compare the obtained parameters, considering the p-value ($p < 0.05$) as statistically significant.

3. Results and Discussion

3.1. Development of DEX-CSNPs and Their Coating

CSNPs were prepared by ionic gelation, wherein self-aggregation of CS and sodium-TPP resulted in ionic crosslinking. Continuous magnetic stirring (at 500 rpm for 2 h) at low TPP: CS weight ratios produced stable NPs. The TPP: CS ratio of 0.4:0.6 (mg/mL) produced NPs of an optimal size suitable for ocular application. They had high EE, DL, and appropriate drug release properties that made them ideal for HA-coating and further characterization [24,40].

The optimum CSNPs were coated with a 2% (w/v) solution of HA in diluted acetic acid according to the previous reports [24,31]. We coated CSNPs with HA because it enhances cellular targeting and interacts with CD-44 receptors to regenerate corneal and conjunctival epithelia [17], which in turn supports receptor-mediated transportation and hyaluronan biodegradation [55]. Hyaluronic acid-coating reversed the surface charge of NPs from highly positive to negative. This could be attributed to the effective adsorption of negatively charged HA molecules to positively charged CSNPs. A reversal in surface charge can result in a high negative charge density around HA-coated CSNPs, which in turn increases their hydrodynamic diameters [56]. Furthermore, HA-coating also was able to protect against the pH-dependent endosomal-mediated disruption of CS [30]. Thus, HA-coating of CSNPs is key for CSNP stability over time, particularly, under low pH conditions within the lysosomes.

3.2. Characterization of HA-Coated DEX-CSNPs

The representative TEM images (Figure 1a,b) indicated that DEX-loaded CSNPs were evenly distributed and did not aggregate. They were found to have solid, dense, spherical morphology with a smooth surface (in the case of HA-coated ones), while the surfaces of uncoated CSNPs were slightly rough, which was also reported previously [57]. Apart from the surface modification, HA-coating increased the particle size, which was further confirmed by DLS measurement as represented in Figure 2. Here, Figure 2a,b represents the particle size and zeta potential distributions of the DEX-loaded CSNPs (uncoated), whereas Figure 2c,d represents the particle size and zeta potential distributions of the DEX-loaded CSNPs coated with HA.

Particle size, polydispersity index (PDI), and zeta potentials are important parameters for preventing eye irritation as well as for prolonging drug retention in the conjunctiva and cornea. Particles must be small (ranging from a few nm to 900 nm), since larger particulates may cause ocular irritation and discomfort and possibly negatively affect patient compliance [58]. In our study, the size of CSNPs was 310.4 ± 12.4 nm before lyophilization and without HA coating, and 368.5 ± 14.4 nm after lyophilization and HA coating. Because human eyes can tolerate particulates up to 10 µm in diameter [58,59], our system of HA-coated CSNPs would be a good candidate for the ocular delivery of DEX.

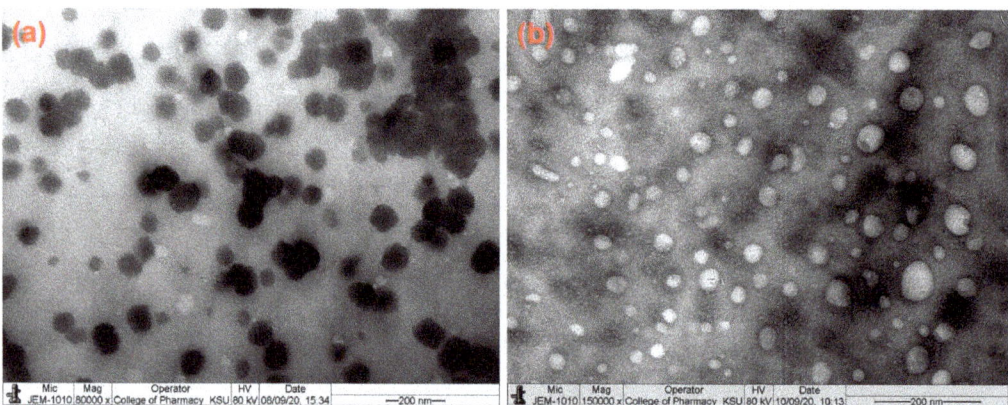

Figure 1. Transmission electron micrographs of DEX-loaded CSNPs: (**a**) uncoated; (**b**) HA-coated.

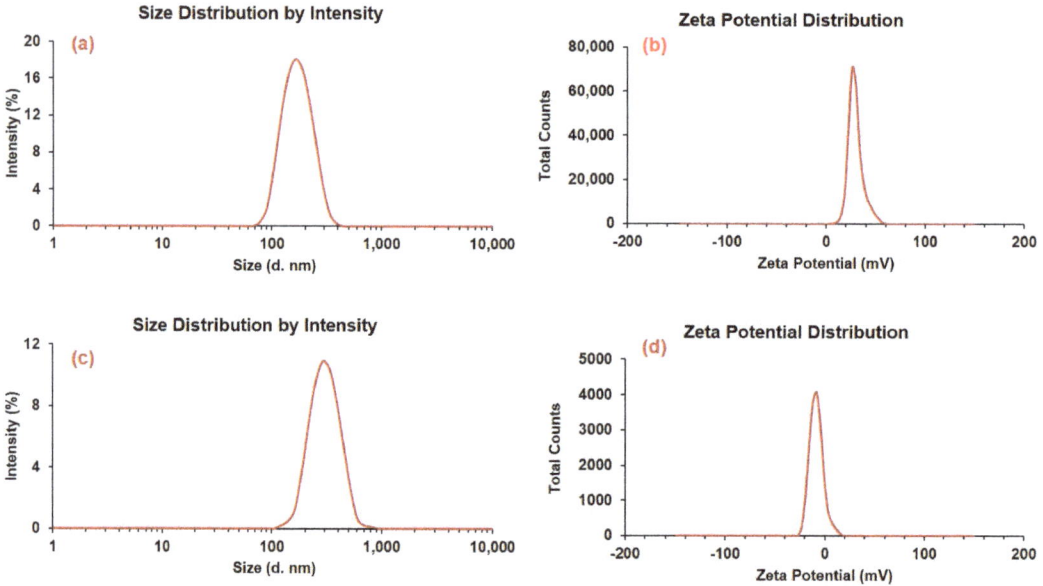

Figure 2. Particle size and zeta potential distributions of DEX-loaded CSNPs; (**a**,**b**) for uncoated; (**c**,**d**) for DEX-loaded CSNPs coated with HA.

Zeta potential and PDI values are summarized in Table 1. High negative or positive zeta potentials would probably lead to a stable colloidal solution, where electrostatic repulsion prevents NP aggregation. Small PDI values also are indicative of stable dispersion and unimodal distribution of CSNPs in the dispersion medium (Table 2). The CSNPs produced by magnetically stirring TPP and CS at a ratio of 0.4:0.6 (mg/mL) for 2 h at 500 rpm had good EE and DL. In order to evaluate the effect of drug concentration on EE and DL, varying amounts of DEX (5, 10, and 15 mg) were added to the DEX-CSNPs formula. We found that 10 mg DEX was optimal for producing DEX-CSNPs with high EE and DL and for which all the physical characteristics were appropriate for ocular application. The values of the obtained parameters are summarized in Table 2.

Table 1. Physical characteristics of uncoated and HA-coated drug-loaded CS-NPs before and after lyophilization without cryoprotectant. The data were presented as the mean of three readings with standard deviations (Mean ± SD, n = 3).

Parameters	Optimized DEX-CS-NPs before Lyophilization		Optimized DEX-CS-NPs after Lyophilization	
	Uncoated	HA-Coated	Uncoated	HA-Coated
Particle size (nm)	310.4 ± 12.4	337.3 ± 14.2	356.8 ± 14.1	368.5 ± 14.4
Polydispersity Index	0.142 ± 0.021	0.179 ± 0.078	0.248 ± 0.041	0.325 ± 0.021
Zeta potential (mV)	+31.4 ± 4.1	−5.7 ± 1.3	+32.2 ± 2.1	−6.2 ± 1.4

Table 2. Physical characteristics of uncoated and HA-coated DEX-loaded CS-NPs after lyophilization with mannitol (2.5%, w/v) as cryoprotectant. The data were presented as the mean of three readings with standard deviations (Mean ± SD, n = 3).

Formulation	Uncoated CS-NPs (0.4:0.6/TPP:CS)	HA-Coated CS-NPs (0.4:0.6/TPP:CS)
Particle size (nm)	361.9 ± 14.3	379.3 ± 13.9
Polydispersity Index (PDI)	0.194 ± 0.075	0.209 ± 0.084
Zeta potential (mV)	+31.2 ± 1.9	−5.6 ± 1.2
Encapsulation (%EE)	73.6 ± 4.6	71.1 ± 3.4
Drug loading (%DL)	6.9 ± 0.4	5.5 ± 0.2
† Aggregation	# #	#

† Aggregation: "#" = low (minimum), and "# #" = intermediate (medium).

The physicochemical characteristics, including clarity, refractive index, pH, and viscosity of the CSNP suspensions were deemed appropriate for ocular application (Table 3). That is, the pH values of CSNP suspensions, which remained virtually unchanged throughout the storage period, were suitable for ocular use (approaching to the normal physiological pH of ocular surfaces in humans, i.e., 7.1 ± 1.5) [60]; and the observed refractive indexes were similar to that of tear fluid. Thus, we anticipate that the formulations would not impair vision and would be comfortable. The viscosity of the nanosuspension affects the proper instillation of ophthalmic medications as well as the ease of sterilization (if by filtration). The observed viscosity of the two nano-formulations was within the range of optimal viscosity (20–30 mPa.s) for ocular preparations [61,62]. Hence, there was no chance of eye discomfort because of blurred vision and foreign particles, and in turn, there was no risk of the elimination of preparations due to reflex tears and frequent eyelid blinking [62–64]. Therefore, the formulations could be retained for prolonged periods without impairing the vision.

3.3. In Vitro Drug Release

Weighed CSNP samples with equivalent amounts of DEX (0.1%, w/v) were used for in vitro release experiments based on encapsulation and initially prepared concentrations of drug and excipients. The in vitro release experiment demonstrated an initial burst release of DEX from the uncoated CSNPs lasting ~3 h, after which there was a sustained release for up to 12 h. On the other hand, there was a sustained release of DEX from the HA-coated CSNPs. We noted that 33.62% of the drug was released at 1 h and around 56.32% at 3 h from the uncoated CSNPs in the rapid release phase, while it was only 13.49% at 1 h and went to 31.54% at 3 h from the HA-coated NPs. The release profile (Figure 3a) indicated slow drug release from the HA-coated NPs, which must be due to the HA-coating of the DEX-loaded CSNPs [24,40]. Although the total amount of released drug from both the NPs was almost comparable, the pattern of drug release from the HA-coated NPs was sustained and consistent over 12 h. In addition, the sustained release of DEX from HA-coated NPs can be explained by Higuchi's square root plot (Figure 3b). It represents the release rate plots for the diffusion of DEX from the CSNPs, where the fraction of the released drug was plotted against the square root of time. The increase in the fraction of DEX released from the HA-coated CSNPs was practically linear (with $R^2 = 0.957$) against the square root of time ($h^{1/2}$) as compared to uncoated CSNPs ($R^2 = 0.695$), which justifies the sustained-release property of HA-coated CSNPs rather than that of the uncoated one [39].

Table 3. Physicochemical characteristics evaluated at ambient temperature of uncoated and HA-coated DEX-loaded CS-NPs after lyophilization with mannitol (2.5%, w/v) as cryoprotectant. The data were presented as the mean of three readings with standard deviations (Mean ± SD, n = 3).

Parameters	Time Points	Uncoated NPs	HA-Coated NPs
Clarity	Initially	Clear and transparent	Clear and transparent
	After 3 months	Clear and translucent	Clear and transparent
Refractive index	Initially	1.34 ± 0.07	1.35 ± 0.12
	After 3 months	1.35 ± 0.09	1.35 ± 0.31
pH	Initially	6.69 ± 0.34	6.81 ± 0.21
	After 3 months	7.15 ± 0.23	7.21 ± 0.03
Viscosity (mPa.s)	Initially	30.74 ± 1.49	33.76 ± 3.12
	After 3 months	34.73 ± 2.19	37.54 ± 2.09

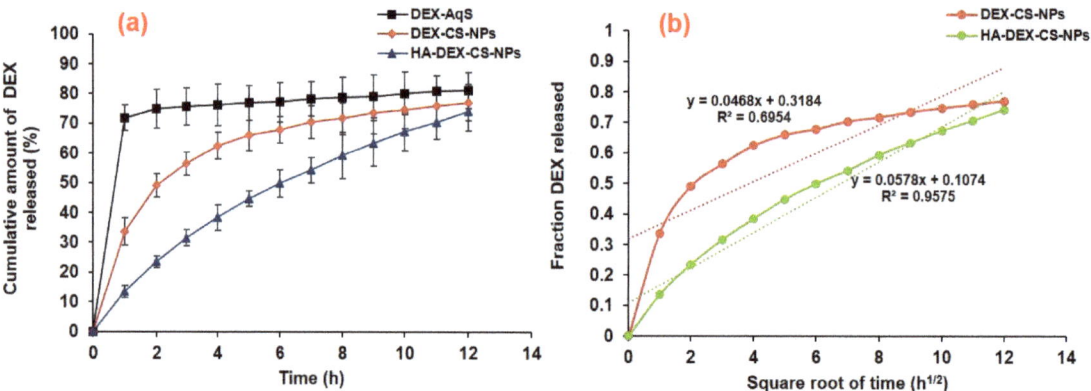

Figure 3. Cumulative amount of drug released versus time profile (**a**) and Higuchi's square root plot (**b**). The data were expressed as the mean of three measurements with standard deviations (Mean ± SD, n = 3).

The initial rapid release of DEX from the uncoated CSNPs could be attributable to a desorption phenomenon, i.e., the rapid dissolution and diffusion of the surface-adsorbed loosely bound drug from the surface of NPs [65], while the release rate of DEX from HA-coated NPs was slower during the initial hours due to the HA-coating. One explanation is that the HA-coating hindered the rapid dissolution and diffusion of the drug from the CSNP core in the release medium (STF). The slow and sustained release of DEX from the HA-coated NPs is owing to the changes in the release mechanism (including liberation and diffusion of drug from the polymer matrix). Another possibility for such an outcome may be due to the polymer degradation in STF or even the combined effects of both drug diffusions from the polymer matrix and polymer degradation in STF.

3.4. Transcorneal Permeation

The permeation flux and P_{app} values of different formulations were calculated (Table 4). The uncoated CSNPs were able to permeate around 28.4 μgcm^{-2} of drug, while it was only 11.8 μgcm^{-2} for the HA-coated CSNPs at 30 min. The HA-coated CSNPs achieved a sustained transcorneal permeation of DEX starting from 30 min until 6 h (Figure 4), which reached a maximum of 69.32 μgcm^{-2} at 6 h. There was around a 4.7-fold and 10.1-fold enhanced flux for uncoated and HA-coated CSNPs, respectively, as compared to DEX-AqS. Due to high mucoadhesiveness and HA interaction with hyaluronan receptors on corneal surfaces, our nano-formulation exploits this property of surface targeting [28] that could potentially enhance cellular uptake through receptor-mediated endocytosis [18]. This could explain the improved permeation of the HA-coated CSNPs compared to the uncoated CSNPs.

Table 4. Corneal permeation parameters of DEX-containing formulations. The data were presented as the mean of three readings with standard deviations (Mean ± SD, $n = 3$).

Corneal Permeation Parameters	DEX-AqS (0.1%, w/v)	Uncoated CS-NPs	HA-Coated CS-NPs
Cumulative amount of DEX permeated (μgcm^{-2} at 0.5 h)	58.44 ± 3.04	28.36 ± 2.05	11.86 ± 3.12
Cumulative amount of DEX permeated (μgcm^{-2} in 6 h)	66.86 ± 3.51	59.52 ± 3.67	69.32 ± 4.58
pH	7.12 ± 0.08	6.69 ± 0.34	6.81 ± 0.21
Steady-state flux, J (μgcm^{-2}h^{-1})	1.76 ± 0.13	8.27 ± 0.49	17.81 ± 0.43
Enhancement ratio	---	4.70 ± 0.39	10.14 ± 0.92
Permeability coefficient, P (cmh^{-1})	$(3.52 ± 0.25) \times 10^{-3}$	$(16.53 ± 0.99) \times 10^{-3}$	$(35.62 ± 0.86) \times 10^{-3}$

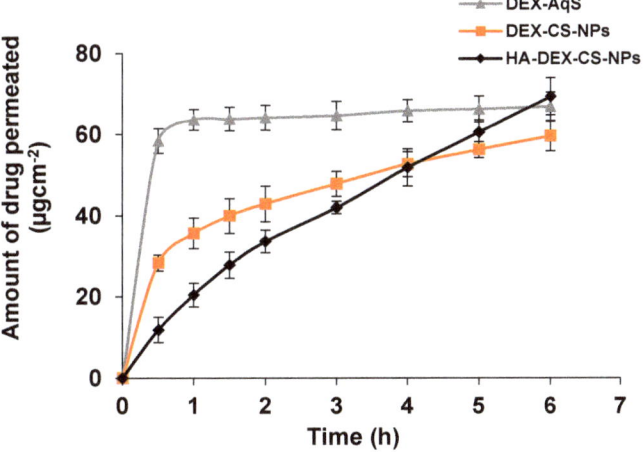

Figure 4. Transcorneal permeation of DEX from CSNPs and DEX−aqueous solution (0.1%, w/v). The data were presented as the mean of three readings with standard deviations (Mean ± SD, $n = 3$).

A neutral pH plays an important role in DEX permeation through the cornea. The first pK$_a$ of DEX is 1.89, at which point the ratio of neutral: monoanion is 50:50. At the second pK$_a$ (6.4), the monoanion: dianion ratio is 50:50. Because DEX has maximum mobility at pH 7, the second pK$_a$ provides high water solubility with sufficient buffering capacity to the formulations for ocular use [66]. In our study, the pH of CSNP suspensions was almost neutral (equivalent to that of tears), whereby a large amount of DEX remained in the unionized state to promote high corneal permeation. The observed additional DEX permeation in the initial hours of the experiment (Figure 4) could be potentially due to the large fraction of unionized DEX at the neutral pH (7.11 ± 0.12) of DEX-AqS [18,67].

3.5. Ocular Irritation

The ocular irritation of CSNPs suspensions in rabbit eyes was assessed against NaCl solution (0.9%, w/v). We have shown in a previous study that recurrent instillation of uncoated and HA-coated CSNPs resulted in slight eye irritation in some rabbits [18]. In contrast, none of the animals in our current study displayed acute or long-term signs of discomfort (Grade 0), which might be due to the immune variability of the animals. Moreover, irritation levels for the conjunctiva, cornea, and eyelids were Grade 0 among rabbits receiving coated and uncoated DEX-CSNPs. The results of this experiment support that DEX-CSNPs are safe and nonirritating for ocular use.

3.6. Ocular Pharmacokinetics

The previously validated UPLC-UV method is effective for the analysis of DEX in aspirated AH samples after the topical application of DEX-containing formulations [18]. The measured concentrations of drug in AH samples at different time points are represented in Figure 5, and the pharmacokinetic parameters calculated using PK-Solver are summarized in Table 5.

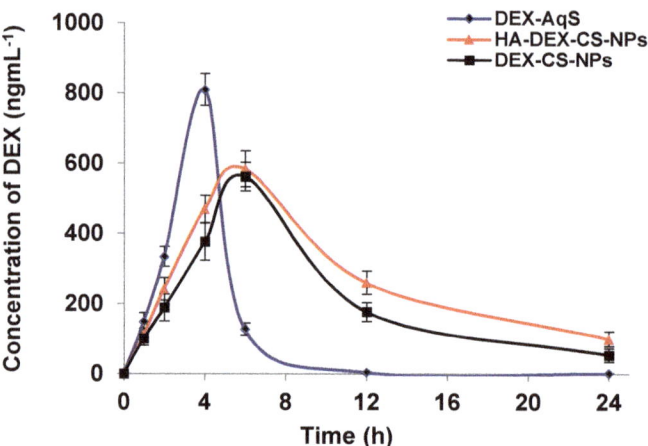

Figure 5. Aqueous humor (AH) drug concentration-time profile of DEX following topical ocular instillation of different formulations containing DEX in rabbits. The data were presented as the mean of three readings with standard deviations (Mean ± SD, n = 3).

The concentrations of DEX in the AH samples were easily quantified for up to 6 h in Group-C (DEX-AqS group); but afterward, the drug was not detectable, demonstrating the relatively faster precorneal loss of DEX from aqueous solution. In contrast, DEX was easily quantified for up to 24 h in animals treated with uncoated (Group-A) and HA-coated (Group-B) drug formulations. The ocular bioavailability of DEX was significantly (p < 0.005) higher in the DEX-CSNPs formulations compared to DEX-AqS. The difference in AUC_{0-24h} was approximately 1.87- and 2.36-fold greater in uncoated and HA-coated DEX-CSNPs compared to that of DEX-AqS, respectively. The biological $t_{1/2}$ of DEX from uncoated and HA-coated DEX-CSNPs was 2.49- and 3.36-fold higher, while the C_{max} of the drug from uncoated and HA-coated DEX-CSNPs was 1.44- and 1.38-fold lower than that of DEX-AqS, respectively. Mean residence time to infinity (MRT_{0-inf}) of the drug in the ocular area was 2.47- and 3.15-fold greater for uncoated and HA-coated DEX-CSNPs as compared to DEX-AqS. The strong mucoadhesive nature of CS and HA is known to support ocular bioadhesion of the DEX-loaded NPs [17]; hence, extending drug retention in the eyes thereby enhances drug availability to ocular tissues [68]. Similarly, we believe that the strong interaction between HA and CD44/hyaluronan receptors on the epithelial surface of ocular tissues is responsible for the improved pharmacokinetic parameters of the HA-coated CSNPs.

Table 5. Pharmacokinetics of dexamethasone in aqueous humor following topical application of different formulations. The data were presented as the mean of three readings with standard deviations (Mean ± SD, n = 3).

Pharmacokinetic Parameters	Numerical Values for		
	DEX-AqS (0.1%, w/v)	DEX-CSNPs	HA-Coated DEX-CSNPs
$t_{1/2}$ (h)	2.18 ± 0.37	5.44 * ± 0.70	7.34 * ± 1.22
T_{max} (h)	4.00 ± 0.00	6.00 ± 0.00	6.00 ± 0.00
C_{max} (ngmL^{-1})	809.26 ± 45.51	561.79 ± 40.51	584.32 ± 50.74
AUC_{0-24} (ngmL^{-1}.h)	2826.71 ± 219.84	5294.19 * ± 687.36	6691.48 * ± 570.10
AUC_{0-inf} (ngmL^{-1}.h)	2830.95 ± 224.12	5727.33 * ± 897.67	7774.81 * ± 489.53
$AUC_{0-24/0-inf}$	0.99 ± 0.001	0.93 ± 0.02	0.86 ± 0.04
$AUMC_{0-inf}$ (ngmL^{-1}.h^2)	11,458.50 ± 1239.01	57,896.82 * ± 14,377.82	99,040.13 * ± 15,826.01
MRT_{0-inf} (h)	4.04 * ± 0.12	10.01 * ± 0.89	12.73 * ± 1.77

* p < 0.005 versus DEX-AqS.

Indeed, our computed pharmacokinetic parameters suggest the bioadhesion of DEX-CSNPs to the corneal and conjunctival epithelium, which enhanced ocular retention and maintained a high transcorneal DEX flux exceeding that of DEX-AqS. In the case of HA-coated DEX-CSNPs, and consistent with previous reports, we believe that such a response is due to the direct interaction with hyaluronan receptors on corneal and conjunctival epithelia [18,27], leading to improved drug retention of the HA-coated DEX-CSNPs on ocular surfaces and an associated transcorneal flux and permeability of the drug.

The HA is known to improve cellular targeting and accelerate cellular uptake of the HA-coated NPs through receptor-mediated endocytosis [18,69]. The high ocular bioavailability of DEX in the HA-coated DEX-CSNPs might have been reinforced by the phagocytic propensity of conjunctival and corneal epithelial cells for HA-coated CSNPs [18,68]. Since the pharmacokinetic parameters of DEX preparations had low variability and were consistent throughout the in vivo, this suggests promising potentials of CSNPs in the topical or intravitreal delivery of DEX to the eyes.

3.7. Ocular Pharmacodynamics

Intravitreal LPS injections induced inflammatory reactions with a marked cellular flare in all LPS-treated rabbit groups. Treatment of LPS-induced uveitis (LIU) with DEX-AqS, DEX-CSNPs, and HA-coated DEX-CSNPs significantly suppressed ocular inflammation in rabbits, as evidenced by visual inspection (i.e., grading in a blinded fashion 24 h after LPS injection). The clinical signs of ocular inflammation, on a scale of 0 to 4 according to a previously published scoring system [49] are presented in Figure 6a. Lipopolysaccharide treatment induced severe inflammation, such that the clinical score for ocular inflammation (3.732 ± 0.053; 100%) was several folds higher in LIU rabbits than in the normal control group. Ocular treatment with DEX-AqS, DEX-CSNPs, or HA-coated DEX-CSNPs significantly reduced those clinical scores to 2.67 ± 0.085 (28.45%), 1.578 ± 0.048 (57.71%), and 0.93 ± 0.053 (75.08%), respectively. Importantly, the clinical scores clearly demonstrated that improving the bioavailability and sustained-release characteristics of DEX help in suppressing ocular inflammation. Topical steroids have been highly effective at mitigating ocular inflammation in several uveitis models [70,71]. In our study, intravitreal injections of LPSs increased cellular infiltration of polymorphonuclear (PMN) cells and monocytes into the AH of rabbits by 775% (LIU). However, this was significantly suppressed through DEX treatment to 533.33% with DEX-AqS, 416.67% with DEX-CSNPs, and 308.33% with HA-coated DEX-CSNPs. Accordingly, our findings demonstrate that HA-coated DEX-CSNPs might exhibit improved clinical outcomes as manifested by suppression of PMN infiltration to the aqueous humor (AH). Turk's staining further illustrated the level of cellular infiltration in LIU rabbits, demonstrating that DEX formulations inhibit the augmentation of cellular infiltrations (Figure 6b). To confirm such an improved protective effect of our HA-coated DEX-CSNP platform compared to other formulations and DEX-AqS, we quantified the protein levels in AH of the formulations studied; HA-coated DEX-CSNPs were the strongest inhibitors of ocular inflammation, as evidenced by reductions in cellular infiltration and clinical scores. To investigate the mechanism by which the formulations inhibited inflammation, we evaluated the effect of various DEX formulations on AH protein concentrations, which we estimated using Lowry's method [52]. As shown in Figure 6c, the protein concentration in the AH of LIU rabbits was 801.47% (5.05 ± 0.40 to 45.61 ± 1.63 mg·mL^{-1}) higher than that of normal rabbits, owing to the cellular infiltration, cytokines, and chemokines at the site of ocular inflammation. The effectiveness of treatment in order of the percentage reduction in the protein concentration with respect to that of untreated LIU rabbits was as follows: HA-coated DEX-CSNPs (64.3%; 45.61 ± 1.63 to 16.27 ± 0.46) > DEX-CSNPs (52.9%; 45.61 ± 1.63 to 21.48 ± 0.66) > DEX-AqS (38.4%; 45.61 ± 1.63 to 28.08 ± 1.09) > LIU (0%; 45.61 ± 1.63 to 45.61 ± 1.63) (Figure 6c). These results suggest that HA-coated DEX-CSNPs and uncoated DEX-CSNPs significantly attenuated ocular inflammation as is evident from the reduction in protein concentrations in AH.

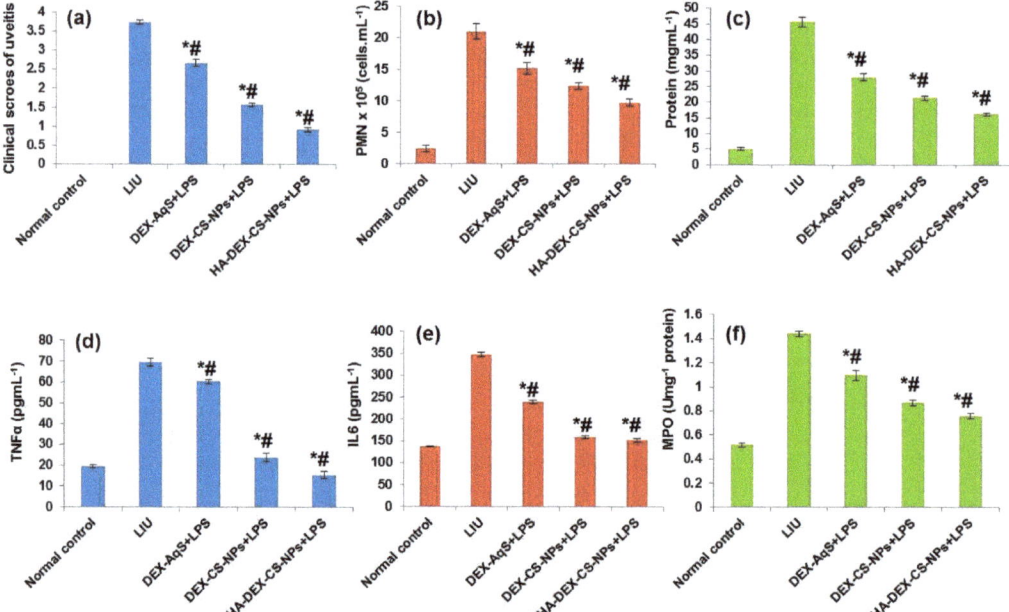

Figure 6. Effects of DEX treatment on LPS-induced uveitis in rabbits: (**a**) clinical scores of uveitis; (**b**) infiltrations of polymorphonuclear (PMN) cells; (**c**) protein concentrations; (**d**) tumor necrosis factor-α; (**e**) interleukin-6; (**f**) and myeloperoxidase (MPO) in the AH of rabbits after intravitreal injection of LPS. Compared to normal control (*)/to LPS control (#), but the effect did not reach significance ($p > 0.05$). All the data were expressed as the mean of three measurements with standard deviations (Mean $\pm$ SD, n = 3).

In the LIU model for acute inflammation, researchers have shown that PMN cells, neutrophils, and monocytes migrate from the iris venules and infiltrate the surrounding ocular tissues [72,73]. Our study also evaluated the levels of TNFα, IL-6, and MPO following intravitreal injection of LPS and in response to the different drug formulation. Our results demonstrated that LPS treatment induced the influx of all cytokines (i.e., TNFα, IL-6, and MPO). However, the drug formulations have suppressed these levels as Figure 6d–f show, which were all statistically significant. The effectiveness of treatment based in the percentage reduction in TNF-α levels with respect to that of untreated LIU rabbits was as follows: HA-coated DEX-CSNPs (77.7%) > DEX-CSNPs (65.6%) > DEX-AqS (13.2%). The effectiveness of treatment in order of the percentage reduction in IL6 levels with respect to that of the untreated LIU rabbits was as follows: HA-coated DEX-CSNPs (56.3%) > DEX-CSNPs (54.3%) > DEX-AqS (31.2%). Also, the effectiveness of treatment in order of the percentage reduction in MPO levels with respect to that of the untreated LIU rabbits was as follows: HA-coated DEX-CSNPs (47.4%) > DEX-CSNPs (39.4%) > DEX-AqS (23.7%). Thus, the results indicate that the DEX formulations have significantly ameliorated ocular inflammation by inhibiting the release of cytokines and reducing cellular infiltration. These results might be owed to the superior pharmacokinetic parameters exhibited by the DEX-CSNP, including the drug bioavailability and sustained-release efficacy.

Lipopolysaccharides are known inducers of redox-sensitive transcription factor NF-κB, which plays a key role in eliciting a cascade of pro-inflammatory genes, such as TNF-α, IL-1β, IL-6, and COX-2, in different inflammatory conditions, including uveitis [74–76]. Under physiological conditions, the p65 subunit of NF-κB is bound with its inhibitor to form a trimetric complex (IκB-NF-κBp50/p65). Upon exposure to LPS, for instance, p65 is released to translocate to the nucleus to induce gene transcription. Exposure of THP-1 monocytes to LPS for 24 h enhances p65 protein levels in the cytosol and nucleus [77] and causes the number of NF-κB p65-positive cells in iris ciliary bodies to gradually increase over a period of 3–24 h [78,79]. In our study, NF-κB p65 proteins were overexpressed in the LIU group (Group-2) compared to the normal control group (Group-1) at 24 h after the LPS injection. Treatment with DEX-CSNPs and HA-coated DEX-CSNPs inhibited NF-κB p65 expression and alleviated ocular inflammation in the LIU rabbits as illustrated in Figure 7. Lipopolysaccharides induce TNF-α–dependent apoptosis in inflammatory tissues of the eye [80]. In turn, TNF-α induces host cell destruction by stimulating caspase-3, a downstream cysteine proteinase, through various apoptotic pathways [81,82]. Immunoblot analysis revealed that expression of the pro-apoptotic protein caspase-3 was enhanced and expression of the anti-apoptotic B-cell lymphoma 2 (BCL2) protein was reduced in LIU tissues compared to that of normal control tissues. Treatment with DEX formulations significantly mitigated the extent of apoptosis by down-regulation of caspase-3 and up-regulation of BCL2 proteins. The effectiveness of the treatment in order of the extent of reduction in apoptosis was as follows: HA-coated-DEX-CSNPs > DEX-CSNPs > DEX-AqS. These results further established that HA-coated DEX-CSNPs and DEX-CSNPs significantly attenuate LPS-induced apoptotic injuries in uveal tissues, as illustrated in Figure 7a–c.

Finally, histological examination of the LIU group (Group-2) showed substantial cell infiltration, primarily into the anterior chamber, compared to that of the normal control group. Histological scoring and pathology revealed that amelioration of LIU reduced the inflammatory cell infiltration into the anterior chamber of cells. The effectiveness of the treatment in order of the extent of reduction in cellular infiltration was as follows: HA-coated DEX-CSNPs > DEX-CSNPs > DEX-AqS > LIU. The results of the present investigation as shown in Figure 8 are in accordance with previously published reports [72,82].

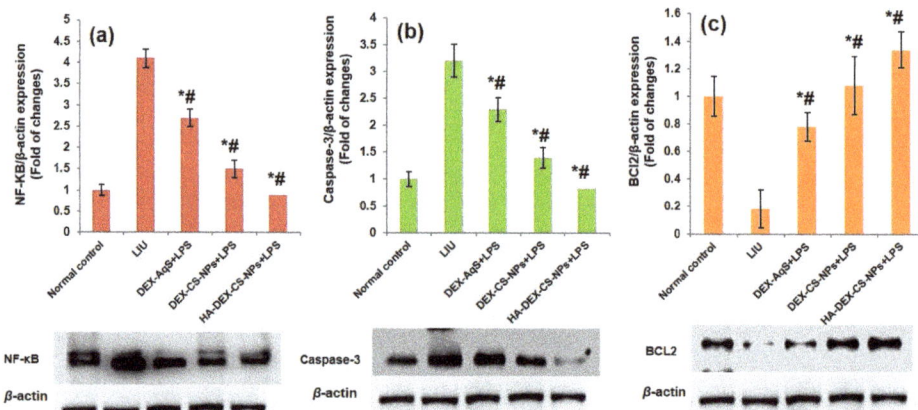

Figure 7. Effect of DEX treatment on LPS-induced uveitis alteration in inflammatory and apoptotic markers in uveal tissues of LIU rabbits. Western blot analysis of apoptotic markers: (**a**) nuclear NF-κB [p65], (**b**) Caspase-3, and (**c**) BCl2, compared to normal control (*)/to LPS control (#), but the effect did not reach significance ($p > 0.05$). All the data were expressed as the mean of three measurements with standard deviations (Mean ± SD, n = 3).

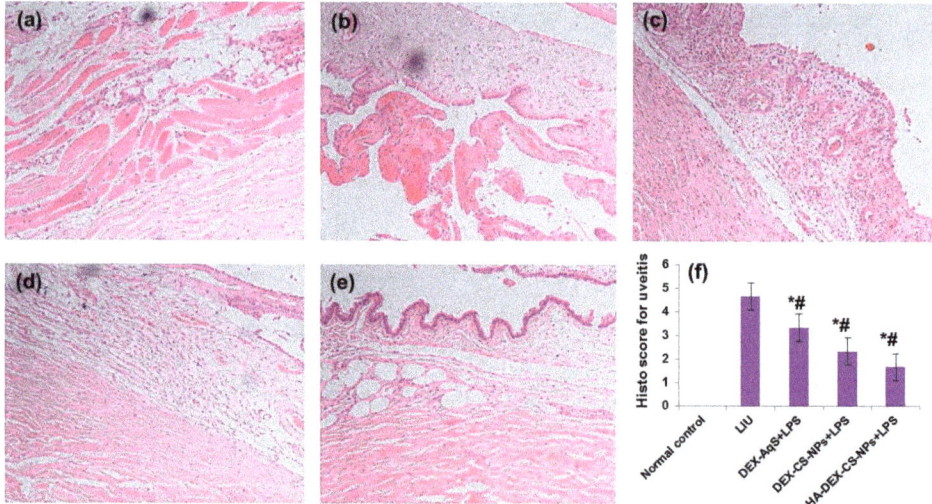

Figure 8. Effects of DEX treatment on the histopathological changes of intraocular inflammation of LIU rabbits. (**a**) Infiltrations of PMN cells were displayed in normal control rabbits. (**b**) Highest PMN cells infiltrated the extravascular uveal tissue in the vehicle + LIU rabbits. (**c**) Slight reduction in PMN cells infiltrated the extravascular uveal tissue in the DEX-loaded CS-NPs + LIU rabbits. (**d**) Moderate reduction in PMN cells infiltration in the extravascular uveal tissue in the DEX-loaded CS-NPs + LIU rabbits. (**e**) Maximum reduction in PMN cells infiltration in the extravascular uveal tissue in the DEX-loaded HA-coated CS-NPs + LIU rabbits. (**e**) Histopathological scores of LIU rabbits. Compared to normal control (*)/to LPS control (#), but the effect did not reach significance ($p > 0.05$). The data in (**f**) were expressed as mean with standard deviations three measurements. Tissues were stained with hematoxylin and eosin and viewed under 200× magnification.

4. Conclusions

Our findings demonstrate that DEX release from HA-coated DEX-CSNPs could be sustained in vitro for 12 h, and the physicochemical characteristics (pH, clarity, refractive index, and viscosity) of the nano-formulation were suitable for topical ocular delivery, such that uncoated and HA-coated DEX-CSNPs were only mildly irritating to rabbit eyes. The Transcorneal passage of DEX from the CSNPs through the excised rabbit cornea was improved, and the ocular bioavailability of DEX from the CSNPs was higher than DEX-AqS. Importantly, coating the CSNPs' surfaces with HA might improve cellular uptake of nanocarriers and improve corneal and conjunctival healing. In comparison to the topical administration of DEX-AqS, uncoated and HA-coated DEX-CSNPs markedly reduced signs and symptoms of LIU, inflammatory cell counts, protein concentration, and the levels of TNFα, IL-6, and MPO in AH. We believe that the DEX-mediated inhibition of apoptosis in uveal tissues is due to an increase in drug bioavailability over time (i.e., sustain release efficacy) afforded by the use of HA-coated and uncoated nanocarriers. In conclusion, our findings suggest that CSNPs have great potential for drug delivery, particularly, for the topical treatment of various inflammatory eye conditions. This nano-formulation may also be administered intravitreally, for instance, in the treatment of retinal disease; however, further investigations are warranted to understand the pharmacokinetics and safety profile of this administration.

Author Contributions: Conceptualization, A.A. (Aws Alshamsan), M.A.K. and M.A.; methodology, M.R., R.A., M.A.A., N.B.A. and A.A. (Aliyah Almomen); software, M.A.K. and M.R.; validation, R.A., M.A. and M.A.K.; formal analysis, A.A. (Aliyah Almomen); investigation, M.A.K., M.R. and R.A.; resources, M.A., M.A.K. and A.A. (Aws Alshamsan); data curation, M.A.K. and M.R., N.B.A.; writing—original draft preparation, M.A., M.A.K., M.R., R.A. and M.A.A.; writing—review and editing, M.A., M.A.K, M.R., M.A.A. and M.A.K.; supervision, A.A. (Aws Alshamsan); project administration, M.A.K., M.A. and A.A. (Aws Alshamsan). All authors have read and agreed to the published version of the manuscript.

Funding: This work was funded by the Deputyship for Research and Innovation, Ministry of Education in Saudi Arabia for funding this research work through the project number (DRI-KSU-1075).

Institutional Review Board Statement: The protocol for animal use was approved by the Research Ethics Committee (REC) at King Saud University (protocol approval number: SE-19-90; 20 November 2019).

Informed Consent Statement: Not applicable.

Data Availability Statement: The data presented in this study are available on request from the corresponding author.

Acknowledgments: The authors extend their appreciation to the Deputyship for Research and Innovation, Ministry of Education in Saudi Arabia for funding this research work through the project number (DRI-KSU-1075).

Conflicts of Interest: The authors declare no conflict of interest.

Abbreviations

DEX	Dexamethasone sodium phosphate
CS	Chitosan
TPP	Tripolyphosphate sodium
NPs	Nanoparticles
CSNPs	Chitosan nanoparticles
DEX-CSNPs	DEX-loaded chitosan nanoparticles
AqS	Aqueous suspension
ZP	Zeta potential
PDI	Polydispersity index

AH	Aqueous humor
HA	Hyaluronic acid
LPS	Lipopolysaccharide
LIU	Lipopolysaccharide-induced uveitis
PMN	Polymorphonuclear
BCL2	B-cell lymphoma 2
MPO	Myeloperoxidase
NF-κB	Nuclear factor kappa B
TNFα	Tumor necrosis factor α
IL	Interleukin
COX-2	Cyclooxygenase-2
REC	Research Ethics Committee

References

1. Chan, C.-C.; Goldstein, D.A.; Davis, J.L.; Sen, H.N. Gender and Uveitis. *J. Ophthalmol.* **2014**, *2014*, 818070. [CrossRef]
2. Acharya, N.R.; Tham, V.M.; Esterberg, E.; Borkar, D.S.; Parker, J.V.; Vinoya, A.C.; Uchida, A. Incidence and prevalence of uveitis: Results from the Pacific Ocular Inflammation Study. *JAMA Ophthalmol.* **2013**, *131*, 1405–1412. [CrossRef] [PubMed]
3. Chan, A.Y.; Conrady, C.D.; Ding, K.; Dvorak, J.D.; Stone, D.U. Factors associated with age of onset of herpes zoster ophthalmicus. *Cornea* **2015**, *34*, 535–540. [CrossRef] [PubMed]
4. Cheng, C.K.; Berger, A.S.; Pearson, P.A.; Ashton, P.; Jaffe, G.J. Intravitreal sustained-release dexamethasone device in the treatment of experimental uveitis. *Investig. Ophthalmol. Vis. Sci.* **1995**, *36*, 442–453.
5. Eom, Y.; Lee, D.Y.; Kang, B.R.; Heo, J.H.; Shin, K.H.; Kim, H.M.; Song, J.S. Comparison of aqueous levels of inflammatory mediators between toxic anterior segment syndrome and endotoxin-induced uveitis animal models. *Investig. Ophthalmol. Vis. Sci.* **2014**, *55*, 6704–6710. [CrossRef]
6. De Vos, A.F.; van Haren, M.A.; Verhagen, C.; Hoekzema, R.; Kijlstra, A. Kinetics of intraocular tumor necrosis factor and interleukin-6 in endotoxin-induced uveitis in the rat. *Investig. Ophthalmol. Vis. Sci.* **1994**, *35*, 1100–1106.
7. Planck, S.R.; Huang, X.N.; Robertson, J.E.; Rosenbaum, J.T. Cytokine mRNA levels in rat ocular tissues after systemic endotoxin treatment. *Investig. Ophthalmol. Vis. Sci.* **1994**, *35*, 924–930.
8. Tsuji, F.; Sawa, K.; Mibu, H.; Shirasawa, E. 16 β-Methyl-17 α,21-diesterified glucocorticoids as partial agonists of glucocorticoid in rat endotoxin-induced inflammation. *Inflamm. Res.* **1997**, *46*, 193–198. [CrossRef]
9. Tanito, M.; Hara, K.; Takai, Y.; Matsuoka, Y.; Nishimura, N.; Jansook, P.; Loftsson, T.; Stefansson, E.; Ohira, A. Topical dexamethasone-cyclodextrin microparticle eye drops for diabetic macular edema. *Invest. Ophthalmol. Vis. Sci.* **2011**, *52*, 7944–7948. [CrossRef]
10. Ohira, A.; Hara, K.; Johannesson, G.; Tanito, M.; Asgrimsdottir, G.M.; Lund, S.H.; Loftsson, T.; Stefansson, E. Topical dexamethasone gamma-cyclodextrin nanoparticle eye drops increase visual acuity and decrease macular thickness in diabetic macular oedema. *Acta Ophthalmol.* **2015**, *93*, 610–615. [CrossRef]
11. Carnahan, M.C.; Goldstein, D.A. Ocular complications of topical, peri-ocular, and systemic corticosteroids. *Curr. Opin. Ophthalmol.* **2000**, *11*, 478–483. [CrossRef]
12. Fardet, L.; Flahault, A.; Kettaneh, A.; Tiev, K.P.; Genereau, T.; Toledano, C.; Lebbe, C.; Cabane, J. Corticosteroid-induced clinical adverse events: Frequency, risk factors and patient's opinion. *Br. J. Dermatol.* **2007**, *157*, 142–148. [CrossRef]
13. Satyanarayanasetty, D.; Pawar, K.; Nadig, P.; Haran, A. Multiple Adverse Effects of Systemic Corticosteroids: A Case Report. *J. Clin. Diagn. Res.* **2015**, *9*, FD01–FD02. [CrossRef] [PubMed]
14. Wong, G.K.; Poon, W.S.; Chiu, K.H. Steroid-induced avascular necrosis of the hip in neurosurgical patients: Epidemiological study. *ANZ J. Surg.* **2005**, *75*, 409–410. [CrossRef] [PubMed]
15. Rafii, B.; Sridharan, S.; Taliercio, S.; Govil, N.; Paul, B.; Garabedian, M.J.; Amin, M.R.; Branski, R.C. Glucocorticoids in laryngology: A review. *Laryngoscope* **2014**, *124*, 1668–1673. [CrossRef]
16. Fangueiro, J.F.; Andreani, T.; Fernandes, L.; Garcia, M.L.; Egea, M.A.; Silva, A.l.M.; Souto, E.B. Physicochemical characterization of epigallocatechin gallate lipid nanoparticles (EGCG-LNs) for ocular instillation. *Colloids Surf. B Biointerfaces* **2014**, *123*, 452–460. [CrossRef] [PubMed]
17. De la Fuente, M.; Seijo, B.; Alonso, M.J. Novel Hyaluronic Acid-Chitosan Nanoparticles for Ocular Gene Therapy. *Investig. Opthalmol. Vis. Sci.* **2008**, *49*, 2016. [CrossRef] [PubMed]
18. Kalam, M.A. The potential application of hyaluronic acid coated chitosan nanoparticles in ocular delivery of dexamethasone. *Int. J. Biol. Macromol.* **2016**, *89*, 559–568. [CrossRef] [PubMed]
19. Uccello-Barretta, G.; Nazzi, S.; Zambito, Y.; Di Colo, G.; Balzano, F.; Sansò, M. Synergistic interaction between TS-polysaccharide and hyaluronic acid: Implications in the formulation of eye drops. *Int. J. Pharm.* **2010**, *395*, 122–131. [CrossRef]
20. Rafie, F.; Javadzadeh, Y.; Javadzadeh, A.R.; Ghavidel, L.A.; Jafari, B.; Moogooee, M.; Davaran, S. In vivo evaluation of novel nanoparticles containing dexamethasone for ocular drug delivery on rabbit eye. *Curr. Eye Res.* **2010**, *35*, 1081–1089. [CrossRef] [PubMed]

21. Johannesson, G.; Moya-Ortega, M.D.; Asgrimsdottir, G.M.; Lund, S.H.; Thorsteinsdottir, M.; Loftsson, T.; Stefansson, E. Kinetics of γ-cyclodextrin nanoparticle suspension eye drops in tear fluid. *Acta Ophthalmol.* **2014**, *92*, 550–556. [CrossRef]
22. Sigurdsson, H.H.; Konraosdottir, F.; Loftsson, T.; Stefensson, E. Topical and systemic absorption in delivery of dexamethasone to the anterior and posterior segments of the eye. *Acta Ophthalmol. Scand.* **2007**, *85*, 598–602. [CrossRef]
23. Hickey, T.; Kreutzer, D.; Burgess, D.J.; Moussy, F. Dexamethasone/PLGA microspheres for continuous delivery of an anti-inflammatory drug for implantable medical devices. *Biomaterials* **2002**, *23*, 1649–1656. [CrossRef]
24. Kalam, M.A. Development of chitosan nanoparticles coated with hyaluronic acid for topical ocular delivery of dexamethasone. *Int. J. Biol. Macromol.* **2016**, *89*, 127–136. [CrossRef] [PubMed]
25. Hosseinnejad, M.; Jafari, S.M. Evaluation of different factors affecting antimicrobial properties of chitosan. *Int. J. Biol. Macromol.* **2016**, *85*, 467–475. [CrossRef]
26. Lerner, L.; Schwartz, D.; Hwang, D.; Howes, E.; Stern, R. Hyaluronan and CD44 in the Human Cornea and Limbal Conjunctiva. *Exp. Eye Res.* **1998**, *67*, 481–484. [CrossRef] [PubMed]
27. Zhu, S.-N.; Nolle, B.; Duncker, G. Expression of adhesion molecule CD44 on human corneas. *Br. J. Ophthalmol.* **1997**, *81*, 80–84. [CrossRef]
28. Vanbeek, M.; Jones, L.; Sheardown, H. Hyaluronic acid containing hydrogels for the reduction of protein adsorption. *Biomaterials* **2008**, *29*, 780–789. [CrossRef] [PubMed]
29. Calvo, P.; Remunan Lopez, C.; Vila-Jato, J.L.; Alonso, M.J. Chitosan and chitosan/ethylene oxide-propylene oxide block copolymer nanoparticles as novel carriers for proteins and vaccines. *Pharm. Res.* **1997**, *14*, 1431–1436. [CrossRef]
30. Nasti, A.; Zaki, N.M.; de Leonardis, P.; Ungphaiboon, S.; Sansongsak, P.; Rimoli, M.G.; Tirelli, N. Chitosan/TPP and Chitosan/TPP-hyaluronic Acid Nanoparticles: Systematic Optimisation of the Preparative Process and Preliminary Biological Evaluation. *Pharm. Res.* **2009**, *26*, 1918–1930. [CrossRef]
31. Almalik, A.; Donno, R.; Cadman, C.J.; Cellesi, F.; Day, P.J.; Tirelli, N. Hyaluronic acid-coated chitosan nanoparticles: Molecular weight-dependent effects on morphology and hyaluronic acid presentation. *J. Control. Release* **2013**, *172*, 1142–1150. [CrossRef]
32. Grenha, A.; Seijo, B.a.; Serra, C.; Remunán-López, C. Chitosan Nanoparticle-Loaded Mannitol Microspheres: Â Structure and Surface Characterization. *Biomacromolecules* **2007**, *8*, 2072–2079. [CrossRef]
33. Almalik, A.; Alradwan, I.; Kalam, M.A.; Alshamsan, A. Effect of cryoprotection on particle size stability and preservation of chitosan nanoparticles with and without hyaluronate or alginate coating. *Saudi Pharm. J.* **2017**, *25*, 861–867. [CrossRef]
34. Kalam, M.A.; Alkholief, M.; Badran, M.; Alshememry, A.; Alshamsan, A. Technology. Co-encapsulation of metformin hydrochloride and reserpine into flexible liposomes: Characterization and comparison of in vitro release profile. *J. Drug Deliv. Sci. Technol.* **2020**, *57*, 101670. [CrossRef]
35. Kwak, H.W.; D'Amico, D.J. Determination of dexamethasone sodium phosphate in the vitreous by high performance liquid chromatography. *Korean J. Ophthalmol.* **1995**, *9*, 79. [CrossRef] [PubMed]
36. Abul Kalam, M.; Sultana, Y.; Ali, A.; Aqil, M.; Mishra, A.K.; Aljuffali, I.A.; Alshamsan, A. Part I: Development and optimization of solid-lipid nanoparticles using Box-Behnken statistical design for ocular delivery of gatifloxacin. *J. Biomed. Mater. Res. A* **2013**, *101*, 1813–1827. [CrossRef]
37. Pignatello, R.; Bucolo, C.; Ferrara, P.; Maltese, A.; Puleo, A.; Puglisi, G. Eudragit RS100 nanosuspensions for the ophthalmic controlled delivery of ibuprofen. *Eur. J. Pharm. Sci.* **2002**, *16*, 53–61. [CrossRef]
38. Tsai, M.-L.; Chen, R.-H.; Bai, S.-W.; Chen, W.-Y. The storage stability of chitosan/tripolyphosphate nanoparticles in a phosphate buffer. *Carbohydr. Polym.* **2011**, *84*, 756–761. [CrossRef]
39. Alkholief, M.; Kalam, M.A.; Almomen, A.; Alshememry, A.; Alshamsan, A. Thermoresponsive sol-gel improves ocular bioavailability of Dipivefrin hydrochloride and potentially reduces the elevated intraocular pressure in vivo. *Saudi Pharm. J.* **2020**, *28*, 1019. [CrossRef] [PubMed]
40. Abul Kalam, M.; Khan, A.A.; Khan, S.; Almalik, A.; Alshamsan, A. Optimizing indomethacin-loaded chitosan nanoparticle size, encapsulation, and release using Box-Behnken experimental design. *Int. J. Biol. Macromol.* **2016**, *87*, 329–340. [CrossRef] [PubMed]
41. Kumari, A.; Sharma, P.K.; Garg, V.K.; Garg, G. Ocular inserts—Advancement in therapy of eye diseases. *J. Adv. Pharm. Technol. Res.* **2010**, *1*, 291–296. [CrossRef]
42. Box, J.A.; Sugden, J.K.; Younis, N.M.T. An Examination of the Sterilization of Eye Drops Using Ultra-Violet Light. *J. Pharm. Sci. Technol.* **1984**, *38*, 115–121.
43. Draize, J.H.; Woodard, G.; Calvery, H.O. Methods for the study of irritation and toxicity of substances applied topically to the skin and mucous membranes. *J. Pharmacol. Exp. Ther.* **1944**, *82*, 377–390.
44. Diebold, Y.; Jarrin, M.; Saez, V.; Carvalho, E.L.S.; Orea, M.; Calonge, M.; Seijo, B.; Alonso, M.J. Ocular drug delivery by liposome-chitosan nanoparticle complexes (LCS-NP). *Biomaterials* **2007**, *28*, 1553–1564. [CrossRef]
45. Liu, Y.; Liu, J.; Zhang, X.; Zhang, R.; Huang, Y.; Wu, C. In Situ Gelling Gelrite/Alginate Formulations as Vehicles for Ophthalmic Drug Delivery. *AAPS PharmSciTech* **2010**, *11*, 610–620. [CrossRef] [PubMed]
46. Reddy, D.B.; Reddanna, P. Chebulagic acid (CA) attenuates LPS-induced inflammation by suppressing NF-kappaB and MAPK activation in RAW 264.7 macrophages. *Biochem. Biophys. Res. Commun.* **2009**, *381*, 112–117. [CrossRef]
47. Toguri, J.T.; Lehmann, C.; Laprairie, R.B.; Szczesniak, A.M.; Zhou, J.; Denovan-Wright, E.M.; Kelly, M.E. Anti-inflammatory effects of cannabinoid CB(2) receptor activation in endotoxin-induced uveitis. *Br. J. Pharmacol.* **2014**, *171*, 1448–1461. [CrossRef]

48. Gupta, S.K.; Agarwal, R.; Srivastava, S.; Agarwal, P.; Agrawal, S.S.; Saxena, R.; Galpalli, N. The anti-inflammatory effects of Curcuma longa and Berberis aristata in endotoxin-induced uveitis in rabbits. *Investig. Ophthalmol. Vis. Sci.* **2008**, *49*, 4036–4040. [CrossRef] [PubMed]
49. Ruiz-Moreno, J.M.; Thillaye, B.; de Kozak, Y. Retino-choroidal changes in endotoxin-induced uveitis in the rat. *Ophthalmic Res.* **1992**, *24*, 162–168. [CrossRef]
50. Lennikov, A.; Kitaichi, N.; Noda, K.; Mizuuchi, K.; Ando, R.; Dong, Z.; Fukuhara, J.; Kinoshita, S.; Namba, K.; Ohno, S.; et al. Amelioration of endotoxin-induced uveitis treated with the sea urchin pigment echinochrome in rats. *Mol. Vis.* **2014**, *20*, 171–177. [PubMed]
51. Kanai, K.; Hatta, T.; Nagata, S.; Sugiura, Y.; Sato, K.; Yamashita, Y.; Kimura, Y.; Itoh, N. Luteolin attenuates endotoxin-induced uveitis in Lewis rats. *J. Vet. Med. Sci.* **2016**, *78*, 1229–1235. [CrossRef]
52. Lowry, O.H.; Rosebrough, N.J.; Farr, A.L.; Randall, R.J. Protein measurement with the Folin phenol reagent. *J. Biol. Chem.* **1951**, *193*, 265–275. [CrossRef]
53. Rossi, S.; Di Filippo, C.; Gesualdo, C.; Potenza, N.; Russo, A.; Trotta, M.C.; Zippo, M.V.; Maisto, R.; Ferraraccio, F.; Simonelli, F.; et al. Protection from endotoxic uveitis by intravitreal Resolvin D1: Involvement of lymphocytes, miRNAs, ubiquitin-proteasome, and M1/M2 macrophages. *Mediat. Inflamm.* **2015**, *2015*, 149381. [CrossRef]
54. Almomen, A.; Jarboe, E.A.; Dodson, M.K.; Peterson, C.M.; Owen, S.C.; Janat-Amsbury, M.M. Imiquimod Induces Apoptosis in Human Endometrial Cancer Cells In Vitro and Prevents Tumor Progression In Vivo. *Pharm. Res.* **2016**, *33*, 2209–2217. [CrossRef] [PubMed]
55. Knudson, W.; Chow, G.; Knudson, C.B. CD44-mediated uptake and degradation of hyaluronan. *Matrix Biol.* **2002**, *21*, 15–23. [CrossRef]
56. Almalik, A.; Day, P.J.; Tirelli, N. HA-Coated Chitosan Nanoparticles for CD44-Mediated Nucleic Acid Delivery. *Macromol. Biosci.* **2013**, *13*, 1671–1680. [CrossRef] [PubMed]
57. Chiesa, E.; Dorati, R.; Conti, B.; Modena, T.; Cova, E.; Meloni, F.; Genta, I. Hyaluronic Acid-Decorated Chitosan Nanoparticles for CD44-Targeted Delivery of Everolimus. *Int. J. Mol. Sci.* **2018**, *19*, 2310. [CrossRef] [PubMed]
58. Zimmer, A.; Kreuter, J. Microspheres and nanoparticles used in ocular delivery systems. *Adv. Drug Deliv. Rev.* **1995**, *16*, 61–73. [CrossRef]
59. Kalam, M.A.; Alshamsan, A.; Aljuffali, I.A.; Mishra, A.K.; Sultana, Y. Delivery of gatifloxacin using microemulsion as vehicle: Formulation, evaluation, transcorneal permeation and aqueous humor drug determination. *Drug Deliv.* **2016**, *23*, 896–907. [CrossRef]
60. Coles, W.H.; Jaros, P.A. Dynamics of ocular surface pH. *Br. J. Ophthalmol.* **1984**, *68*, 549–552. [CrossRef]
61. Di Colo, G.; Zambito, Y.; Zaino, C.; Sansò, M. Selected polysaccharides at comparison for their mucoadhesiveness and effect on precorneal residence of different drugs in the rabbit model. *Drug Dev. Ind. Pharm.* **2009**, *35*, 941–949. [CrossRef]
62. Salzillo, R.; Schiraldi, C.; Corsuto, L.; D'Agostino, A.; Filosa, R.; De Rosa, M.; La Gatta, A. Optimization of hyaluronan-based eye drop formulations. *Carbohydr. Polym.* **2016**, *153*, 275–283. [CrossRef]
63. Oescher, M.; Keipert, S. Polyacrylic acid/polyvinylpyrrolidone biopolymeric systems: I. Rheological and mucoadhesive properties of formulations potentially useful for the treatment of dry-eye-syndrome. *Eur. J. Pharm. Biopharm.* **1999**, *47*, 113–118. [CrossRef]
64. Pires, N.R.; Cunha, P.L.; Maciel, J.S.; Angelim, A.L.; Melo, V.M.; de Paula, R.C.; Feitosa, J.P. Sulfated chitosan as tear substitute with no antimicrobial activity. *Carbohydr. Polym.* **2013**, *91*, 92–99. [CrossRef]
65. Agnihotri, S.A.; Mallikarjuna, N.N.; Aminabhavi, T.M. Recent advances on chitosan-based micro- and nanoparticles in drug delivery. *J. Control. Release* **2004**, *100*, 5–28. [CrossRef]
66. Jansook, P.; Ritthidej, G.C.; Ueda, H.; Stefansson, E.; Loftsson, T. γCD/HPγCD mixtures as solubilizer: Solid-state characterization and sample dexamethasone eye drop suspension. *J. Pharm. Pharm. Sci.* **2010**, *13*, 336–350. [CrossRef]
67. Cohen, A.E.; Assang, C.; Patane, M.A.; From, S.; Korenfeld, M. Evaluation of dexamethasone phosphate delivered by ocular iontophoresis for treating noninfectious anterior uveitis. *Ophthalmology* **2012**, *119*, 66–73. [CrossRef]
68. Contreras-Ruiz, L.; de la Fuente, M.; Parraga, J.E.; Lopez-Garcia, A.; Fernandez, I.; Seijo, B.; Sanchez, A.; Calonge, M.; Diebold, Y. Intracellular trafficking of hyaluronic acid-chitosan oligomer-based nanoparticles in cultured human ocular surface cells. *Mol. Vis.* **2011**, *17*, 279–290.
69. Bernatchez, S.F.; Tabatabay, C.; Gurny, R. Sodium Hyaluronate 0.25-Percent Used as a Vehicle Increases the Bioavailability of Topically Administered Gentamicin. *Graefes Arch. Clin. Exp. Ophthalmol.* **1993**, *231*, 157–161. [CrossRef]
70. Denniston, A.K.; Tomlins, P.; Williams, G.P.; Kottoor, S.; Khan, I.; Oswal, K.; Salmon, M.; Wallace, G.R.; Rauz, S.; Murray, P.I.; et al. Aqueous humor suppression of dendritic cell function helps maintain immune regulation in the eye during human uveitis. *Investig. Ophthalmol. Vis. Sci.* **2012**, *53*, 888–896. [CrossRef] [PubMed]
71. Goncu, T.; Oguz, E.; Sezen, H.; Kocarslan, S.; Oguz, H.; Akal, A.; Adibelli, F.M.; Cakmak, S.; Aksoy, N. Anti-inflammatory effect of lycopene on endotoxin-induced uveitis in rats. *Arq. Bras. Oftalmol.* **2016**, *79*, 357–362. [CrossRef] [PubMed]
72. Chen, C.L.; Chen, J.T.; Liang, C.M.; Tai, M.C.; Lu, D.W.; Chen, Y.H. Silibinin treatment prevents endotoxin-induced uveitis in rats in vivo and in vitro. *PLoS ONE* **2017**, *12*, e0174971. [CrossRef] [PubMed]
73. Bhattacherjee, P.; Williams, R.N.; Eakins, K.E. An evaluation of ocular inflammation following the injection of bacterial endotoxin into the rat foot pad. *Investig. Ophthalmol. Vis. Sci.* **1983**, *24*, 196–202.
74. Srivastava, S.K.; Ramana, K.V. Focus on molecules: Nuclear factor-kappaB. *Exp. Eye Res.* **2009**, *88*, 2–3. [CrossRef] [PubMed]

75. Ghosn, C.R.; Li, Y.; Orilla, W.C.; Lin, T.; Wheeler, L.; Burke, J.A.; Robinson, M.R.; Whitcup, S.M. Treatment of experimental anterior and intermediate uveitis by a dexamethasone intravitreal implant. *Investig. Ophthalmol. Vis. Sci.* **2011**, *52*, 2917–2923. [CrossRef] [PubMed]
76. Hunter, R.S.; Lobo, A.M. Dexamethasone intravitreal implant for the treatment of noninfectious uveitis. *Clin. Ophthalmol.* **2011**, *5*, 1613–1621. [CrossRef]
77. Cordle, S.R.; Donald, R.; Read, M.A.; Hawiger, J. Lipopolysaccharide induces phosphorylation of MAD3 and activation of c-Rel and related NF-kappa B proteins in human monocytic THP-1 cells. *J. Biol. Chem.* **1993**, *268*, 11803–11810. [CrossRef]
78. Li, A.; Leung, C.T.; Peterson-Yantorno, K.; Mitchell, C.H.; Civan, M.M. Pathways for ATP release by bovine ciliary epithelial cells, the initial step in purinergic regulation of aqueous humor inflow. *Am. J. Physiol. Cell Physiol.* **2010**, *299*, C1308–C1317. [CrossRef] [PubMed]
79. Yadav, U.C.; Srivastava, S.K.; Ramana, K.V. Aldose reductase inhibition prevents endotoxin-induced uveitis in rats. *Investig. Ophthalmol. Vis. Sci.* **2007**, *48*, 4634–4642. [CrossRef]
80. Yang, W.; Li, H.; Chen, P.W.; Alizadeh, H.; He, Y.; Hogan, R.N.; Niederkorn, J.Y. PD-L1 Expression on Human Ocular Cells and Its Possible Role in Regulating Immune-Mediated Ocular Inflammation. *Investig. Ophthalmol. Vis. Sci.* **2009**, *50*, 273–280. [CrossRef]
81. Joussen, A.M.; Doehmen, S.; Le, M.L.; Koizumi, K.; Radetzky, S.; Krohne, T.U.; Poulaki, V.; Semkova, I.; Kociok, N. TNF-alpha mediated apoptosis plays an important role in the development of early diabetic retinopathy and long-term histopathological alterations. *Mol. Vis.* **2009**, *15*, 1418–1428. [PubMed]
82. Xaus, J.; Comalada, M.; Valledor, A.F.; Lloberas, J.; Lopez-Soriano, F.; Argiles, J.M.; Bogdan, C.; Celada, A. LPS induces apoptosis in macrophages mostly through the autocrine production of TNF-α. *Blood* **2000**, *95*, 3823–3831. [CrossRef] [PubMed]

Disclaimer/Publisher's Note: The statements, opinions and data contained in all publications are solely those of the individual author(s) and contributor(s) and not of MDPI and/or the editor(s). MDPI and/or the editor(s) disclaim responsibility for any injury to people or property resulting from any ideas, methods, instructions or products referred to in the content.

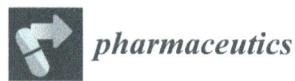 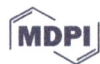

Article

Development of Blueberry-Derived Extracellular Nanovesicles for Immunomodulatory Therapy

Tuong Ngoc-Gia Nguyen [1], Cuong Viet Pham [1], Rocky Chowdhury [1], Shweta Patel [1], Satendra Kumar Jaysawal [1], Yingchun Hou [2], Huo Xu [3], Lee Jia [3], Andrew Duan [4], Phuong Ha-Lien Tran [1,*] and Wei Duan [1,*]

[1] School of Medicine, Faculty of Health, Deakin University, Geelong Waurn Ponds Campus, Geelong, VIC 3216, Australia; nnguyen9@nymc.edu (T.N.-G.N.); cuong.pham@baker.edu.au (C.V.P.); chowdhuryro@deakin.edu.au (R.C.); patelshw@deakin.edu.au (S.P.); sjaysawal@deakin.edu.au (S.K.J.)
[2] Laboratory of Tumor Molecular and Cellular Biology, College of Life Sciences, Shaanxi Normal University, 620 West Chang'an Avenue, Xi'an 710119, China; ychhou@snnu.edu.cn
[3] College of Materials and Chemical Engineering, Minjiang University, Fuzhou 350108, China; 2627@mju.edu.cn (H.X.); leejia2000@mju.edu.cn (L.J.)
[4] School of Medicine, Faculty of Medicine, Nursing and Health Sciences, Monash University, Clayton, VIC 3800, Australia; adua0001@student.monash.edu
* Correspondence: phuong.tran1@deakin.edu.au (P.H.-L.T.); wei.duan@deakin.edu.au (W.D.)

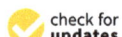

Citation: Nguyen, T.N.-G.; Pham, C.V.; Chowdhury, R.; Patel, S.; Jaysawal, S.K.; Hou, Y.; Xu, H.; Jia, L.; Duan, A.; Tran, P.H.-L.; et al. Development of Blueberry-Derived Extracellular Nanovesicles for Immunomodulatory Therapy. *Pharmaceutics* 2023, 15, 2115. https://doi.org/10.3390/pharmaceutics15082115

Academic Editor: Hugo Agostinho Machado Fernandes

Received: 19 June 2023
Revised: 3 August 2023
Accepted: 4 August 2023
Published: 10 August 2023

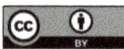

Copyright: © 2023 by the authors. Licensee MDPI, Basel, Switzerland. This article is an open access article distributed under the terms and conditions of the Creative Commons Attribution (CC BY) license (https://creativecommons.org/licenses/by/4.0/).

Abstract: Over the past decade, there has been a significant expansion in the development of plant-derived extracellular nanovesicles (EVs) as an effective drug delivery system for precision therapy. However, the lack of effective methods for the isolation and characterization of plant EVs hampers progress in the field. To solve a challenge related to systemic separation and characterization in the plant-derived EV field, herein, we report the development of a simple 3D inner filter-based method that allows the extraction of apoplastic fluid (AF) from blueberry, facilitating EV isolation as well as effective downstream applications. Class I chitinase (PR-3) was found in blueberry-derived EVs (BENVs). As Class I chitinase is expressed in a wide range of plants, it could serve as a universal marker for plant-derived EVs. Significantly, the BENVs exhibit not only higher drug loading capacity than that reported for other EVs but also possess the ability to modulate the release of the proinflammatory cytokine IL-8 and total glutathione in response to oxidative stress. Therefore, the BENV is a promising edible multifunctional nano-bio-platform for future immunomodulatory therapies.

Keywords: plant EV; biomarker; pathogen-related proteins; class I chitinase; drug delivery; immunomodulatory

1. Introduction

Plant-derived extracellular vesicles (EVs) have emerged as an unconventional means of self-protection from invasion by pathogens [1]. In addition, plant-derived EVs can block fungal growth by generating papillae and encasements using cargos contained in the EVs, namely antifungal peptides and small RNAs [1]. For the pharmaceutical industry, plant-derived EVs are an attractive alternative to mammalian-derived EVs due to their human-friendly characteristics such as their non-immunogenic properties [2].

Concerns have been raised regarding the safety of mammalian-derived EVs since they might transfer hazardous materials such as zoonotic or human pathogens [2] or pro-cancerous elements [3] from the parental cancer or immortalized cells to the recipient human cells. In contrast, plant-derived EVs are less immunogenic, contain intrinsic therapeutic abilities, display better cellular uptake, and are able to withstand the harsh environment of the gastrointestinal tract [2]. Furthermore, the preparation of plant-derived EVs is less complex than that of animal-derived EV platforms [2]. In addition, plant-derived EVs provide better protection of their cargoes, securely concealing the cargoes from proteinases and nucleases to minimize enzymatic decomposition [4]. Therefore, the development of plant-derived EVs as effective therapeutic and delivery platforms provides a new weapon to the armamentarium for cancer therapeutics, including cancer immunotherapy. However, compared to their mammalian EV counterparts, the field of plant-derived EVs faces a series of technical challenges, including techniques for isolation and characterization, the ability to carry a high quantity of payload, and the evaluation of internalization into and interaction with targeted cells [2].

Currently, plant-derived EV-like nanoparticles are commonly isolated from juices generated by grinding or squeezing methods. The collected plant-derived EVs from these methods do not come from the extracellular space only, but are contaminated by microsomal fragments during the grinding and juicing processes [5]. To protect the plasma membrane from collapsing and to retain cell wall-bound proteins, several approaches have been introduced such as vacuum infiltration–centrifugation [6–9], pressure dehydration with careful temperature adjustment [10,11], filtration using appropriate simulated apoplastic solutions [12], vacuum perfusion [13], and elution [14]. Nevertheless, these techniques have some limitations. For example, the elution method is unable to discriminate between apoplastic fluids and protoplasts, resulting in more than 30% contamination from the protoplast fluids present in the collected solution. Moreover, the ratio between the cutting surface and tissue volume determines the level of contamination of released intracellular solutes [10]. On the other hand, the vacuum perfusion and pressure dehydration techniques require complicated and cumbersome instruments, rendering them unsuitable for large-scale production. Although perfusion and infiltration methods are fast and inexpensive, there is a possibility of altering the ionic composition, pH value, and metabolite concentration of apoplastic fluid due to additive-stimulated apoplastic solutions or water infiltration [15]. In addition, it is impractical to evaluate the physiological concentration of distinct metabolites and molecules in the apoplastic fluid ex situ [15]. Finally, the vacuum infiltration–centrifugation method generates a low amount of apoplastic proteins in waxy-coated leaves (e.g., rice and maize), hence reducing the extracted proteome [16]. Therefore, there is an urgent unmet pharmaceutical need for effective methods to extract plant-derived EVs from extracellular fluid outside the plasma membrane to achieve high-quality plant-derived EVs for clinical therapy.

Another challenge that impedes the development of plant-derived EVs is the lack of suitable and reliable biomarkers for plant-derived EVs. The development of plant EV biomarkers will contribute to the advancement of all aspects in the field, including isolation and characterization techniques, classifications, and downstream applications. So far, only a few plant-derived EV proteomes from apoplasts have been analyzed, such as those from olive pollen grains [17], *A. thaliana* (thale cress) leaves [18,19], sunflower seedlings [20], and *N. benthamiana* leaves [18]. In addition, no commercial antibodies against biomarkers for plant-derived EVs are available, hindering further progress in the field. Pinedo et al. suggested that there are three possible EV markers that were presented in both plant and mammalian proteomes, including heat shock protein 70 (HSP70), S-adenosyl-homocysteinase, and glyceraldehyde 3 phosphate dehydrogenase (GAPDH) [21]. Other possible cytosolic proteins in plant-derived EVs include native Pattelin-1 and -2 (PATL-1 and PATL-2), which participate in membrane-trafficking activities [21]. Unfortunately, these protein families are also found in plant-derived nanoparticles that might have been contaminated by destructive processes, together with proteins originating from plant-derived EVs such as glutathione S-transferase and annexin [22–25]. Pinedo et al. also suggested that plant-derived EV biomarkers should persist across different plant species and accumulate at high levels in EVs instead of in whole cells [21]. However, the diversity of plant proteomes poses a major challenge for the development of biomarkers for plant-derived EVs.

In this study, we aimed to address several challenges in the development of plant-derived EVs. Firstly, we established a comprehensive EV isolation system for succulent fruits using blueberry (BB) as a model plant source, followed by extensive characterization and an attempt to identify specific biomarkers for blueberry-derived EVs (BENVs) as well as plant-derived EVs in general. We have identified a general biomarker for plant-derived EVs from different edible fruits and showed that BENVs have a much higher drug loading capacity than other types of EVs. The confirmation of the presence of anthocyanins in blueberry-derived EVs supports their potential health benefits, such as antioxidant properties, protection against cardiovascular diseases, cancers, diabetes, and UV-B radiation [26]. Our results suggest that the isolated BENVs retain the antioxidant properties of the whole fruit and are thus a promising next generation of edible drug delivery vehicle with intrinsic anti-inflammatory capacity.

2. Materials and Methods

2.1. Materials

Aspirin (Sigma-Aldrich, St. Louis, MO, USA, Cat #5376) and curcumin (Sigma-Aldrich, Cat #C1386) were purchased from Sigma Aldrich (USA). The solvents were used at HPLC grade and other analytical grade chemicals were utilized without further purification.

2.2. Cell Culture

Human colon adenocarcinoma epithelial cell line (Caco-2) and human colorectal adenocarcinoma cell line (HT-29) were acquired from American Type Culture Collection (ATCC) (Manassas, VA, USA). All cells were grown in Dulbecco's modified Eagle's medium (DMEM, Invitrogen, Waltham, MA, USA, Cat #12800-017) supplemented with 12–15% fetal bovine serum (FBS, Hyclone, Logan, Utah, Cat #A50111-5039), 100 U/mL penicillin and 100 µg/mL streptomycin (Invitrogen^{TM}, Cat #15070-063). Cells were kept at 37 °C and 5% CO_2 in an incubator.

2.3. Preparation of Plant-Derived Nanovesicles

Blueberries were directly purchased from Tuckerberry Hill Blueberry Farm (Drysdale Victoria, Australia), or from Coles Supermarket (Waurn Ponds, VIC, Australia). Blueberries were washed 3 times with Milli-Q water. The unripe and rotten fruits were eliminated. After that, the blueberries were frozen and stored at −20 °C for further use.

Apoplastic fluid (AF) was extracted from blueberries using the centrifugation method modified from a study by Wada et al. [27]. Briefly, each blueberry was cut with a disposable blade and 2 mm of the pericarp from the stylar (distal) was removed as the residual part. The flat cut surface was immediately placed onto a homemade, reusable filter tube produced by 3D printing technique (Figure S1). Subsequently, the filter tube was put into the 50 mL conical tube. Next, the tube was centrifuged at 30× g for 10 min at 4 °C and the solution at the bottom of the tube was discarded to eliminate symplast contamination from the cutting method and damaged cells [28]. The filter tube containing blueberry was transferred into a clean 50 mL conical tube and then centrifuged at 200× g, 4 °C for another 10 min to collect the apoplastic fluid. The apoplastic fluid was filtered through a 0.8 µm mixed cellulose esters membrane to remove cellular debris and unwanted organelles before being stored at −20 °C for further use.

In this study, BENVs were isolated from AF using differential centrifugation approaches modified from a method described by Regente et al. [20]. Briefly, 13 mL of AF was centrifuged at 2000× g at 4 °C for 20 min and then 10,000× g for 30 min at 4 °C to eliminate cells and cellular debris in the pellet. The supernatants were collected for EV collection using differential ultracentrifugation. Minced juices (MJs) of different fruits were prepared as follows: Blueberry juice was produced by homogenizing frozen blueberries in a blender for 5 min to collect juice; grapefruits with skin removed were cut in half before squeezing in a cold room to collect juice. In the case of grapes, after removal of the skin, they were homogenized in a blender for 2 min. The grape juice was diluted with cold PBS (1:1) and centrifuged at 2000× g for 10 min at 4 °C to collect the supernatant. The collected juices were filtered through a 0.45 µm mixed cellulose esters syringe filter. Subsequently, all filtered juices were centrifuged at 2000× g for 20 min followed by centrifuged at 10,000× g for 30 min to eliminate cells and cellular debris in the pellets. Finally, the supernatants collected from AF and juices were centrifuged at 40,000× g and 100,000× g, respectively, for 6 h at 4 °C using the Beckman Coulter Optima L-90K Ultracentrifuge, and the pellets were suspended in 400 µL PBS.

2.4. Attenuated Total Reflection Fourier-Transform Infrared Spectroscopy (ATR-FTIR)

Solution samples were directly examined on the "Gold Gate" single reflection diamond ATR accessory using a Bruker Vertex 70 FTIR spectrometer at a resolution of 4 cm^{-1}. The instrument was performed with an average of 32 scans and in the wavelength range of 600–4000 cm^{-1}. The FTIR data was analyzed as described by Mihály et al. [29].

2.5. Nanoparticle Tracking Analysis (NTA)

NTA analysis was performed as described in our previous study [30]. In brief, 1 mL of diluted sample was loaded into the chamber of NTA equipment, and three videos were recorded in 60 s. The average size and number of particles from three recorded videos were then determined.

2.6. Transmission Electron Microscopy (TEM)

Ten microliters of BENVs collected at the centrifugal force of 40,000× g or 100,000× g was fixed in 50 µL of 2% paraformaldehyde (Sigma-Aldrich). Then, 5 µL of the mixed solution was transferred onto a Formvar carbon-coated electron microscopy grid and incubated for 20 min in a closed petri dish. The grid was subsequently washed by 100 µL of PBS for 2 min and transferred with 50 µL of 1% glutaraldehyde for 5 min, followed by washing with milli-Q water for 2 min. Next, the grid was negatively stained with 2% phosphotungstic acid (Sigma-Aldrich) for 2 min, and the excess staining solution was removed by a piece of filter paper before allowing to dry for 15 min in air. The TEM images were obtained using JEOL JEM 2100 TEM at 100 kV.

2.7. Protein Extraction of Plant Samples

Plant proteins were extracted using Kikuchi's method with minor modification [31]. Briefly, one mL of sample (containing either 1.8 mg/mL or 0.9 mg/mL of total protein) was mixed with 10 mL of extraction buffer (8 M urea, 50 mM Tris–HCl, pH 7.6, 2% (w/v) Triton X-100, 5 mM EDTA, 10 mM dithiothreitol (DTT) and protease inhibitor mixture tablet (Roche, Basel, Switzerland, Cat #11697498001)) for 5 min at 25 °C. The mixture was centrifuged at 16,000× g, for 10 min at 4 °C. Proteins in the supernatants were precipitated by adding 40 mL of acetone and incubation at −20 °C overnight. The suspension was centrifuged at 2300× g for 5 min at 4 °C. The pellets were washed twice with 75% acetone and dissolved in protein extract solution (1.2% (w/v) sodium dodecyl sulfate (SDS), 50 mM Tris-HCl, pH 6.8, 1% (v/v) β-mercaptoethanol, 20% glycine, and 0.001% (w/v) bromophenol blue), at 95 °C for 5 min. Insoluble proteins were eliminated by a brief centrifugation at 10,000× g for 1 min at 4 °C. The final protein concentration in samples were determined using BCA protein assay kit (Thermo Scientific, Waltham, MA, USA) and stored at −80 °C for further analysis.

2.8. Aptamer Binding Assay Using Fluorescence Polarization

Modified SYL3C aptamer labelled with FAM (FAM-anti-EpCAM-Chol aptamer) [32] (25 nM) was synthesized from IDT. The aptamers were folded by denaturing at 85 °C for 5 min in binding buffer (PBS containing 5 mM of MgCl$_2$), followed by returning to room temperature over 10 min and a refolding at 37 °C for at least 15 min.

BENVs were lysed by incubating isolated BENVs with 0.05% Triton X-100 for 30 min at room temperature. An equal volume of intact BENVs or lysed BENVs (1.56 × 10^8 particles/mL) was added into a 96-well black plate and mixed with 5 nM of modified SYL3C aptamer in PBS at different ratios to obtain a total reaction volume of

100 µL. The plate was placed onto an orbital shaking incubator for 15 or 30 min at room temperature in the dark, with gentle shaking at 30 rpm. Subsequently, the fluorescence polarization values were measured with an excitation at 485 nm and an emission at 528 nm using VICTORTM X5 Plate Reader.

2.9. DiD-Labeled Aptamer-Conjugated BENVs

The labeling of aptamer-conjugated BENVs (Apt-BENVs) with Vybrant DiD solution (Thermo Fisher, Waltham, MA, USA, Cat #V22887) was performed as follows: 1 mL of aptamer-conjugated BENVs (1.56×10^7 particles/mL) was incubated with 6 µL of Vybrant DiD solution for 30 min, followed by two washes with 1 mL of PBS followed by ultracentrifugation at 4 °C, $100,000 \times g$ for 1 h each to remove free dyes. The pellet was resuspended in filtered PBS and stored at -80 °C for further analysis.

2.10. Cellular Uptake

Caco-2 cells and HT-29 cells were seeded on 8-chamber slides (Thermo Fisher, Cat #154534PK) at 4000 cells/well and 3000 cells/well, respectively. After culturing for 48 h at 37 °C, the cells were washed twice with Hank's balanced salt solution (HBSS, Sigma-Aldrich). Then, 200 µL of fresh culture media containing DiD-BENVs-Apt (3×10^6 particles/mL) was added to each well and incubated for 6 h at 37 °C. Prior to analyzing by microscope, cells were extensively washed with 0.5 mL of HBSS for three times to remove the non-internalizing DiD-BENVs-Apt. Next, cells were treated with 50 µL of nucleic indicator Hoechst 33342 (2 µg/mL) and incubated at room temperature in the dark for 10 min. Subsequently, cells were washed extensively with HBSS to remove the DiD-BENVs-Apt bound on the cell surface. The uptake of DiD-BENVs-Apt was analyzed using ECLIPSE Ti2 inverted microscope and flow cytometry.

2.11. Transport Study

Caco-2 cells were seeded onto Corning Transwell inserts (0.4 µm pore diameter, 1.12 cm^2) for 21 days prior to studying of drug transportation. Before analysis, the inserts were washed twice and equilibrated with transport medium (i.e., 25 mM HEPES in HBSS (pH 7.4)). An addition of 1% DMSO in the transport buffer served as co-solvent. The integrity of the Caco-2 cells monolayer and their differentiation were evaluated by measuring the trans-epithelial electrical resistance (TEER) using the Millicell® ERS-2. The resistance value is presented as Ω (electric resistance), and the TEER value was calculated as:

$$\text{TEER } (\Omega \cdot \text{cm}^2) = (\Omega_{\text{cell insert}} - \Omega_{\text{cell-free insert}}) \times 1.12 \text{ cm}^2$$

Next, 0.5 mL of DiD-labeled BENVs (10^8 particles/mL) in transport buffer were added on the apical side of the chamber and 1.5 mL of transport buffer was added on the basolateral side. After incubation in an orbital shaking incubator at 37 °C, 150 µL of media was collected from the basolateral side at different intervals of incubation (i.e., 0, 1, and 3 h), and fresh media was added to maintain the volume at the lower chamber. At the end of the experiment, the TEER was measured again to examine the intact BENVs of the Caco-2 cell monolayer. Moreover, the transported DiD-BENVs in the basolateral chamber were determined by fluorescence microscopy.

2.12. Preparation of Drug-Loaded BENVs

Drug-loaded BENVs were prepared by conventional incubation method. BENVs at different concentrations (i.e., 500 µg/mL or 1000 µg/mL of total proteins) after thawing were immediately kept at different temperatures (i.e., 4 °C or 25 °C) for 5 min or 10 min to determine the effects of conditions before drug loading. Next, payload, either 120 µM aspirin or 100 µM curcumin in absolute ethanol, was incubated with the designed amounts of BENVs at different temperature (i.e., 25 °C and 37 °C), shaking condition (i.e., 150 rpm and 200 rpm), and incubation time (i.e., 15, 20, 30, 45, and 60 min). All the experiments with curcumin were performed in the dark. After the incubation, the mixture was centrifuged at a low speed of 5000× g for 10 min at 4 °C to remove the unbound precipitated drugs. Supernatants were collected and designated as W1 samples, and the pellets were suspended in 1 mL of filtered PBS. Subsequently, drug-loaded BENVs were washed twice in filtered PBS solution by a centrifugation at 100,000× g for 45 min at 4 °C. The collected supernatants were designated as W2 and W3 for unbound drugs in the solution and on the BENV surface, respectively. The final pellets were resuspended in 200 µL of filtered PBS and stored at −20 °C for further experiments. Drug concentrations were determined by HPLC [33]. The percentage of drug loading and entrapment efficiency were calculated as follow:

$$\text{Drug loading (\%)} = \frac{\text{Amount of drug in drug} - \text{loaded BENVs}}{\text{Amount of exosomal proteins in drug} - \text{loaded BENVs}} \times 100$$

$$\text{Entrapment efficiency (\%)} = \frac{(\text{Drug added} - W1 - W2 - W3)}{\text{Drug added}} \times 100$$

2.13. Cell Viability Assay

MTT assay was used to determine cell viability. Caco-2 cells were seeded at 5000 cells/well in a 96-well plate and incubated at 37 °C and 5% CO_2 in an incubator for 24 h. Then, the medium was removed, and cells were treated with 100 µL of fresh culture medium containing either free curcumin, BENVs, or curcumin-loaded BENVs at various concentrations, followed by an incubation for 48 or 72 h at 37 °C. Non-treatment cells and culture medium only served as the negative controls and were designated as cells without test compound and medium control, respectively. Next, 20 µL of MTT in PBS (5 mg/mL) was added into each well and incubated for another 4 h at 37 °C, followed by the addition of 150 µL of DMSO to solubilize MTT. The absorbance was measured at 570 nm by a VICTOR TM X5 Plate Reader. The viability of cells was calculated as follows:

$$\text{Viability (\%)} = \left(\frac{\overline{M}_{\text{treated cells}} - \overline{M}_{\text{medium control}}}{\overline{M}_{\text{control cells without test compound}} - \overline{M}_{\text{medium control}}} \right) \times 100$$

2.14. Evaluation of BENVs' Capability in Immune Modulation

The capability in modulating immune systems was evaluated based on the release of pro-inflammatory cytokines IL-8 in Caco-2 cells during hydrogen peroxide (H_2O_2)-induced oxidative stress. IL-8 release in supernatants were measured by a Human IL-8/CXCL8 ELISA Kit as per the manufacture's instruction (Sigma-Aldrich, Cat #RAB0319-1KT). Total glutathione was measured to evaluate the intrinsic cellular antioxidant responses during the anthocyanin-rich treatments [34]. Post-treatment Caco-2 cells were washed with cold PBS three times and immersed in cold PBS before being collected by scraping method using Falcon™ Cell Scrapers. The collected samples were centrifuged at 600× g for 5 min at 4 °C and the pellets were suspended in 500 µL of ice cold 5% aqueous 5-sulfosalicylic acid dihydrate (SSA). Cells were disrupted by sonicating in ice-water bath for 5 min, followed by an incubation at 4 °C for 10 min. Subsequently, samples were centrifuged at 14,000× g for 10 min at 4 °C, and the supernatants were collected and stored at −80 °C for further analysis. The total GSH was measured by a Glutathione Fluorescent Detection Kit (Invitrogen, Cat #EIAGSHF) following the manufacturer's instructions.

2.15. Immunoblotting Analysis

The collected plant proteins were separated on SDS-PAGE gel and blotted onto nitrocellulose membranes (Whatman, Maidstone, UK, Cat. 10401196). Goat anti-rabbit HRP-conjugated secondary antibody (Thermo Fisher Scientific, Waltham, MA, USA; Cat #31460) was used to detect PR-3/CHN I Class I chitinase (Agrisera, Vännäs, Sweden, Cat #AS07 207) and PR-2 I GLU I I Class I beta-1,3-glucanase (Agrisena, Vännäs, Sweden, Cat #AS07 208).

2.16. Statistical Analysis

All samples were prepared in triplicate and results were expressed as means ± standard deviations unless otherwise stated. Statistical analysis was executed by GraphPad PRISM

8 with one-way analysis of variance (ANOVA) for differences among multiple groups and two-sided paired Student's *t*-test for differences between two specific groups. A *p* value ≤ 0.05 was considered statically significant.

3. Results

3.1. Preparation and Characterization of Blueberry-Derived Extracellular Nanovesicles (BENVs)

In 1990, Welbaum and Meinzer et al. proposed a method to extract apoplastic fluid (AF) from sugarcane using serial low-speed centrifugation accompanied with a 0.8 μm cellulose acetate filter in a 5 mL tube [28]. However, this method can only be applied to watery plants because the viscosity sap will block the filter as soon as they are in contact. In addition, low-speed centrifugation is unable to force the high viscosity AF through the filter. Therefore, we introduced a new strategy for the preparation of BENVs in which a tube holder with small holes (0.5–1.5 mm) separated the AF out of the fruit at low-speed centrifugation. Subsequently, the collected AF was filtered through a 0.8 μm mixed cellulose esters membrane using a vacuum filter apparatus to remove cellular debris and unwanted organelles. The strategy of serial low-speed centrifugation allows AF to be collected at its purest form as the symplastic contaminations from the cutting process and damaged cells are eliminated [28] (Figure S1).

For the analysis of BENVs thus prepared, we employed a FTIR technique as it is efficient in identifying biomarkers in different biological species, particularly for extracellular vesicles, based on the "spectroscopic" protein-to-lipid ratio (P/L ratio) [29]. Specifically, it was utilized to distinguish between apoplastic fluid (AF), blueberry minced juice (MJ) collected at $2000\times g$ and $10,000\times g$ (i.e., MJ 2k and MJ 10k, respectively), and blueberry-derived extracellular vesicles collected at $40,000\times g$ and $100,000\times g$ (i.e., BENV 40k and BENV 100k, respectively) (Figure S2). To facilitate the analysis, all input samples were adjusted to the same protein concentration prior to FTIR study. As shown in Figure 1A, MJ and BENVs showed higher P/L ratio compared to that in AF, indicating the lower lipid concentrations in these samples. It is most likely that the AF is enriched with the cell wall's lipids when it flows through the 3D filter [35]. Moreover, the lipid contents in the MJ could be influenced by damaged cells or fragmented cells generated from the grinding or juicing process. Thus, BENVs contained lower lipid concentrations than the intact fruit, resulting in a higher P/L ratio at the same input concentration, indicative of the success of our novel 3D filter-based isolation method.

Next, the total anthocyanin content in each sample, including AF, MJ 10k, and BENV 40k, was determined by HPLC (Figure S3). Interestingly, AF and BENV were found to contain anthocyanin, which was mainly comprised of malvidin, approximately 88% of the total anthocyanins (Figure 1B). Meanwhile, malvidin accounted for more than half of the total anthocyanins in MJ (53.65%), followed by peonidin (18.73%) and petunidin (18.28%). The presence of delphinidin and cyanidin in all three samples was hardly noticeable. The higher percentage of anthocyanin compounds in BENVs compared to that in AF might result from the sedimentation of the smallest non-EV structures (e.g., exomeres and high-density lipoprotein) upon extended high-speed centrifugation [36]. This hypothesis was supported by NTA data in which an abundance of uncharacterized small particles ranging from 10 nm to 30 nm was detected in BENV samples collected at $40,000\times g$ and $100,000\times g$ (Figure 1C). Remarkably, the particle numbers of the BENVs isolated from apoplastic fluid at different centrifugal forces were significantly enriched to $7.77 \times 10^9 \pm 2.24 \times 10^8$ particles/mL and $9.08 \times 10^9 \pm 6.22 \times 10^7$ particles/mL for BENVs collected with a centrifugal force of $40,000\times g$ and $100,000\times g$, respectively (Figure 1C). A small number of BENV particles ranging from 300–450 nm was also counted as EVs, corresponding to a study by Xiao et al. [37]. The 2D and 3D morphology of BENVs were studied by TEM and AFM, respectively (Figures 1D and S4). BENVs exhibited a lipid bilayer typical of extracellular nanovesicles and were surrounded by a network of extravesicular channels. This is consistent with a study performed by Sharma et al., in which the AFM image of saliva EVs displayed a similar channel network [38]. Moreover, the protein content of BENVs was found to be 6174.04 ± 68.58 mg per liter, which is 18-fold higher than those collected from milk EVs and 3000-fold higher than EVs collected from cell culture supernatant (Table S1), indicating a high yield of our isolation method for drug delivery purposes [39,40].

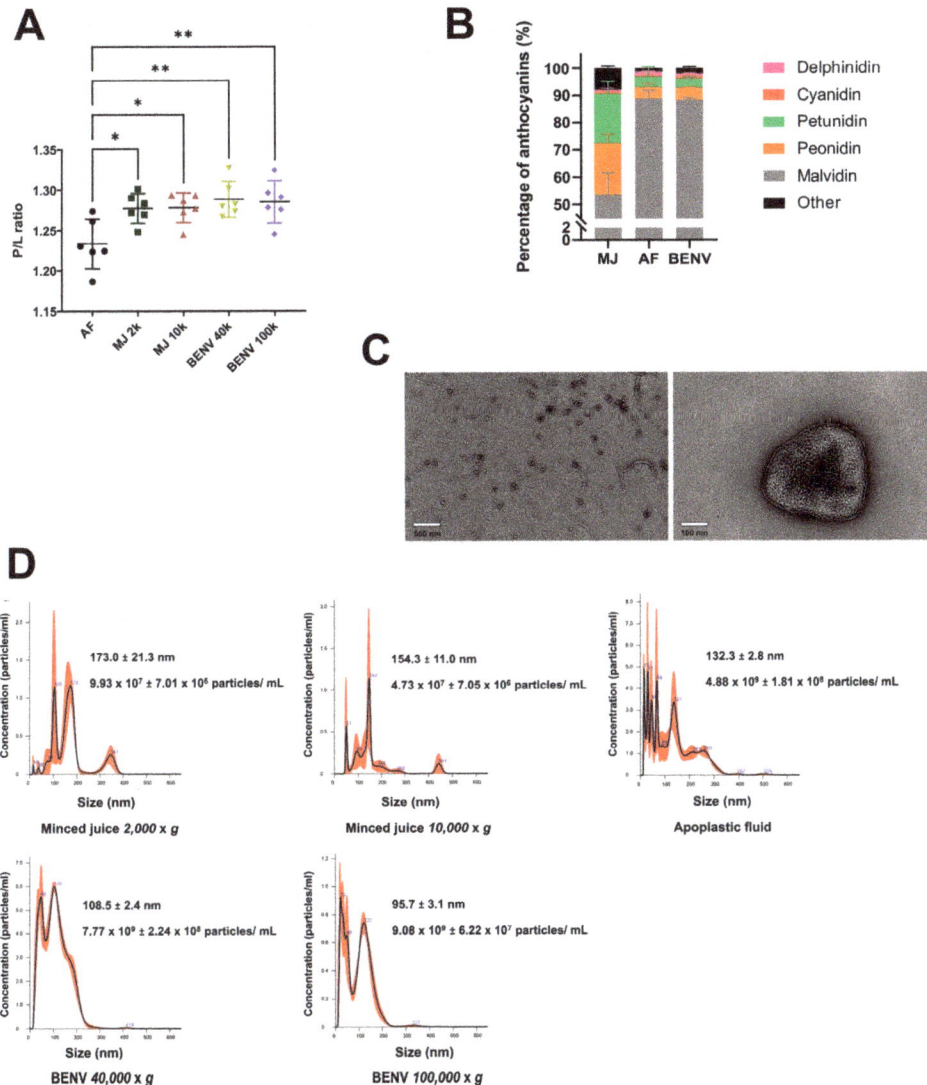

Figure 1. Characterization of blueberry-derived extracellular nanovesicles. (**A**) FTIR spectroscopic protein-to-lipid ratio (P/L ratio) calculated by the relative intensities of amide I to CH_2/CH_3 stretching of apoplastic fluid (AF), minced juices (MJ) collected at different centrifugation forces ($2000\times g$ and $10,000\times g$), and BENVs collected at different centrifugation forces ($40,000\times g$ and $100,000\times g$). Mean values are represented by horizontal lines, and the standard deviation of the mean is shown as error bars (n = 6). (**B**) Anthocyanin contents in anthocyanin-rich extracts identified by HPLC (n = 3). (**C**) The BENVs collected at $40,000\times g$ were stained with phosphotungstic acid to obtain TEM images. (**D**) Particle sizes of anthocyanin-rich extracts collected from different centrifugation forces using NanoSight NS300 (n = 3). *, $p < 0.05$ and **, $p < 0.01$.

3.2. A putative "Universal" Biomarker of Plant-Derived Extracellular Nanovesicles

To the best of our knowledge, there are only a handful putative plant-derived EV biomarkers described so far, including Helija [41,42], TET8 [43], and AtTET8-GFP [44]. However, there is no commercial antibody available for those putative biomarkers, hindering the progression of plant-derived EV research and development. Therefore, we set out to investigate biomarker(s) for plant-derived EVs in general and for BENVs in particular. To this end, the protein species in various fractions of blueberry EV preparation were initially visualized in Coomassie blue-stained gel (Figure 2A). The nature of the proteins of interest found in AF, MJ, and BENVs were investigated further by mass spectrometry to identify possible protein sequences (Supporting Information, Materials and Methods). Based on the mass spectrometry results, the protein of 28 kDa was identified as acidic endochitinase, which is a defensive protein released upon the invasion of fungal pathogens. Previous studies on exosome-like nanovesicles isolated from ginger [45], shiitake [46], and citrus [47] also reported the presence of a protein with similar molecular weight in the SDS-PAGE analysis, though the identity of such protein remains elusive. As EVs are originally attributed to the interactions between plants and pathogens, we hypothesized that pathogen-related (PR) proteins could be sorted onto the EV surface and thus serve as biomarkers for plant-derived EVs. To test this hypothesis, we proceeded to examine the presence of pathogen-related (PR) proteins such as class I β-1,3-glucanase (PR-2), class I chitinase (PR-3), pathogenesis-related protein 5 (PR-5), and isoflavone reductase (IFR) in different fruit samples (i.e., blueberry, grapefruit, and grape) to identify possible biomarkers. A complete blot of the SDS-PAGE analysis is shown in Figure 2. Among them, class I chitinase (PR-3) was present in all samples and highly accumulated in EV samples, either at the position of 25 kDa or 38 kDa upon Western blot analysis (Figure 2B–D). However, grapefruit EVs extracted at $40,000\times g$ displayed a very faint band of PR-3 (Figure 2C), which could be explained by the fact that, although the protein concentration of grapefruit EVs is similar to that in other samples, the juicy nature and the contaminated fragments generated during the squeezing method might affect the protein composition of collected EVs. Moreover, grapefruits were reported as cold-sensitive species that developed chilling injury symptoms under low-temperature storage conditions (i.e., lower than 8–10 °C) [48]. In addition, Porat et al. described low levels of chitinase in flavedo tissue of grapefruit in nontreatment conditions in comparison with stress conditions such as wounding and UV treatment, whereas β-1,3-glucanase (PR-2) expression remained stable with or without stress conditions [49]. This could account for the low chitinase expression in all grapefruit samples. Notably, in all samples, there was an accumulation of PR-3 in EVs extracted at $40,000\times g$ in comparison with MJ at different molecular weights because they exist in different isozymes (black arrow). For instance, at $40,000\times g$, blueberry EVs and grape EVs showed a prominent protein at 25 kDa, while grapefruit displayed a major protein at 38 kDa. All EVs isolated at $100,000\times g$ contained proteins similar to those of the original MJ and/or AF. Another PR protein that was detected in grape and grapefruit-derived EV samples is class I β-1,3-glucanase (PR-2). With an apparent molecular mass of 30 kDa [50], PR-2 was accumulated in grape-derived EVs isolated at $40,000\times g$, while PR-2 isozyme located at approximately 33 kDa [51,52] was observed as faint bands in both grape-derived EVs extracted at $40,000\times g$ and grapefruit-derived EVs extracted at $100,000\times g$. This concords with a previous study in which only trace amounts of PR-2 and PR-3 were detected in intracellular and intercellular sites of healthy plants, and the increased expression of PR proteins frequently relates to pathogen attack [20,51,53]. Hence, pathogen-related proteins, such as PR-2 and PR-3 identified here, could be utilized as promising plant-derived EV biomarkers and be used for tracking biogenesis pathways that drive plant-derived EVs to designed locations.

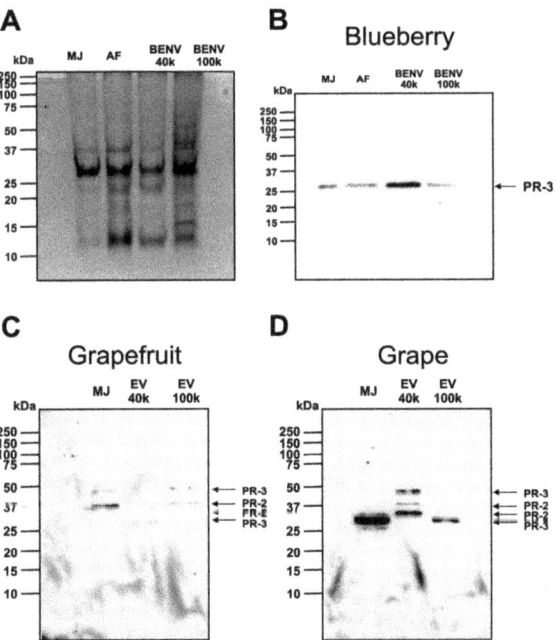

Figure 2. Analysis of proteins in blueberry-derived extracellular nanovesicles. (**A**) Coomassie staining of 12% SDS-PAGE gels of protein extracts (17.3 µg/lane) prepared from anthocyanin-rich extracts. Immunodetection of extracellular vesicles extracted from different succulent fruits such as blueberry (**B**), grapefruit (**C**), and grape (**D**) using class I β-1,3-glucanase (PR-2) and class I chitinase (PR-3) antibodies. The isozyme of PR-2 and PR-3 are identified by black arrows. A total of 16.2 µg protein was loaded into each lane. Data shown are representative of three independent experiments.

3.3. BENVs as a Nanocarrier for Drug Delivery

Due to the absence of biomarkers, the application of plant-derived EVs in the pharmaceutical industry is hampered by the inability to identify and detect the plant-derived EV itself and demonstrate the binding of plant-derived EVs to target cells or tissues. Herein, we used anti-EpCAM aptamer (SYL3C) as a model EV tracker to investigate the incorporation of modified aptamers to the lipid bilayer membrane of BENVs (Figure S5). The SYL3C aptamer was labelled with 6-FAM (6-Carboxyfluorescein) at the 5′- end to generate a fluorescently tagged version of the aptamer for the BENV trafficking study. The 3′ end of the aptamer was conjugated with TEG-cholesterol, allowing it to insert into the BENV membrane through hydrophobic interactions between the lipid-PEG linker and the phospholipid bilayer [54]. Furthermore, cholesterol-PEG possesses superior characteristics for drug delivery systems (DDS), such as enhanced fluorescence intensity of labeled cells, prevention of the self-assembly of micelles/liposomes, and higher rigidity and stability [54]. Fluorescence polarization (FP) was used to investigate the binding capacity of the anti-EpCAM aptamer and BENVs as the bound and the free form of fluorescently labelled aptamer can easily be analyzed in solution using FP. As shown in Figure 3A, when the aptamer concentration was higher than 5 nM, the FP value was constant (approximately 185 mP), indicating a stable conjugation of the aptamer into BENVs [55]. Encouragingly, ΔFP increased when the BENV concentration increased from 1.2×10^7 particles/mL to 3×10^8 particles/mL (Figure 3B). Moreover, a higher ΔFP was observed after a 30-min incubation compared to that with a 15-min incubation, indicating time-dependent binding, as aptamers had sufficient time to insert into the BENV membrane. At a BENV concentration of 3×10^8 particles/mL, the binding reached its plateau with minimal difference in ΔFP between the two incubation times. To demonstrate that the increase in ΔFP was derived from the decoration of aptamers onto the EV surface and not from the attachment of aptamers to non-vesicle particles in the detection buffer, BENVs were treated with 0.05% Triton X-100 to lyse the vesicles. Indeed, the intact BENVs presented a high ΔFP value because the binding between aptamer and BENV decelerates the rotation speed of the aptamer (Figure 3C). On the contrary, lysed BENVs contained numerous small fragments and exhibited a low ΔFP value, which revealed either no binding or fast diffusion motion of the aptamer-bound fragments, as the molecular mass of lysed BENV fragments treated by detergent have minimal impact on the molecular mass/volume ratio of the aptamer.

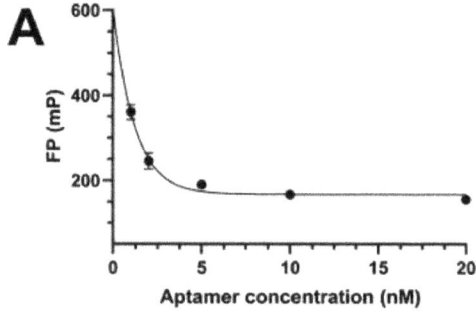

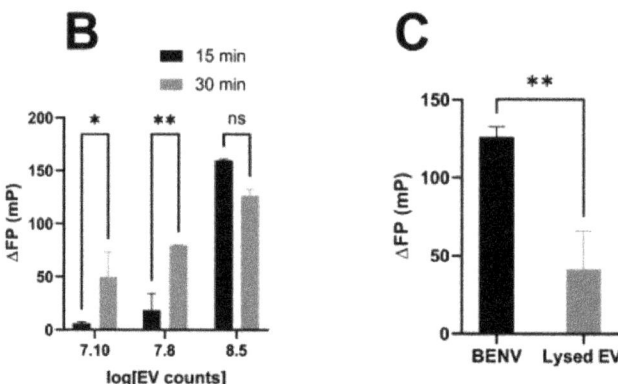

Figure 3. Characterization of conjugation of FAM-labelled EpCAM aptamer with BENV surface using fluorescence polarization. (**A**) Fluorescence polarization of FAM-labelled EpCAM aptamer at different concentrations. (**B**) Effect of incubation time on ΔFP. (**C**) Comparison of the conjugation of FAM-labelled EpCAM aptamer BENV surface to that of BNEV lysed by 0.05% Triton X-100. ns, a statistically non-significant difference. Data shown are means ± S.D., n = 3, *, $p < 0.05$, and **, $p < 0.01$.

Next, we investigated the cellular uptake of BENVs. To this end, lipophilic carbocyanine membrane dye DiD (red) was incorporated into the BENV membrane and the FAM-anti-EpCAM-Chol aptamer (green) was conjugated onto the BENV surface to produce a dual-fluorescence label. The dual-labelled BENVs were found to be completely internalized into Caco-2 and HT-29 cells (Figure 4A,B) after 6 h of incubation. The colocalization of red (DiD, for BENV's lipid bilayer membrane) and green (FAM, for EpCAM aptamer) indicates the integrity of BENVs after internalization. Interestingly, BENVs tended to accumulate in the cytoplasm of Caco-2 cells, suggesting that BENVs might be taken up by Caco-2 cells via receptor-mediated internalization [56]. Remarkably, BENVs were found to selectively distribute to the nuclear region of HT-29 cells. Since Caco-2 cells exhibit low cancer phenotypes in comparison with bona fide high grade colorectal adenocarcinoma cells such as HT-29, it would be interesting to explore if BENVs could preferentially target susceptible cells [57]. The cellular uptake results were also confirmed by flow cytometry in which all human cancer cells contained fluorescence-labelled BENVs after 6 h (Figure 4C,D). Additional studies are planned to explore the mechanism of uptake.

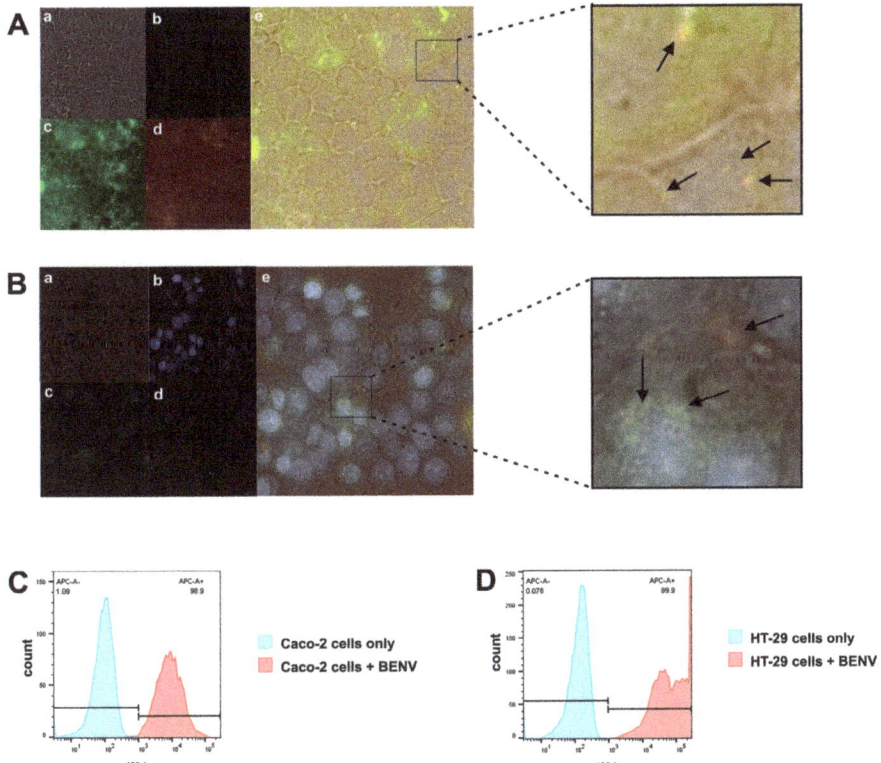

Figure 4. Cellular uptake of dual labelled BENVs in Caco-2 cells and HT-29 cells: (**a**) Bright field, (**b**) Hoechst 33342-stained cells, (**c**) FAM-labelled BENVs uptake by cells, (**d**) DiD-labelled BENV uptake by cells, and (**e**) I merged images. BENVs are labelled with lipophilic carbocyanine membrane dye—DiD (red) and FAM-cholesterol EpCAM aptamer (green). Caco-2 and HT-29 cells were incubated with dual labelled BENVs for 6 h at 37 °C, prior to analysis by Nikon Ti2 microscope (Magnification: 100×) (**A,B**) and flow cytometry (**C,D**). Data are representative of three independent experiments. Arrows: endocytosed BENVs.

Generally, the small size of BENVs, i.e., approximately 100 nm, allows them to extravasate and translocate through physical barriers as well as travel through the extracellular matrix [58]. We performed a transport study to examine the capability of BENVs to deliver payload across epithelial cell barriers. Figure 5A presents the TEER values of Caco-2 cell monolayers before and after being exposed to CUR-loaded BENVs labeled with DiD (red) for 1 h and 3 h. TEER values before treatment were found to be 570 ± 80 $\Omega \cdot cm^2$, which is indicative of a good barrier integrity of the Caco-2 cell monolayer (>260 $\Omega \cdot cm^2$) [59]. Cell monolayers with TEER values lower than 260 $\Omega \cdot cm^2$ were discarded. As shown in Figure 5A, there were only minor changes in the TEER value after 1 h of incubation with BENVs, indicating that BENVs could be transported across the epithelial monolayer without compromising the integrity of the epithelial cell barrier. Nevertheless, 3 h of incubation with a high concentration of BENVs (10^8 particles/mL) resulted in a disruption of tight junction integrity leading to leakage of BENVs. Intact BENVs with a spherical shape were detected in the lower chamber after 1 h of incubation. Additionally, observation revealed the presence of more BENVs in the lower chamber after 3 h of incubation, confirming the opening of tight junctions. The disruption of tight junctions could occur during reversible tight junction opening to facilitate the transcellular permeability, which could be recovered after the removal of BENV solution. Based on the results from the cytotoxicity test, it is unlikely that BENVs caused the irreversible disruption on Caco-2 cells as cell viability remained at high values after 24- and 48-h incubation (Section 3.4). Although the appropriate amount of BENVs per specific area (cm^2) was yet to be determined in this study, the transport study revealed that BENVs could retain the encapsulated materials after crossing the epithelial barrier without causing membrane disruption for 1 h.

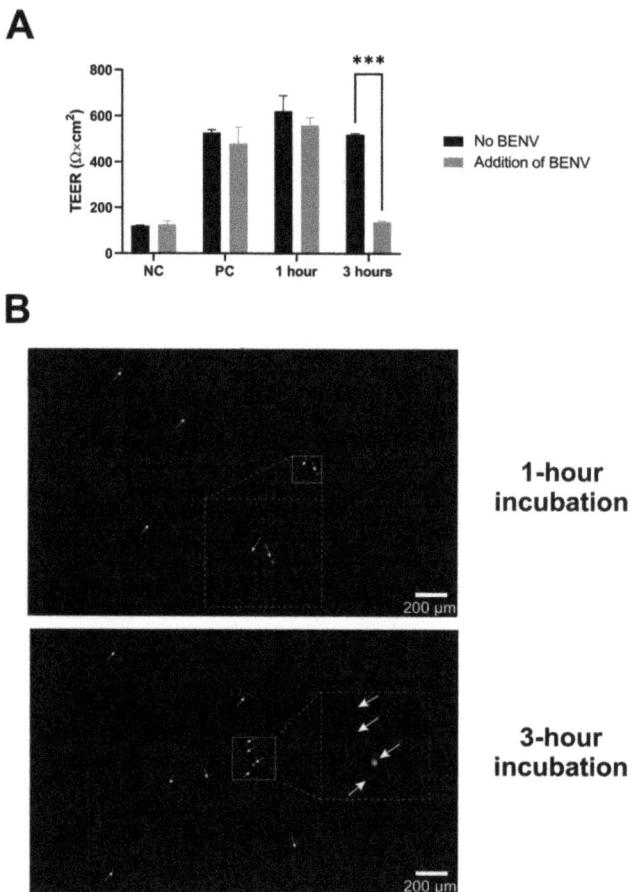

Figure 5. Time-dependent translocation of intact BENVs across Caco-2 cells monolayer. (**A**) Transepithelial electrical resistance (TEER) values of Caco-2 cell monolayers before and after exposure to CUR-loaded BENVs labelled with DiD (red) for 1 h and 3 h. NC, the membrane filter without cells as a negative control. PC, the Caco-2 cell monolayer without CUR-loaded BENV's treatment as a positive control for TEER. Data are shown as means ± SD (n = 3). ***, $p < 0.001$. (**B**) Visualization of DiD-labelled BENVs collected from the basal compartment after 1-h (up panel) and 3-h (bottom panel) incubation using epifluorescence microscopy. Arrows: DiD-labelled BENVs. Data are representative of three independent experiments.

Next, we evaluated the loading capacity of BENVs. In these studies, aspirin and curcumin, well-known hydrophobic drugs that possess cancer chemopreventive and therapeutic effects, were utilized as a model payload. Different factors (such as carrier condition, shaking power, and incubation time) that influenced drug loading efficiency during incubation were examined to determine the optimal loading conditions for BENVs (Figure S6). Even though the encapsulation efficiency increased over time, however, there was only a moderate increase in drug loading from 5 min incubation to 30 min incubation. As shown in Figure 6A, BENVs possessed a high EE for curcumin (approximately 82.76% after 5 min of incubation), which had a tendency of increasing over time, i.e., from 89.41% at 15 min to 92.68% at 30 min. This was a remarkable result because the current loading efficiency of EVs for curcumin is reported to be 18–24% by conventional incubation methods [60]. However, it is clear that the encapsulation efficiency of curcumin is significantly higher than that of aspirin despite of the comparable input amount, namely 120 µM of curcumin and 100 µM of aspirin per 10^{11} BENV particles. The amount of drug loaded into BENVs is significantly higher than those in recent studies on drug-loaded EVs, in which the amounts of doxorubicin and paclitaxel loaded were approximately 0.03 µM and 0.03 µM per 10^{11} EV particles, respectively [61].

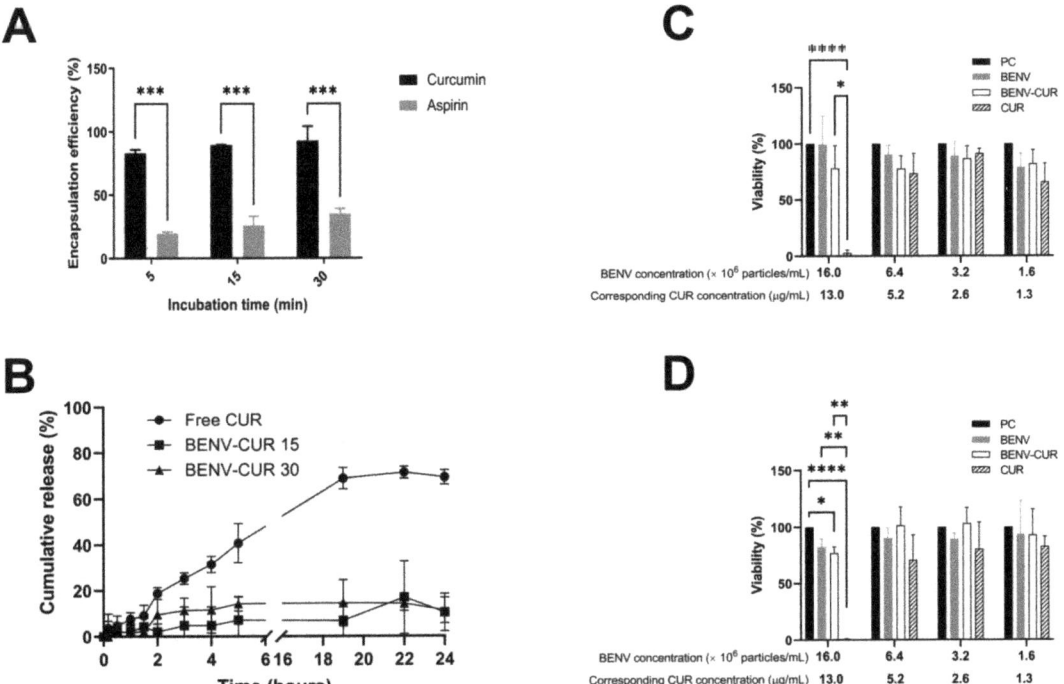

Figure 6. Drug release and safety profile of curcumin-loaded BENVs. (**A**) Encapsulation efficiency of BENVs loaded with curcumin and aspirin over different incubation times. (**B**) Drug release profiles of free curcumin (Free CUR), CUR-loaded BENVs for 15 min (BENV-CUR 15), and CUR-loaded BENVs for 30 min (BENV-CUR 30) in vitro. Samples were incubated in a buffer of pH 1.2 for 2 h before transferring to a buffer of pH 6.8 for 22 h. Cytotoxicity assay (MTT assay) for Caco-2 cells treatment were identified after incubating Caco-2 cells with free curcumin (CUR), BENVs, and curcumin-loaded BENVs (BENV-CUR) for 48 h (**C**) and 72 h (**D**). The concentration of free CUR was equivalated to the CUR concentration encapsulated in BENVs. PC: cells without drug treatment. Data shown as means ± S.D., n = 3. (*, $p < 0.05$; **, $p < 0.01$, ***, $p < 0.001$, ****, $p < 0.0001$).

Oral administration is the route used for approximately 60% of commercial drug products [62]. The main challenges associated with oral DDSs are the harsh environment of the gastrointestinal tract (GIT) and the residence time required for complete absorption [63]. In fact, the GIT confronts oral controlled release formulations with its unique physiological properties, leading to a fast release rate, drug degradation, or pre-systemic clearance [64]. To demonstrate that BENVs can serve as nanocarrier platforms, we investigated their stability at different pH levels, drug release profiles, and cytotoxicity. As shown in Figure S7, the particle sizes of BENVs were found to remain stable in simulated gastric fluid for 2 h, followed by simulated intestinal fluid for the following 22 h. However, particles were prone to aggregation when incubated in water. The zeta potential in simulated gastric fluid increased from −15.6 mV to −2.05 mV, whereas in the simulated intestinal fluid, the zeta potential was greatly reduced to −52.3 mV (Figure S7). Figure 6B shows the in vitro drug release profile of free curcumin and curcumin loaded BENVs at 24 h. During the first 2 h in simulated gastric fluid, 18.82% of the free curcumin passed through a dialysis membrane and was detected in the dialysate. On the other hand, curcumin was slowly liberated and dialysed from BENV-CUR 15 and BENV-CUR 30, approximately 2.02% and 9.53%, respectively. After being transferred to simulated small intestinal fluid, free CUR was gradually released and reached a plateau after 24 h (approximately 71.37%). However, BENVs released curcumin slowly at approximately 7.1% and 14.3% for BENV-CUR 15 and BENV-CUR 30 after 19 h, respectively. Interestingly, curcumin incubated with BENVs for 30 min exhibited a higher percentage of drug release than that achieved with the shorter incubation time (15 min). This result could be explained by the different curcumin-to-lipid (C/L) molar ratios. Curcumin molecules tend to associate with the glycerol group at low C/L, whereas at higher C/L, they accumulate closer to the headgroup of the lipids in the membrane leaflet [65]. We speculated that the increase in C/L after a 30-min incubation reorients curcumin molecules towards the headgroup of the leaflet, facilitating the liberation of curcumin from BENV. Nevertheless, unlike the properties demonstrated in the releasing profile of free CUR, BENVs were able to retain most of its payload, facilitating sustained release and accumulation of curcumin at the intended sites of targeted drug delivery. As for their potential toxicity, BENV and CUR-loaded BENV were found to be largely nontoxic to cells (Figure 6C,D and Figure S8). However, the viability of CaCo-2 cells and HT-29 cells was reduced with the increase in free curcumin levels. In addition, HT-29 cells displayed more resistance to curcumin than that of Caco-2 cells, evident from the fact that 13 µg/mL curcumin caused 96.4% and 65.8% loss of cell viability in Caco-2 and HT-29 cells, respectively. Although curcumin at the concentrations of 2.5 and 5 µg/mL induces DNA damage to human hepatoma G2 cells both in the mitochondrial and nuclear genomes [66], cancer cells do not die unless they are exposed to 5–50 µM curcumin for several hours [67–69]. In our study, HT-29 cells were able to maintain their viability when they were treated with either BENV or CUR-loaded BENV for 48–72 h. This result could be explained by the ability of BENV to hold its payload once encapsulated, with only 14.3% of curcumin released from BENVs over a period of 72 h. A slow leak of a small amount of encapsulated CUR is insufficient to cause cell death in HT-29 cells. In addition, it is possible that the intrinsic contents of BENVs may counteract the effects of curcumin.

3.4. Immunomodulatory Effects of BENVs

Oxidative stress upregulates the production of inflammatory cytokines in cells [70]. The gastrointestinal tract (GIT) is vulnerable to exogenous oxidant effects as it serves as the primary digestive system. The GIT is directly affected by various stimuli, such as pollutants, smoking, drugs, xenobiotics, food toxins, heavy metal ions, and intestinal microflora [71]. Although monocytic cells are commonly used to evaluate the immunomodulatory effects, Caco-2 (Cancer Coli-2) was chosen as a cellular model to study the ability of BENVs to regulate inflammation-associated colorectal cancer because of their ability to mimic the intestinal barrier and high sensitivity to H_2O_2-induced oxidative stress. Proinflammatory cytokine IL-8 is well-known as an oxidative stress indicator in Caco-2 cells. We hypothesized that the production of IL-8 protein caused by oxidative stress will be suppressed by pre-incubating Caco-2 cells with anthocyanin-rich extracts. Indeed, preincubation of Caco-2 cells with AF and BENVs significantly reduced the IL-8 level caused by H_2O_2, whereas MJ only suppressed IL-8 release after 8 h of incubation (Figure 7A). This could be attributed by the malvidin contents in AF and BENVs, which facilitates a faster transportation across the Caco-2 cell monolayer [72]. A short pre-incubation time with MJ (i.e., 1 h or 5 h) had no effect on oxidative stress modulation nor increased IL-8 release (Figure 7A).

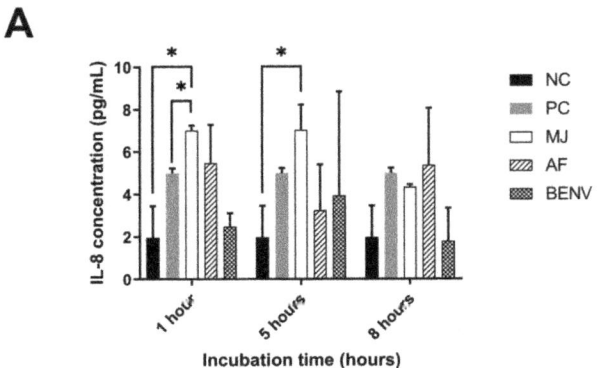

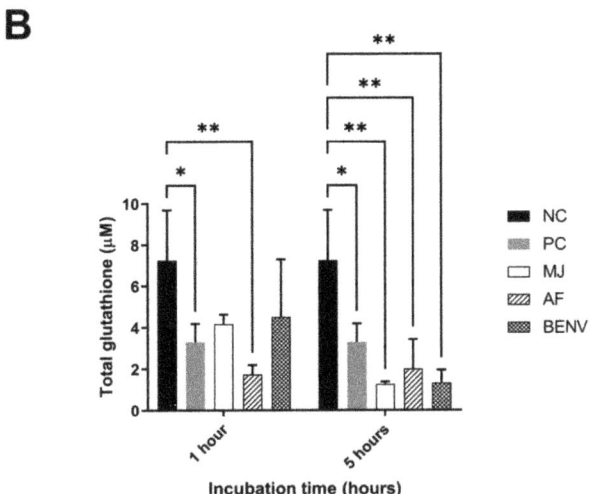

Figure 7. Immunomodulatory effects of anthocyanin-rich extracts. Caco-2 cells were pre-treated with 500 µg/mL extracts as indicated for 1, 5, and 8 h, followed by incubation with 2 mM of H_2O_2 for 6 h. The IL-8 released into the supernatant (**A**) or total GSH production in treated Caco-2 cells (**B**) were analyzed. MJ: minced juice; AF: apoplastic fluid, BENV: blueberry-derived EVs; NC: at the end of the 14-h experiment, the supernatant of the control wells containing cell culture medium/PBS without the treatment of fruit extract nor H_2O_2 was collected and used for the determination of basal IL-8. For the determination of basal level of GSH, the cells treated with medium/PBS only were collected by the scraping method (Section 2.14); and PC: cells treated with H_2O_2 only as a positive control. Data shown as means ± S.D., n = 3. (*, $p < 0.05$ and **, $p < 0.01$).

Total glutathione (GSH) is an important indicator of the intrinsic cellular antioxidant response and thus we studied the GSH level to explore the biochemical mechanism underlying the antioxidant effects of BENVs. As shown in Figure 7B, treatment of Caco-2 cells with MJ and BENVs resulted in an elevation of the total GSH after 1 h of preincubation, of approximately 57.5% and 61.6%, respectively, in comparison with that in the control Caco-2 cells. On the other hand, treatment with AF retained a low total GSH level (23.7%) under oxidative stress, which was even lower than that in the positive control cells (54.8%) (Figure 7B). However, pre-treatment of Caco-2 cells by incubating with BENVs or blueberry extracts (i.e., MJ and AF) for 5 h was unable to provoke anti-oxidative activity, evident from the low GSH level. The percentages of recovery of total glutathione of MJ, AF, and BENVs after 5 h of preincubation were 17.1%, 27.4%, and 17.8%, respectively. The low level of GSH in Caco-2 cells after 5 h incubation with anthocyanin-rich extracts compared to that after 1-h incubation could be attributed to the degradation of anthocyanins in culture medium. In addition, although 5-h incubation of anthocyanin-rich extracts such as AF and BENVs could suppress H_2O_2-induced oxidative stress, total GSH remained at a low level, indicating that anthocyanin contents in anthocyanin-rich extracts might modulate inflammatory processes at the cytokine level but not at the enzymatic level. It also remains possible that the immunomodulatory effects derive from the combined effects of different constituents that are co-extracted with anthocyanins.

4. Discussion

Currently, the conventional approach for extracting AF from seeds or leaves employs the infiltration method. This method has several limitations, such as bulky installation, tissue shearing, contamination, and unknown impacts of filtration buffers on the obtained EV samples [21]. Herein, we proposed a straightforward method to extract AF and designed a laboratory-scale tool to facilitate the extraction process. We have been successful in isolating BENVs from AF, paving the way to collect EVs with minimal destruction of cells, improving the purity of EVs and facilitating downstream applications. The isolated BENVs exhibited small particle size with remarkably high concentrations of plant-based proteins that could facilitate a plant-based oral drug delivery system [39,40].

The discovery of biomarkers for plant-derived EVs constitutes one of the bottlenecks in plant EV research. Our immunoblotting assays revealed the presence of PR proteins in all EV samples (Figure 2), implying that PR proteins could be sorted into EV membranes and fused to the plasma membrane. To test our hypothesis, we investigated the linkage between PR proteins and the EV's trafficking pathways. In plants, EVs are formed from the TGN (also known as early endosomes), where sorting occurs to release, recycle, and transport the vacuolar membrane [73]. The ESCRT-independent pathway has been implicated in the sorting, revealing that the formation of EVs in the multivesicular body (MVB) lumen continues without the presence of all four ESCRT complexes [74]. Here, we employed an indirect approach to study the EV secretion in which the essential membrane trafficking components participating in MBV formation were investigated [1]. In the conventional pathway, MVBs are fused with the tonoplast or engulfed by the tonoplast, and subsequently release their cargo into the vacuole for degradation. In the unconventional pathway, MVBs are fused with the plasma membrane followed by the releasing of EVs. In this context, the plant EV biomarker proteins might be able to guide EVs either to the vacuole or the pathogenic attack sites. Defense-related proteins, which account for a majority of the proteins of the basal apoplastic proteome, are known to play different roles in plant survival [75]. Among defense-related proteins, pathogen-related proteins are most abundant, accounting for approximately 23–33% of such proteins. However, only 10–15% of the pathogen-related proteins are released into apoplastic fluid under biotic stress [76–78]. In susceptible conditions, pathogen-related proteins participate in various defense-related activities, including antifungal [79,80] and cryoprotective functions [81,82]. In healthy plants, pathogen-related proteins are employed to maintain various physiological processes such as material trafficking, flower formation, seed maturation, and ripening [83–87]. It is well-known that PR-3 is involved in the plant defense system alone or in combination with PR-2 [81,88], as well as contributing to growth and developmental processes. Hence, they are present in all organs and plant tissues, including the apoplast and vacuole [88].

Furthermore, class I β-1,3-glucanase and class I chitinase have been shown to be essential determinants for vacuolar sorting machinery [82,89–91]. In addition, pathogen-related proteins are transported from the endoplasmic reticulum (ER) to the vacuole thanks to their special peptide structures [89,90]. Family 19 chitinases (i.e., class I, II, and IV chitinases) possess a peculiar C-terminal extension that is crucial for transport to the vacuole [91]. The C-terminal pro-peptides of vacuolar class I chitinase were able to effortlessly enter the sorting machinery and could be eliminated by endo- or exosome-peptidases [91]. On the other hand, class I β-1,3-glucanases contain both an N-terminal hydrophobic signal peptide and an N-glycosylated C-terminal extension at a single site, facilitating the targeting activity of the protein to the vacuole [82,92]. Therefore, the presence of PR-2 and PR-3 proteins in MVB or its pinching EVs could improve vacuolar targeting. Furthermore, pathogen-related proteins participate in the defense system and plant metabolism [75], in which they guide the released EVs to be fused with the plasma membrane and transported through apoplastic fluid to their destinations. Based on the data presented in Figure 2, we proposed that these pathogen-related proteins are sorted onto the EV surface through the ESCRT-independent pathways. Subsequently, the pathogen-related proteins containing EVs either follow the fusion of MVBs to the plasma membrane and are transported to pathogenic sites/neighboring plant cells through the apoplastic pathway or are guided to vacuoles for degradation.

Although EV-based drug delivery possesses various attractive characteristics as cancer therapeutics, two challenges remain in the clinical approach, including low yield and labor-intensive preparation procedures to produce targeted EVs [54]. Until now, there has been only one study that fabricated arrow-tail pRNA-3 WJ and folic acid onto plant-derived EV surfaces for targeted delivery to the tumor site [93]. Herein, we introduce an aptamer design that is straightforward and suitable for large-scale production. Moreover, the characterization of the binding assay was facilitated by the FP technique, which greatly enhances the effectiveness of the procedure. The FP assay showed a significant increase in the FP value in the presence of BENVs, indicating strong binding between the FAM-anti-EpCAM-Chol aptamer and BENVs (Figure 3). To the best of our knowledge, this is the first time that an FP assay has been applied to demonstrate the binding between aptamers and plant-derived EVs, paving the way for investigating the surface engineering of plant-derived EVs, especially when biomarkers of plant-derived EVs remain scant. As the use of plant-derived EVs is still in its infancy, the surface functionalized aptamers would play dual functions: not only targeting cancer cells but also tracking plant-derived EVs along with lipophilic dyes.

It has been shown that there are at least four different transport mechanisms underlying the uptake and transportation of macromolecules through the epithelial monolayer, including paracellular transport, passive diffusion, vesicle-mediated transcytosis, and carrier-mediated uptake and diffusion [94]. Vashisht et al. visualized the uptake of curcumin-loaded milk-derived EVs in Caco-2 cells using fluorescence microscopy, demonstrating the accumulation of curcumin-loaded milk-derived EVs in the cytosol [95]. Interestingly, we found that BENVs tend to accumulate in the cytoplasm of Caco-2 cells, suggesting that BENVs were taken up by Caco-2 cells via receptor-mediated internalization [56]. Additionally, BENVs are specifically distributed in the nuclear region of HT-29 cells. Therefore, we propose that BENVs might be able to selectively distribute to different subcellular locations depending on the cell type. Previous studies proposed several mechanisms for EV uptake. Tian et al. indicated that actin is involved in EV endocytosis [96]. Actin polymerization participates in various endocytosis pathways including phagocytosis, macropinocytosis, clathrin-mediated endocytosis (CME), clathrin-independent carrier/GPI-anchored protein enriched endosomal compartment (CLIC/GEEC) endocytosis, fast endophilin-mediated endocytosis (FEME) and interleukin-2 receptor (IL2R) endocytosis [96,97]. The latest studies added two endocytic pathways into the system, namely fast endophilin-mediated endocytosis (FEME, a clathrin-independent but dynamin-dependent pathway for rapid ligand-driven endocytosis of specific membrane proteins) and caveolar endocytosis [98].

However, additional experiments are required to demonstrate the uptake mechanisms and endocytosis pathways. The enterocytes account for 90–95% of cell lining in the GIT [99]. The enterocyte barrier-forming Caco-2 cells could facilitate the investigation of BENV absorption through the intestinal wall, and subsequently evaluate the capability of BENVs to enter the systemic circulation and travel to the targeted cancer site. Our results showed that CUR-loaded BENVs could pass through the epithelial monolayer after 1 h without causing disruption to the membrane, demonstrating the potential of BENVs as a promising next generation oral drug delivery system. The potential application of BENVs as nanocarriers to deliver therapeutic substances was further evaluated based on their stability, encapsulation efficiency, and cytotoxicity. One of the prerequisites for BENVs to serve as a nanocarriers for oral DDS is the ability to withstand the harsh environment of orally administered drugs in the GIT. As shown in Figure S7, the isolated BENVs were highly stable in the simulated gastrointestinal tract and displayed a zeta potential value similar to those of previous studies [24,100]. Our BENVs are likely to maintain their particle size despite the change in surface charge, as indicated through experiments performed in simulated gastric solution, simulated intestinal solution, and PBS solution (Figure S7).

The BENVs exhibited high encapsulation efficiency when the conventional incubation method was used, with values of approximately 36.79% and 82.76% for aspirin and curcumin, respectively. In contrast, recent research has reported that the highest encapsulation efficiency for drug-loaded EVs is 18%, depending on specific drugs as well as the sources of EVs [30,60,61]. Notably, 10^{11} BENV particles can load up to 120 µM of curcumin and 100 µM of aspirin, considerably higher than that achieved with other EV-based drug carriers. For instance, Haney et al. reported that only 0.027 µM of paclitaxel and 0.025 µM of doxorubicin were loaded into 10^{11} macrophage-derived EVs [61]. Intriguingly, curcumin-loaded BENVs had relatively higher encapsulation efficiency than that of currently used curcumin-loaded liposomes, with only 5 min of incubation [101,102]. When inserted into the lipid bilayer, curcumin stays in the lipid tail region, also called the glycerol region, which is near the interface of the lipid head and lipid tail, [103]. Ileri Ercan et al. investigated the distribution of curcumin at different C/L ratios [65]. Curcumin is normally located within the glycerol group at lower C/L; however, an increase in C/L causes the relocation of curcumin towards the headgroup of the lipids [65]. Furthermore, the adjustment of the density distribution in the presence of a higher concentration of CUR likely initiates an energy barrier, which facilitates the penetration of molecules through the bilayers [65]. A previous study showed that 95% of curcumin remained intact in the CUR-DMPC liposome complex after 2 days at pH 6, implying that curcumin is stable in the lipid bilayer [104]. Nevertheless, the loading capacity and encapsulation efficiency are also influenced by the lipophilic characteristics of the drug and concentration gradient [105,106], which require further experiments to optimize. Previous studies showed that the maximum solubility of aspirin in saturated lipid bilayers was 50 mol% aspirin, in which each lipid molecule "hosts" one aspirin molecule to form a non-physiological 2D crystal-like state. Hence, in this study we started with a low dose of aspirin which was 100 µM of aspirin per 10^{11} BENV particles to preserve the lipid bilayer membrane. On the other hand, the mechanism underlying the interaction between curcumin and the BENV lipid bilayer membrane is likely to be similar to that of cholesterol, in which a lower curcumin concentration (<1%) significantly remodels the overall order of the membrane, while a higher curcumin concentration (>1%) induces a decline in the ordering of the glycerol region, followed by the formation of acyl chains [104].

We observed that 7.1% and 14.3% of encapsulated curcumin was released in the pH 6.8 buffer after 19 h for BENV-CUR 15 and BENV-CUR 30, respectively (Figure 6B). A longer incubation time apparently promoted a higher amount of curcumin release, possibly because the high concentration of curcumin caused high disorder in the lipid bilayer over time. Additionally, the increase in curcumin concentration also improved its mobility within the bilayer and created an energy barrier, allowing curcumin molecules to be exposed to more water molecules and thus increasing solvation. High loading capacity, in combination with a prolonged release profile, allows BENVs to become an ideal edible plant-based carrier that reduces dosing cycles and minimizes cytotoxicity [107]. Our MTT results suggest that the encapsulation of curcumin considerably shielded BENVs from the cytotoxicity of free curcumin in both Caco-2 and HT-29 cells (Figures 6C,D and S8).

Anthocyanin-rich phenolic compounds have been reported as immunomodulatory agents in the human colon adenocarcinoma cell line Caco-2 [34]. In this study, we investigated the effects of BENVs on H_2O_2-induced oxidative stress, demonstrating its capability to modulate the immune system. Our results revealed that BENVs suppressed more than 94% of IL-8 release, which is associated with the restoration of cell viability after 6 h of treatment. Long-term exposure to ROS could trigger chronic inflammation and cancerous features in Caco-2 cells. Hence, the suppression of IL-8 by BENVs allows Caco-2 cells to recover with minimal aggressive tumor phenotypes. In previous studies, long-term preincubation was deemed to likely degrade phenolic compounds or convert phenolic-rich compounds into less effective metabolites [34]. However, our results showed that BENVs might overcome the instability of phenolic compounds in cell culture media, resulting in higher cell viability and improved IL-8 suppression (Figure 7). Previous studies showed the intake of approximately 50 to 150 g of fresh blueberries, could contribute to the prevention of type 2 diabetes, neurological decline, and cardiovascular disease [108,109]. In our study, 500 μg/mL BENV proteins extracted from approximately 50 g of fresh blueberry were adequate for the inhibition of IL 8 overproduction, implying that the BENVs could preserve the bioactive properties of blueberries. A previous study showed that the amount of anthocyanin extracted from blueberry transported through a Caco-2 cell monolayer was minimal, approximately 3–4% for averaged transport efficiency [72]. Among them, delphinidin glucoside (Dp-glc) had the lowest transportation/absorption efficiency (<1%), whereas malvidin glucoside (Mv-glc) had the highest. This might explain the greater immunomodulatory effects of AF and BENVs in comparison with MJ, as the malvidin groups were significantly elevated in the obtained AF and BENV, resulting in better transportation and absorption. Although MJ contained a very high amount of peonidin, which would help it absorb through the Caco-2 layer, the anthocyanins extracted from blueberry were drastically degraded in cell culture media (approximately 60% retained in the first hour) [72]. This finding implies that BENVs shelter anthocyanin compounds from degradation, providing long-term proinflammatory effects that none of the current anthocyanin-rich extracts can achieve.

5. Conclusions

In this study, we designed an in-tube 3D filter-based approach to extract apoplastic fluid from succulent fruits, using blueberry as a model of edible fruits. This extraction approach is simple, straightforward, and requires no specialized technical skills. Our results demonstrated that apoplastic fluid is successfully extracted from blueberry and the obtained blueberry-derived extracellular nanovesicles contained a significantly higher amount of total proteins in comparison with that in current extracellular nanovesicles extracted from milk and supernatant of mammalian cell culture. Furthermore, plant-based proteins have been shown to assist drug delivery on multiple fronts, enabling future development of BENVs as a novel edible nanocarrier. Additionally, this method preserves the purity of the plant sources and eliminates the interference from extraction buffers or detergents, thus facilitating downstream analysis and applications. Notably, we discovered that pathogen-related proteins (i.e., class I β-1,3-glucanase and class I chitinase) are fused with plant-derived EVs in the transport process, suggesting that these proteins could be used as a potential general biomarker for plant-derived EVs. We show that BENVs possess attractive features of a nanocarrier for drug delivery system, such as incredible stability, low toxicity, low immunogenic effect, high immunomodulatory effect, high cellular uptake, and ability to be transported through the intestinal epithelial barrier. Interestingly, BENVs are able to prolong treatment efficacy by sheltering anthocyanin compounds from degradation caused by culture medium. This characteristic surpasses current anthocyanin-rich extracts.

Future optimization of BENVs is likely to make this edible plant EV a multifunctional nanoplatform for targeted drug delivery in immunomodulatory therapy.

Supplementary Materials: The following supporting information can be downloaded at: https://www.mdpi.com/article/10.3390/pharmaceutics15082115/s1, Figure S1: An illustration of apoplastic fluid extraction method using homemade in-tube filter to prevent disruption of cell membrane. Figure S2: (A) FTIR spectra of apoplastic fluid (AF), minced juices (MJ) collected at 2000× g (MJ 2k) and 10,000× g (MJ 10k), and BENVs collected at 40,000× g (BENV 40k) and 100,000× g (BENV 100k). (B,C) Illustration of selected wavenumber regions for spectral evaluation based on spectroscopic protein-to-lipid ratio (P/L) protocol of Mihaly et al. [29]: (B) Amide group at wavenumber region (1770–1470 cm^{-1}) deconvoluted by curve fitting with Lorentz-function (band denoted by dotted lines), (C) C-H stretching region (3040–2700 cm^{-1}) indicative for lipid components. The FTIR areas represented amide group and lipid group were calculated by a formula followed Mihaly et al. Figure S3: FTIR profiles of functional groups in 15 possible anthocyanin compounds in the study. Figure S4: Topography of BENVs. Figure S5: Schematic of cancer cell targeting with BENV functionalized with EpCAM aptamer (SYL3C). Figure S6: The effect of experimental conditions on the encapsulation efficiency of BENVs with poorly water-soluble aspirin. Figure S7: The in vitro stability of BENVs under physiological mimetic conditions. Figure S8: Cytotoxicity of BENV and curcumin-loaded BENV in HT-29 cells. Figure S9: Effect of H_2O_2 concentration on IL-8 protein secretion in Caco-2 cells. Table S1: Comparison of the protein concentrations in EV samples isolated from different sources. References [29,39,110–113] are cited in the supplementary materials.

Author Contributions: Conceptualization, P.H.-L.T.; methodology, P.H.-L.T., T.N.-G.N., C.V.P. and R.C.; validation, P.H.-L.T. and T.N.-G.N.; investigation, P.H.-L.T. and T.N.-G.N.; resources, P.H.-L.T. and W.D.; data curation, P.H.-L.T. and T.N.-G.N.; formal analysis, C.V.P., S.P., S.K.J., Y.H., H.X. and L.J.; writing—original draft preparation, T.N.-G.N. and P.H.-L.T.; writing—review and editing, T.N.-G.N., P.H.-L.T., R.C., S.P., S.K.J., Y.H., H.X., L.J., A.D. and W.D.; visualization, T.N.-G.N. and C.V.P.; supervision, P.H.-L.T. and W.D.; project administration, P.H.-L.T., T.N.-G.N. and W.D.; funding acquisition, P.H.-L.T. All authors have read and agreed to the published version of the manuscript.

Funding: T.N.-G.N. was supported by a Deakin University Postgraduate Research Scholarship. P.H.-L.T. was supported by a Discovery Early Career Researcher Award from the Australian Research Council.

Institutional Review Board Statement: The use of human cell lines was approved by the Deakin University Human Research Ethics Committee, # 2019-175 (24 July 2019).

Informed Consent Statement: Not applicable.

Data Availability Statement: Data are available upon request.

Acknowledgments: The technical support from the Deakin Medical School is acknowledged.

Conflicts of Interest: The authors declare no conflict of interest.

References

1. Hansen, L.L.; Nielsen, M.E. Plant exosomes: Using an unconventional exit to prevent pathogen entry? *J. Exp. Bot.* **2018**, *69*, 59–68. [CrossRef] [PubMed]
2. Dad, H.A.; Gu, T.-W.; Zhu, A.-Q.; Huang, L.-Q.; Peng, L.-H. Plant exosome-like nanovesicles: Emerging therapeutics and drug delivery nanoplatforms. *Mol. Ther.* **2021**, *29*, 13–31. [CrossRef] [PubMed]
3. Schillaci, O.; Fontana, S.; Monteleone, F.; Taverna, S.; Di Bella, M.A.; Di Vizio, D.; Alessandro, R. Exosomes from metastatic cancer cells transfer amoeboid phenotype to non-metastatic cells and increase endothelial permeability: Their emerging role in tumor heterogeneity. *Sci. Rep.* **2017**, *7*, 4711. [CrossRef] [PubMed]
4. Wang, Q.; Ren, Y.; Mu, J.; Egilmez, N.K.; Zhuang, X.; Deng, Z.; Zhang, L.; Yan, J.; Miller, D.; Zhang, H.-G. Grapefruit-derived nanovectors use an activated leukocyte trafficking pathway to deliver therapeutic agents to inflammatory tumor sites. *Cancer Res.* **2015**, *75*, 2520–2529. [CrossRef] [PubMed]
5. Rutter, B.D.; Innes, R.W. Extracellular vesicles as key mediators of plant–microbe interactions. *Curr. Opin. Plant Biol.* **2018**, *44*, 16–22. [CrossRef]
6. Turhan, E.; Karni, L.; Aktas, H.; Deventurero, G.; Chang, D.; Bar-Tal, A.; Aloni, B. Apoplastic anti-oxidants in pepper (*Capsicum annuum* L.) fruit and their relationship to blossom-end rot. *J. Hortic. Sci. Biotechnol.* **2006**, *81*, 661–667. [CrossRef]
7. Kim, S.G.; Wang, Y.; Lee, K.H.; Park, Z.-Y.; Park, J.; Wu, J.; Kwon, S.J.; Lee, Y.-H.; Agrawal, G.K.; Rakwal, R. In-depth insight into in vivo apoplastic secretome of rice-Magnaporthe oryzae interaction. *J. Proteomics* **2013**, *78*, 58–71. [CrossRef]

8. Witzel, K.; Shahzad, M.; Matros, A.; Mock, H.-P.; Mühling, K.H. Comparative evaluation of extraction methods for apoplastic proteins from maize leaves. *Plant Methods* **2011**, *7*, 48. [CrossRef]
9. Lohaus, G.; Pennewiss, K.; Sattelmacher, B.; Hussmann, M.; Hermann Muehling, K. Is the infiltration-centrifugation technique appropriate for the isolation of apoplastic fluid? A critical evaluation with different plant species. *Physiol. Plant.* **2001**, *111*, 457–465. [CrossRef]
10. Ruan, Y.; Mate, C.; Patrick, J.; Brady, C. Non-destructive collection of apoplast fluid from developing tomato fruit using a pressure dehydration procedure. *Funct. Plant Biol.* **1995**, *22*, 761–769. [CrossRef]
11. Almeida, D.P.; Huber, D.J. Apoplastic pH and inorganic ion levels in tomato fruit: A potential means for regulation of cell wall metabolism during ripening. *Physiol. Plant.* **1999**, *105*, 506–512. [CrossRef]
12. Almeida, D.P.; Huber, D.J. Autolysis of cell walls from polygalacturonase-antisense tomato fruit in simulated apoplastic solutions. *Plant Physiol. Biochem.* **2011**, *49*, 617–622. [CrossRef]
13. Bernstein, L. Method for determining solutes in the cell walls of leaves. *Plant Physiol.* **1971**, *47*, 361–365. [CrossRef] [PubMed]
14. Long, J.M.; Widders, I.E. Quantification of apoplastic potassium content by elution analysis of leaf lamina tissue from pea (*Pisum sativum* L. cv Argenteum). *Plant Physiol.* **1990**, *94*, 1040–1047. [CrossRef] [PubMed]
15. Maksimović, J.J.D.; Živanović, B.D.; Maksimović, V.M.; Mojović, M.D.; Nikolic, M.T.; Vučinić, Ž.B. Filter strip as a method of choice for apoplastic fluid extraction from maize roots. *Plant Sci.* **2014**, *223*, 49–58. [CrossRef]
16. Gupta, R.; Lee, S.E.; Agrawal, G.K.; Rakwal, R.; Park, S.; Wang, Y.; Kim, S.T. Understanding the plant-pathogen interactions in the context of proteomics-generated apoplastic proteins inventory. *Front. Plant Sci.* **2015**, *6*, 352. [CrossRef] [PubMed]
17. Prado, N.; de Dios Alché, J.; Casado-Vela, J.; Mas, S.; Villalba, M.; Rodríguez, R.; Batanero, E. Nanovesicles are secreted during pollen germination and pollen tube growth: A possible role in fertilization. *Mol. Plant* **2014**, *7*, 573–577. [CrossRef] [PubMed]
18. Movahed, N.; Cabanillas, D.G.; Wan, J.; Vali, H.; Laliberté, J.-F.; Zheng, H. Turnip mosaic virus components are released into the extracellular space by vesicles in infected leaves. *Plant Physiol.* **2019**, *180*, 1375–1388. [CrossRef]
19. Rutter, B.D.; Innes, R.W. Extracellular vesicles isolated from the leaf apoplast carry stress-response proteins. *Plant Physiol.* **2017**, *173*, 728–741. [CrossRef]
20. Regente, M.; Pinedo, M.; San Clemente, H.; Balliau, T.; Jamet, E.; De La Canal, L. Plant extracellular vesicles are incorporated by a fungal pathogen and inhibit its growth. *J. Exp. Bot.* **2017**, *68*, 5485–5495. [CrossRef]
21. Pinedo, M.; de la Canal, L.; de Marcos Lousa, C. A call for Rigor and standardization in plant extracellular vesicle research. *J. Extracell. Vesicles* **2021**, *10*, e12048. [CrossRef] [PubMed]
22. Raimondo, S.; Naselli, F.; Fontana, S.; Monteleone, F.; Dico, A.L.; Saieva, L.; Zito, G.; Flugy, A.; Manno, M.; Di Bella, M.A. Citrus limon-derived nanovesicles inhibit cancer cell proliferation and suppress CML xenograft growth by inducing TRAIL-mediated cell death. *Oncotarget* **2015**, *6*, 19514. [CrossRef] [PubMed]
23. Ju, S.; Mu, J.; Dokland, T.; Zhuang, X.; Wang, Q.; Jiang, H.; Xiang, X.; Deng, Z.-B.; Wang, B.; Zhang, L. Grape exosome-like nanoparticles induce intestinal stem cells and protect mice from DSS-induced colitis. *Mol. Ther.* **2013**, *21*, 1345–1357. [CrossRef] [PubMed]
24. Wang, B.; Zhuang, X.; Deng, Z.-B.; Jiang, H.; Mu, J.; Wang, Q.; Xiang, X.; Guo, H.; Zhang, L.; Dryden, G. Targeted drug delivery to intestinal macrophages by bioactive nanovesicles released from grapefruit. *Mol. Ther.* **2014**, *22*, 522–534. [CrossRef] [PubMed]
25. Pocsfalvi, G.; Turiák, L.; Ambrosone, A.; Del Gaudio, P.; Puska, G.; Fiume, I.; Silvestre, T.; Vékey, K. Physiochemical and protein datasets related to citrus juice sac cells-derived nanovesicles and microvesicles. *Data Brief* **2019**, *22*, 251–254. [CrossRef]
26. Oancea, S.; Oprean, L. Anthocyanins, from Biosynthesis in Plants to Human Health Benefits. *Acta Univ. Cinbinesis Ser. E Food Technol.* **2011**, *15*, 3–16.
27. Wada, H.; Shackel, K.A.; Matthews, M.A. Fruit ripening in Vitis vinifera: Apoplastic solute accumulation accounts for pre-veraison turgor loss in berries. *Planta* **2008**, *227*, 1351–1361. [CrossRef]
28. Welbaum, G.E.; Meinzer, F.C. Compartmentation of solutes and water in developing sugarcane stalk tissue. *Plant Physiol.* **1990**, *93*, 1147–1153. [CrossRef]
29. Mihály, J.; Deák, R.; Szigyártó, I.C.; Bóta, A.; Beke-Somfai, T.; Varga, Z. Characterization of extracellular vesicles by IR spectroscopy: Fast and simple classification based on amide and C H stretching vibrations. *Biochim. Biophys. Acta (BBA)-Biomembr.* **2017**, *1859*, 459–466. [CrossRef]
30. Tran, P.H.L.; Wang, T.; Yin, W.; Tran, T.T.D.; Barua, H.T.; Zhang, Y.; Midge, S.B.; Nguyen, T.N.G.; Lee, B.-J.; Duan, W. Development of a nanoamorphous exosomal delivery system as an effective biological platform for improved encapsulation of hydrophobic drugs. *Int. J. Pharm.* **2019**, *566*, 697–707. [CrossRef] [PubMed]
31. Kikuchi, T.; Masuda, K. Class II chitinase accumulated in the bark tissue involves with the cold hardiness of shoot stems in highbush blueberry (*Vaccinium corymbosum* L.). *Sci. Hortic.* **2009**, *120*, 230–236. [CrossRef]
32. Song, Y.; Zhu, Z.; An, Y.; Zhang, W.; Zhang, H.; Liu, D.; Yu, C.; Duan, W.; Yang, C.J. Selection of DNA aptamers against epithelial cell adhesion molecule for cancer cell imaging and circulating tumor cell capture. *Anal. Chem.* **2013**, *85*, 4141–4149. [CrossRef]
33. Nguyen, T.N.-G.; Tran, P.H.-L.; Tran, T.V.; Vo, T.V.; Truong-DinhTran, T. Development of a modified–solid dispersion in an uncommon approach of melting method facilitating properties of a swellable polymer to enhance drug dissolution. *Int. J. Pharm.* **2015**, *484*, 228–234. [CrossRef] [PubMed]
34. Zhang, H.; Liu, R.; Tsao, R. Anthocyanin-rich phenolic extracts of purple root vegetables inhibit pro-inflammatory cytokines induced by H_2O_2 and enhance antioxidant enzyme activities in Caco-2 cells. *J. Funct. Foods* **2016**, *22*, 363–375. [CrossRef]

35. Misra, B.B. The black-box of plant apoplast lipidomes. *Front. Plant Sci.* **2016**, *7*, 323. [CrossRef]
36. Mathieu, M.; Martin-Jaular, L.; Lavieu, G.; Théry, C. Specificities of secretion and uptake of exosomes and other extracellular vesicles for cell-to-cell communication. *Nat. Cell Biol.* **2019**, *21*, 9–17. [CrossRef] [PubMed]
37. Xiao, J.; Feng, S.; Wang, X.; Long, K.; Luo, Y.; Wang, Y.; Ma, J.; Tang, Q.; Jin, L.; Li, X. Identification of exosome-like nanoparticle-derived microRNAs from 11 edible fruits and vegetables. *PeerJ* **2018**, *6*, e5186. [CrossRef] [PubMed]
38. Sharma, A.; Choi, H.-K.; Kim, Y.-K.; Lee, H.-J. Delphinidin and Its Glycosides' War on Cancer: Preclinical Perspectives. *Int. J. Mol. Sci.* **2021**, *22*, 11500. [CrossRef] [PubMed]
39. Munagala, R.; Aqil, F.; Jeyabalan, J.; Gupta, R.C. Bovine milk-derived exosomes for drug delivery. *Cancer Lett.* **2016**, *371*, 48–61. [CrossRef] [PubMed]
40. Jao, D.; Xue, Y.; Medina, J.; Hu, X. Protein-Based Drug-Delivery Materials. *Materials* **2017**, *10*, 517. [CrossRef]
41. Regente, M.; Corti-Monzón, G.; Maldonado, A.M.; Pinedo, M.; Jorrín, J.; de la Canal, L. Vesicular fractions of sunflower apoplastic fluids are associated with potential exosome marker proteins. *FEBS Lett.* **2009**, *583*, 3363–3366. [CrossRef] [PubMed]
42. Regente, M.; Pinedo, M.; Elizalde, M.; de la Canal, L. Apoplastic exosome-like vesicles: A new way of protein secretion in plants? *Plant Signal. Behav.* **2012**, *7*, 544–546. [CrossRef] [PubMed]
43. Cui, Y.; Gao, J.; He, Y.; Jiang, L. Plant extracellular vesicles. *Protoplasma* **2020**, *257*, 3–12. [CrossRef] [PubMed]
44. Zhang, J.; Qiu, Y.; Xu, K. Characterization of GFP-AtPEN1 as a marker protein for extracellular vesicles isolated from *Nicotiana benthamiana* leaves. *Plant Signal. Behav.* **2020**, *15*, 1791519. [CrossRef]
45. Chen, X.; Zhou, Y.; Yu, J. Exosome-like nanoparticles from ginger rhizomes inhibited NLRP3 inflammasome activation. *Mol. Pharm.* **2019**, *16*, 2690–2699. [CrossRef] [PubMed]
46. Lu, Y. Inhibitory Effects of Shiitake-Derived Exosome-like Nanoparticles on NLRP3 Inflammasome Activation. Master's Thesis, University of Nebraska, Lincoln, NB, USA, 2019.
47. Pocsfalvi, G.; Turiák, L.; Ambrosone, A.; Del Gaudio, P.; Puska, G.; Fiume, I.; Silvestre, T.; Vákey, K. Dissection of protein cargo of citrus fruit juice sac cells-derived vesicles reveals heterogeneous transport and extracellular vesicles subpopulations. *bioRxiv* **2018**. [CrossRef]
48. Lado, J.; Rodrigo, M.J.; Zacarías, L. Analysis of ethylene biosynthesis and perception during postharvest cold storage of Marsh and Star Ruby grapefruits. *Food Sci. Technol. Int.* **2015**, *21*, 537–546. [CrossRef] [PubMed]
49. Porat, R.; Lers, A.; Dori, S.; Cohen, L.; Weiss, B.; Daus, A.; Wilson, C.; Droby, S. Induction of chitinase and β-1, 3-endoglucanase proteins by UV irradiation and wounding in grapefruit peel tissue. *Phytoparasitica* **1999**, *27*, 233–238. [CrossRef]
50. Velazhahan, R.; Jayaraj, J.; Liang, G.; Muthukrishnan, S. Partial purification and N-terminal amino acid sequencing of a β-1, 3-glucanase from sorghum leaves. *Biol. Plant.* **2003**, *46*, 29–33. [CrossRef]
51. Krishnaveni, S.; Muthukrishnan, S.; Liang, G.; Wilde, G.; Manickam, A. Induction of chitinases and β-1, 3-glucanases in resistant and susceptible cultivars of sorghum in response to insect attack, fungal infection and wounding. *Plant Sci.* **1999**, *144*, 9–16. [CrossRef]
52. Balasubramanian, V.; Vashisht, D.; Cletus, J.; Sakthivel, N. Plant β-1, 3-glucanases: Their biological functions and transgenic expression against phytopathogenic fungi. *Biotechnol. Lett.* **2012**, *34*, 1983–1990. [CrossRef] [PubMed]
53. Boevink, P.C. Exchanging missives and missiles: The roles of extracellular vesicles in plant–pathogen interactions. *J. Exp. Bot.* **2017**, *68*, 5411. [CrossRef] [PubMed]
54. Wan, Y.; Wang, L.; Zhu, C.; Zheng, Q.; Wang, G.; Tong, J.; Fang, Y.; Xia, Y.; Cheng, G.; He, X. Aptamer-conjugated extracellular nanovesicles for targeted drug delivery. *Cancer Res.* **2018**, *78*, 798–808. [CrossRef] [PubMed]
55. Zhang, Z.; Tang, C.; Zhao, L.; Xu, L.; Zhou, W.; Dong, Z.; Yang, Y.; Xie, Q.; Fang, X. Aptamer-based fluorescence polarization assay for separation-free exosome quantification. *Nanoscale* **2019**, *11*, 10106–10113. [CrossRef] [PubMed]
56. Li, W.; Chen, H.; Yu, M.; Fang, J. Targeted Delivery of Doxorubicin Using a Colorectal Cancer-Specific ssDNA Aptamer. *Anat. Rec.* **2014**, *297*, 2280–2288. [CrossRef]
57. Guardamagna, I.; Lonati, L.; Savio, M.; Stivala, L.A.; Ottolenghi, A.; Baiocco, G. An Integrated Analysis of the Response of Colorectal Adenocarcinoma Caco-2 Cells to X-Ray Exposure. *Front. Oncol.* **2021**, *11*, 688919. [CrossRef]
58. van den Boorn, J.G.; Schlee, M.; Coch, C.; Hartmann, G. SiRNA delivery with exosome nanoparticles. *Nat. Biotechnol.* **2011**, *29*, 325. [CrossRef]
59. Hubatsch, I.; Ragnarsson, E.G.; Artursson, P. Determination of drug permeability and prediction of drug absorption in Caco-2 monolayers. *Nat. Protoc.* **2007**, *2*, 2111–2119. [CrossRef] [PubMed]
60. Aqil, F.; Munagala, R.; Jeyabalan, J.; Agrawal, A.K.; Gupta, R. Exosomes for the enhanced tissue bioavailability and efficacy of curcumin. *AAPS J.* **2017**, *19*, 1691–1702. [CrossRef] [PubMed]
61. Haney, M.J.; Zhao, Y.; Jin, Y.S.; Li, S.M.; Bago, J.R.; Klyachko, N.L.; Kabanov, A.V.; Batrakova, E.V. Macrophage-Derived Extracellular Vesicles as Drug Delivery Systems for Triple Negative Breast Cancer (TNBC) Therapy. *J. Neuroimmune Pharmacol.* **2020**, *15*, 487–500. [CrossRef]
62. Alqahtani, M.S.; Kazi, M.; Alsenaidy, M.A.; Ahmad, M.Z. Advances in Oral Drug Delivery. *Front. Pharmacol.* **2021**, *12*, 618411. [CrossRef] [PubMed]
63. Tu, J.; Shen, Y.; Mahalingam, R.; Jasti, B.; Li, X. *Polymers in Oral Modified Release Systems*; John Wiley & Sons Inc.: Hoboken, NJ, USA, 2010.

64. Wen, H.; Park, K. *Oral Controlled Release Formulation Design and Drug Delivery: Theory to Practice*; John Wiley & Sons: Hoboken, NJ, USA, 2011.
65. Ileri Ercan, N. Understanding Interactions of Curcumin with Lipid Bilayers: A Coarse-Grained Molecular Dynamics Study. *J. Chem. Inf. Model.* **2019**, *59*, 4413–4426. [CrossRef] [PubMed]
66. Cao, J.; Jia, L.; Zhou, H.-M.; Liu, Y.; Zhong, L.-F. Mitochondrial and nuclear DNA damage induced by curcumin in human hepatoma G2 cells. *Toxicol. Sci.* **2006**, *91*, 476–483. [CrossRef] [PubMed]
67. López-Lázaro, M. Anticancer and carcinogenic properties of curcumin: Considerations for its clinical development as a cancer chemopreventive and chemotherapeutic agent. *Mol. Nutr. Food Res.* **2008**, *52*, S103–S127. [CrossRef] [PubMed]
68. Syng-Ai, C.; Kumari, A.L.; Khar, A. Effect of curcumin on normal and tumor cells: Role of glutathione and bcl-2. *Mol. Cancer Ther.* **2004**, *3*, 1101–1108. [CrossRef]
69. López-Lázaro, M.; Willmore, E.; Jobson, A.; Gilroy, K.L.; Curtis, H.; Padget, K.; Austin, C.A. Curcumin induces high levels of topoisomerase I– and II– DNA complexes in K562 leukemia cells. *J. Nat. Prod.* **2007**, *70*, 1884–1888. [CrossRef]
70. Bhattacharyya, A.; Chattopadhyay, R.; Mitra, S.; Crowe, S.E. Oxidative stress: An essential factor in the pathogenesis of gastrointestinal mucosal diseases. *Physiol. Rev.* **2014**, *94*, 329–354. [CrossRef]
71. Cross, C.; Halliwell, B.; Allen, A. Antioxidant protection: A function of tracheobronchial and gastrointestinal mucus. *Lancet* **1984**, *323*, 1328–1330. [CrossRef]
72. Yi, W.; Akoh, C.C.; Fischer, J.; Krewer, G. Absorption of anthocyanins from blueberry extracts by caco-2 human intestinal cell monolayers. *J. Agric. Food Chem.* **2006**, *54*, 5651–5658. [CrossRef]
73. Richter, S.; Kientz, M.; Brumm, S.; Nielsen, M.E.; Park, M.; Gavidia, R.; Krause, C.; Voss, U.; Beckmann, H.; Mayer, U. Delivery of endocytosed proteins to the cell-division plane requires change of pathway from recycling to secretion. *eLife* **2014**, *3*, e02131. [CrossRef]
74. Theos, A.C.; Truschel, S.T.; Tenza, D.; Hurbain, I.; Harper, D.C.; Berson, J.F.; Thomas, P.C.; Raposo, G.; Marks, M.S. A luminal domain-dependent pathway for sorting to intralumenal vesicles of multivesicular endosomes involved in organelle morphogenesis. *Dev. Cell* **2006**, *10*, 343–354. [CrossRef]
75. Delaunois, B.; Jeandet, P.; Clément, C.; Baillieul, F.; Dorey, S.; Cordelier, S. Uncovering plant-pathogen crosstalk through apoplastic proteomic studies. *Front. Plant Sci.* **2014**, *5*, 249. [CrossRef] [PubMed]
76. Cheng, F.-y.; Blackburn, K.; Lin, Y.-m.; Goshe, M.B.; Williamson, J.D. Absolute protein quantification by LC/MSE for global analysis of salicylic acid-induced plant protein secretion responses. *J. Proteome Res.* **2008**, *8*, 82–93. [CrossRef] [PubMed]
77. Kaffarnik, F.A.; Jones, A.M.; Rathjen, J.P.; Peck, S.C. Effector proteins of the bacterial pathogen *Pseudomonas syringae* alter the extracellular proteome of the host plant, *Arabidopsis thaliana*. *Mol. Cell. Proteomics* **2009**, *8*, 145–156. [CrossRef]
78. Zhou, L.; Bokhari, S.A.; Dong, C.-J.; Liu, J.-Y. Comparative proteomics analysis of the root apoplasts of rice seedlings in response to hydrogen peroxide. *PLoS ONE* **2011**, *6*, e16723. [CrossRef]
79. Ebrahim, S.; Usha, K.; Singh, B. Pathogenesis-related (PR)-proteins: Chitinase and β-1, 3-glucanase in defense mechanism against malformation in mango (*Mangifera indica* L.). *Sci. Hortic.* **2011**, *130*, 847–852. [CrossRef]
80. Miles, T.D.; Schilder, A.C. Host defenses associated with fruit infection by Colletotrichum species with an emphasis on anthracnose of blueberries. *Plant Health Progress* **2013**, *14*, 30. [CrossRef]
81. Fernandez-Caballero, C.; Romero, I.; Goni, O.; Escribano, M.I.; Merodio, C.; Sanchez-Ballesta, M.T. Characterization of an antifungal and cryoprotective class I chitinase from table grape berries (*Vitis vinifera* Cv. Cardinal). *J. Agric. Food Chem.* **2009**, *57*, 8893–8900. [CrossRef] [PubMed]
82. Romero, I.; Fernandez-Caballero, C.; Goñi, O.; Escribano, M.I.; Merodio, C.; Sanchez-Ballesta, M.T. Functionality of a class I beta-1, 3-glucanase from skin of table grapes berries. *Plant Sci.* **2008**, *174*, 641–648. [CrossRef]
83. Hamel, F.; Bellemare, G. Characterization of a class I chitinase gene and of wound-inducible, root and flower-specific chitinase expression inBrassica napus. *Biochim. Biophys. Acta (BBA)-Gene Struct. Expr.* **1995**, *1263*, 212–220. [CrossRef]
84. Ding, C.-K.; Wang, C.; Gross, K.C.; Smith, D.L. Jasmonate and salicylate induce the expression of pathogenesis-related-protein genes and increase resistance to chilling injury in tomato fruit. *Planta* **2002**, *214*, 895–901. [CrossRef] [PubMed]
85. Neale, A.D.; Wahleithner, J.A.; Lund, M.; Bonnett, H.T.; Kelly, A.; Meeks-Wagner, D.R.; Peacock, W.J.; Dennis, E.S. Chitinase, beta-1, 3-glucanase, osmotin, and extensin are expressed in tobacco explants during flower formation. *Plant Cell* **1990**, *2*, 673–684. [CrossRef] [PubMed]
86. Robinson, S.P.; Jacobs, A.K.; Dry, I.B. A class IV chitinase is highly expressed in grape berries during ripening. *Plant Physiol.* **1997**, *114*, 771–778. [CrossRef] [PubMed]
87. Wu, C.-T.; Leubner-Metzger, G.; Meins, F., Jr.; Bradford, K.J. Class I β-1, 3-glucanase and chitinase are expressed in the micropylar endosperm of tomato seeds prior to radicle emergence. *Plant Physiol.* **2001**, *126*, 1299–1313. [CrossRef] [PubMed]
88. Kasprzewska, A. Plant chitinases-regulation and function. *Cell. Mol. Biol. Lett.* **2003**, *8*, 809–824. [PubMed]
89. Pereira, C.; Pereira, S.; Pissarra, J. Delivering of proteins to the plant vacuole—An update. *Int. J. Mol. Sci.* **2014**, *15*, 7611–7623. [CrossRef]
90. Isayenkov, S. Plant vacuoles: Physiological roles and mechanisms of vacuolar sorting and vesicular trafficking. *Cytol. Genet.* **2014**, *48*, 127–137. [CrossRef]
91. Stigliano, E.; Di Sansebastiano, G.-P.; Neuhaus, J.-M. Contribution of chitinase A's C-terminal vacuolar sorting determinant to the study of soluble protein compartmentation. *Int. J. Mol. Sci.* **2014**, *15*, 11030–11039. [CrossRef]

92. Meins, F.; Sperisen, C.; Neuhaus, J.-M.; Ryals, J. The primary structure of plant pathogenesis-related glucanohydrolases and their genes. In *Genes Involved in Plant Defense*; Springer: Vienna, Austria, 1992; pp. 245–282.
93. Li, Z.; Wang, H.; Yin, H.; Bennett, C.; Zhang, H.-G.; Guo, P. Arrowtail RNA for Ligand Display on Ginger Exosome-like Nanovesicles to Systemic Deliver siRNA for Cancer Suppression. *Sci. Rep.* **2018**, *8*, 14644. [CrossRef]
94. Lea, T. Caco-2 cell line. In *The Impact of Food Bioactives on Health*; Springer: Cham, Switzerland, 2015; pp. 103–111.
95. Vashisht, M.; Rani, P.; Onteru, S.K.; Singh, D. Curcumin encapsulated in milk exosomes resists human digestion and possesses enhanced intestinal permeability in vitro. *Appl. Biochem. Biotechnol.* **2017**, *183*, 993–1007. [CrossRef]
96. Tian, T.; Wang, Y.; Wang, H.; Zhu, Z.; Xiao, Z. Visualizing of the cellular uptake and intracellular trafficking of exosomes by live-cell microscopy. *J. Cell. Biochem.* **2010**, *111*, 488–496. [CrossRef]
97. Chakrabarti, R.; Lee, M.; Higgs, H.N. Multiple roles for actin in secretory and endocytic pathways. *Curr. Biol.* **2021**, *31*, R603–R618. [CrossRef] [PubMed]
98. Rennick, J.J.; Johnston, A.P.; Parton, R.G. Key principles and methods for studying the endocytosis of biological and nanoparticle therapeutics. *Nat. Nanotechnol.* **2021**, *16*, 266–276. [CrossRef] [PubMed]
99. Hua, S. Advances in Oral Drug Delivery for Regional Targeting in the Gastrointestinal Tract—Influence of Physiological, Pathophysiological and Pharmaceutical Factors. *Front. Pharmacol.* **2020**, *11*, 00524. [CrossRef] [PubMed]
100. Ghiasi, M.R.; Rahimi, E.; Amirkhani, Z.; Salehi, R. Leucine-rich Repeat-containing G-protein Coupled Receptor 5 Gene Overexpression of the Rat Small Intestinal Progenitor Cells in Response to Orally Administered Grape Exosome-like Nanovesicles. *Adv. Biomed. Res.* **2018**, *7*, 125.
101. Chen, Y.; Wu, Q.; Zhang, Z.; Yuan, L.; Liu, X.; Zhou, L. Preparation of curcumin-loaded liposomes and evaluation of their skin permeation and pharmacodynamics. *Molecules* **2012**, *17*, 5972–5987. [CrossRef]
102. Jin, H.-H.; Lu, Q.; Jiang, J.-G. Curcumin liposomes prepared with milk fat globule membrane phospholipids and soybean lecithin. *J. Dairy Sci.* **2016**, *99*, 1780–1790. [CrossRef]
103. Lyu, Y.; Xiang, N.; Mondal, J.; Zhu, X.; Narsimhan, G. Characterization of interactions between curcumin and different types of lipid bilayers by molecular dynamics simulation. *J. Phys. Chem. B* **2018**, *122*, 2341–2354. [CrossRef] [PubMed]
104. Barry, J.; Fritz, M.; Brender, J.R.; Smith, P.E.; Lee, D.-K.; Ramamoorthy, A. Determining the effects of lipophilic drugs on membrane structure by solid-state NMR spectroscopy: The case of the antioxidant curcumin. *J. Am. Chem. Soc.* **2009**, *131*, 4490–4498. [CrossRef]
105. Antimisiaris, S.G.; Mourtas, S.; Marazioti, A. Exosomes and exosome-inspired vesicles for targeted drug delivery. *Pharmaceutics* **2018**, *10*, 218. [CrossRef]
106. Sun, D.; Zhuang, X.; Xiang, X.; Liu, Y.; Zhang, S.; Liu, C.; Barnes, S.; Grizzle, W.; Miller, D.; Zhang, H.-G. A novel nanoparticle drug delivery system: The anti-inflammatory activity of curcumin is enhanced when encapsulated in exosomes. *Mol. Ther.* **2010**, *18*, 1606–1614. [CrossRef] [PubMed]
107. Kalaydina, R.-V.; Bajwa, K.; Qorri, B.; Decarlo, A.; Szewczuk, M.R. Recent advances in "smart" delivery systems for extended drug release in cancer therapy. *Int. J. Nanomed.* **2018**, *13*, 4727. [CrossRef] [PubMed]
108. Kalt, W.; Cassidy, A.; Howard, L.R.; Krikorian, R.; Stull, A.J.; Tremblay, F.; Zamora-Ros, R. Recent Research on the Health Benefits of Blueberries and Their Anthocyanins. *Adv. Nutr.* **2019**, *11*, 224–236. [CrossRef] [PubMed]
109. Curtis, P.J.; van der Velpen, V.; Berends, L.; Jennings, A.; Feelisch, M.; Umpleby, A.M.; Evans, M.; Fernandez, B.O.; Meiss, M.S.; Minnion, M. Blueberries improve biomarkers of cardiometabolic function in participants with metabolic syndrome—Results from a 6-month, double-blind, randomized controlled trial. *Am. J. Clin. Nutr.* **2019**, *109*, 1535–1545. [CrossRef] [PubMed]
110. Lätti, A.K.; Riihinen, K.R.; Kainulainen, P.S. Analysis of anthocyanin variation in wild populations of bilberry (*Vaccinium myrtillus* L.) in Finland. *J. Agric. Food Chem.* **2007**, *56*, 190–196. [CrossRef] [PubMed]
111. Sheng, H.; Hassanali, S.; Nugent, C.; Wen, L.; Hamilton-Williams, E.; Dias, P.; Dai, Y.D. Insulinoma-released exosomes or microparticles are immunostimulatory and can activate autoreactive T cells spontaneously developed in nonobese diabetic mice. *J. Immunol.* **2011**, *187*, 1591–1600. [CrossRef] [PubMed]
112. Estelles, A.; Sperinde, J.; Roulon, T.; Aguilar, B.; Bonner, C.; LePecq, J.B.; Delcayre, A. Exosome nanovesicles displaying G protein-coupled receptors for drug discovery. *Int. J. Nanomed.* **2007**, *2*, 751.
113. Mitchell, J.P.; Court, J.; Mason, M.D.; Tabi, Z.; Clayton, A. Increased exosome production from tumour cell cultures using the Integra CELLine Culture System. *J. Immunol. Methods* **2008**, *335*, 98–105. [CrossRef]

Disclaimer/Publisher's Note: The statements, opinions and data contained in all publications are solely those of the individual author(s) and contributor(s) and not of MDPI and/or the editor(s). MDPI and/or the editor(s) disclaim responsibility for any injury to people or property resulting from any ideas, methods, instructions or products referred to in the content.

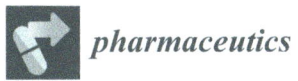

Review

Development of Organs-on-Chips and Their Impact on Precision Medicine and Advanced System Simulation

Ying Luo [1,2,3,†], Xiaoxiao Li [1,2,3,4,†], Yawei Zhao [5,6], Wen Zhong [5], Malcolm Xing [6,*] and Guozhong Lyu [1,2,3,7,*]

1. Burn & Trauma Treatment Center, The Affiliated Hospital of Jiangnan University, Wuxi 214000, China; 7222808005@stu.jiangnan.edu.cn (Y.L.); lxx19971014@163.com (X.L.)
2. Engineering Research Center of the Ministry of Education for Wound Repair Technology, Jiangnan University, Wuxi 214000, China
3. Wuxi School of Medicine, Jiangnan University, Wuxi 214000, China
4. Department of General Surgery, Huai'an 82 Hospital, Huai'an 223003, China
5. Department of Biosystems Engineering, University of Manitoba, Winnipeg, MB R3T 2N2, Canada; zhaoy13@myumanitoba.ca (Y.Z.); wen.zhong@umanitoba.ca (W.Z.)
6. Department of Mechanical Engineering, University of Manitoba, Winnipeg, MB R3T 2N2, Canada
7. National Research Center for Emergency Medicine, Beijing 100000, China
* Correspondence: malcolm.xing@umanitoba.ca (M.X.); luguozhong@jiangnan.edu.cn (G.L.)
† These authors contributed equally to this work.

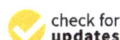

Citation: Luo, Y.; Li, X.; Zhao, Y.; Zhong, W.; Xing, M.; Lyu, G. Development of Organs-on-Chips and Their Impact on Precision Medicine and Advanced System Simulation. *Pharmaceutics* 2023, 15, 2094. https://doi.org/10.3390/pharmaceutics15082094

Academic Editor: Elena Cichero

Received: 4 July 2023
Revised: 28 July 2023
Accepted: 2 August 2023
Published: 7 August 2023

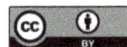

Copyright: © 2023 by the authors. Licensee MDPI, Basel, Switzerland. This article is an open access article distributed under the terms and conditions of the Creative Commons Attribution (CC BY) license (https://creativecommons.org/licenses/by/4.0/).

Abstract: Drugs may undergo costly preclinical studies but still fail to demonstrate their efficacy in clinical trials, which makes it challenging to discover new drugs. Both in vitro and in vivo models are essential for disease research and therapeutic development. However, these models cannot simulate the physiological and pathological environment in the human body, resulting in limited drug detection and inaccurate disease modelling, failing to provide valid guidance for clinical application. Organs-on-chips (OCs) are devices that serve as a micro-physiological system or a tissue-on-a-chip; they provide accurate insights into certain functions and the pathophysiology of organs to precisely predict the safety and efficiency of drugs in the body. OCs are faster, more economical, and more precise. Thus, they are projected to become a crucial addition to, and a long-term replacement for, traditional preclinical cell cultures, animal studies, and even human clinical trials. This paper first outlines the nature of OCs and their significance, and then details their manufacturing-related materials and methodology. It also discusses applications of OCs in drug screening and disease modelling and treatment, and presents the future perspective of OCs.

Keywords: organs-on-chips; drug screening; ADME (absorption, distribution, metabolism, and excretion); maternal–foetal interface; personalised treatment; bone marrow-on-a-chip; AngioChip

1. Introduction

Time and economic challenges limit the use of disease modelling for better treatment. Current animal models allow us to understand pathophysiology and drug screening; however, inconsistencies in findings between animal models and human trials are constantly observed. Many drugs have been screened in vitro and then by using animals; however, when drugs enter the clinical trial stage, they are often suspended due to inadequate efficacy and unexpected side effects [1,2]. Therefore, ideal models and test platforms for better prediction of human responses are urgently required. Current platforms for drug efficacy and toxicity evaluation and disease modelling generally fall into the categories of cell lines, tissue/organ cultures in vitro, organoids, and organs-on-chips (OCs), as shown in Figure 1A. Cell lines are quick and convenient to culture, but cannot mimic numerous phenotypes of cells and tissues in the human body and lack host immunity and tissue- and organ-level responses [3,4]. Although culture methods of in vitro human tissues/organs could produce a highly relevant model for our body system, which is a reasonable approach for various tests, tissue/organs cultured in vitro do not survive well and are expensive; there is also a short supply of their sources. Our body is a combination of complex systems, but human tissues and organs cultured in vitro are independent of those in living organisms. Thus, they cannot be used to study coherent host reaction mechanisms. In addition, large individual differences and poor reproducibility in experimental results limit their in-depth study. Organoids have advanced significantly in recent years. They imitate the growth and interaction of tissues and organs by coculturing various types of cells to form functional tissues with a certain structure, eventually resulting in cellular diversity [5]. Organoids are generalised by the free or well-ordered organisation of cells, and the final formation of the structured tissue is highly correlated to some functions of human organs and tissues [6], but they always neglect the microenvironment, including oxygen gradients and pressure differences, and have insufficient dynamic signals such as those of air flow and blood flow. These signals are crucial for simulating human physiology [7–9].

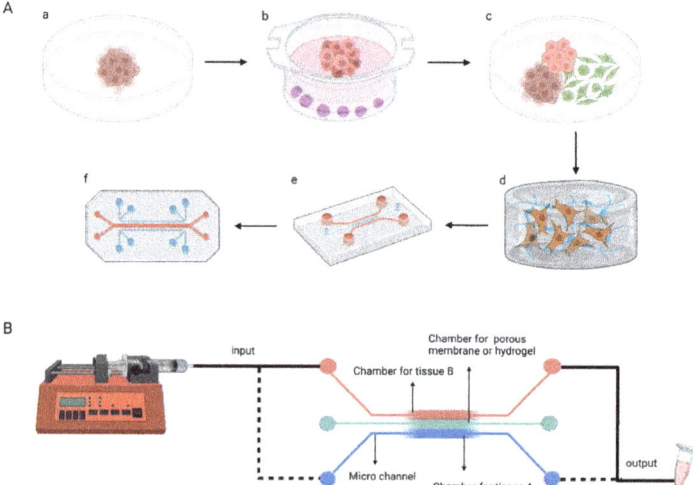

Figure 1. Brief introduction to OCs. (**A**) Drug screening cell models: (**a**) Cells cultured in 2D. (**b,c**) Several types of cells cultured separately and then assembled together. (**d**) Cells cultured in a 3D matrix. (**e,f**) Cells cultured in a microfluid system and distributed by design. (**B**) Primary composition of OCs, including a microfluidic system and cell culture chambers.

OCs, also known as micro physiological systems or tissue chips (Figure 1B), are used to model tissues and organs by simulating physiological and pathological tissue components and arrangement, structural composition, and dynamic components (gas, blood, force, etc.) [2,10]. They employ advanced technologies such as microfabrication, microfluidics, and bioprinting to establish the corresponding structure and dynamic microenvironments on a tiny chip. In addition, OCs can be integrated with a sensor system to achieve continuous and automatic detection of biochemical and physical parameters [2,11,12].

In contrast to the various abovementioned detection and test platforms, OCs have unique properties in terms of tissue arrangement, biomechanical clues, and engineering design. Tissues on an OC platform can be orderly arranged in three dimensions (3D), allowing many types of cells to work together to reflect the physiological balance of cells as well as cells and tissues within a controlled design integration [11]. Specifically, OCs can also include biomechanical clues, such as the tensile and compressive forces of a lung tissue or the haemodynamic shear stress of a vascular tissue. Differences in the simulation of biomechanical forces can cause variations in tissue inflammation and drug absorption [2,13–15]. Creating OCs involves the reverse deduction to human cell system engineering, and the reverse engineering of body tissues and physiological systems is very complex. Consequently, OCs tend to simplify organ complexity by avoiding a comprehensive model. OCs present the main characteristics of human tissues by designing ideal structures; however, these designs can still provide relevant and helpful cues in the formation and development of certain diseases and, thereby, help to treat them [16–19].

This paper first outlines the nature of OCs and their significance. It then discusses their manufacturing-related materials and methodology, and highlights the applications of OCs in drug screening, disease modelling, and treatment. Finally, the future perspective of OCs is presented.

2. Manufacture of OCs

The manufacture of OCs involves a complex process that requires materials that are suitable for microfabrication with essential biocompatibility. When selecting materials for OCs, a confined long-term cell culture microenvironment should be considered, with multiple assays in sequence or synchronisation. Agreeable materials should simulate components to provide a safe and stable framework beneficial to cell growth and migration; they should also enable material exchange and signal communication between cells. These materials are referred to as 'organ materials' or 'chip materials' (Table 1). After the general structure of OCs is created with agreeable materials and advanced technology, the chips are subjected to specific environmental parameters, such as electromechanical stimuli and dynamic microenvironments. This process also can involve biosensing installation. The detecting elements are placed in the OCs, and the transduction components and signal-processing devices are connected to the outside.

2.1. Materials

The materials used in manufacturing and simulating biological components in OCs are referred to as 'organ materials'. They are used mainly in the form of hydrogels and simulate the extracellular matrix of living cells and tissues.

Hydrogels can be of natural, synthetic, or hybrid origin. Natural hydrogels exhibit satisfactory biocompatibility with functional sites for cell adhesion and communication [20,21]. For example, collagen [22] and gelatin exhibit low immunogenicity and extensive structural domains for cell adhesion. They can create a cellular microenvironment similar to tissues [21,23]. As an example, by integrating collagen I hydrogel on polydimethylsiloxane (PDMS) gear, stem cell-derived endothelial cells grow on collagen membrane, and then, with collagenase, morphological changes in membranes and cells with progressive degradation of collagen can be studied [24]. Collagen–elastin (CE) membranes can also be cast onto the surface of PDMS moulds for better culturing of cells, as they have mechanical properties similar to those of in vivo biofilms [25]. Polysaccharides, chitosan, alginate, and hyaluronic acid can be modified in response to light, pH, temperature, and ion concentration. They are commonly used to encapsulate cells and for bioactive factor-controlled releasing [26]. In another study, chitosan was prepared as microspheres loaded with anticancer drugs, and drug release was controlled by two types of cross-linking: tripolyphosphate (TPP) and glutaraldehyde (GTA). Cumulative drug release was greater at lower pH values, demonstrating the pH-responsive nature of chitosan [27]. Alginate is considered an ideal substrate for the in vitro construction of muscle models, which can successfully induce ventricular myocytes and vascular smooth muscle cells to form striated and smooth muscle tissues by specific cues [28]. Natural polymers usually show weak mechanical properties, poorly controlled chemical and physical properties, and fast degradation rates [21,29]. Natural hydrogels can be chemically modified to cross-linkable methacrylate(MA), such as alginate (MAA) [30] and methacryloyl gelatine (GelMA) [31,32]. Synthetic polymers have high reproducibility in synthesis and biological experiments [20,33], such as cell cultures, with stable results [21]. These synthetic hydrogels can be prepared from polyethylene glycol (PEG), polylactic acid (PLA), poly (lactic-co-glycolic acid) (PLGA), polyvinyl alcohol (PVA), polyacrylamide (PAAM), poly (hydroxyethyl methacrylate) (PHEMA), and polyurethane (PU). As a material that mimics natural ECM, researchers have explored the effects of

PAAM's modifiable physical properties on the morphology, skeletal structure, and cell expression of kidney podocytes and have demonstrated them to be suitable for use in building kidney microarray models [34]. However, a significant disadvantage of synthetic polymers is that they lack cell-adhesion ligands and cytocompatibility [20]. Both natural and synthetic materials can be combined and integrated to take advantage of their complementary properties to form a rational design for on-demand physicochemical attributes, such as the combination of poly (ethylene glycol) diacrylate (PEGDA) with GelMA [35] and PEG with fibrinogen [36] for 3D printed scaffolds for cell seeding. Hydrogels can be coated on the surface of a chip channel. PDMS microfluidics have a gel as a cellular adhesive layer material to simulate the tissue environment in channel walls [37–39].

Cells can be of different types, including primary, immortalised, adult stem, embryonic stem cells, and human induced pluripotent stem cells. Among them, primary cells have a cellular phenotype most similar to that of human cells, but they have a limited lifespan and are difficult to obtain and preserve. Phenotypic differences exist between batches of primary cells [40]. Immortalised cells do not suffer from long-term preservation, and phenotypic differences and can be obtained with better reproducibility; however, they undergo genotypic and phenotypic drift modifications, exhibiting different functions from those of the original tissue or organ [41,42]. Stem cells, however, can differentiate into adult cells without phenotypic differences or concerns regarding long-term preservation. One commonly used adult stem cell is the mesenchymal stem cell, which supports differentiation into different types of cells; however, different methods of isolation and culture can likewise lead to phenotypic differences [43]. Embryonic stem cells are suitable for OCs, allowing for unlimited proliferation and differentiation, and are highly relevant to human cells; however, their use is ethically controversial [44]. Currently, human induced pluripotent stem cells are the most commonly used OCs because of their great relevance to humans, and they can be differentiated into human cells without ethical problems [43,45].

Biopsies are also frequently assembled in the design of OCs, and their use brings intercellular integration and overall function of the tissue within the OCs closer to that of living tissue [46,47]. For example, researchers grew mouse colon crypt biopsies on the chip, allowing and designing tissue blocks to proliferate and differentiate within the chip, with the final chip model exhibiting better cellular integration and a specific appearance of the structure [48]. Biopsied human skin tissue was used in a toxicity study in a multi-organs-on-a-chip (MOC) model for drug screening [19]. In addition, in building personalised disease models of patients, many microarray platforms are fitted with the disease site of the patient's biopsy, such as the airway component of a patient with chronic obstructive pulmonary disease (COPD) [49].

However, the effect of cell sex on the results of experiments is often ignored when choosing cell types. Researchers often prefer male cells or tissues because female models are influenced by reproductive hormone levels, which makes results more unpredictable. Moreover, it is usually believed that sex differences have little impact on systems other than the reproductive system and are of little value to study [50]. Nevertheless, an increasing number of studies have revealed sex differences in non-reproductive tissues. For example, the brains of males and females show significant differences in anatomy and physiology, leading to sex differences in neurophysiology and behavior [51]. Males are more biased towards autism spectrum disorders [52], while females are biased towards depression and anxiety disorders [53]. In addition, there are sex-specific differences in the cardiovascular [54] and immune systems [55].

The materials used to create and simulate the non-biological components of OCs can be referred to as "chip materials" or structural materials of the chip, such as microfluidic devices and the barrier membranes between different types of cells. Elastomeric materials, such as PDMS [56–58], poly (octamethylene maleate (anhydride) citrate) (POMaC), thermoplastics, and inorganic materials are commonly used today.

PDMS is economical, low-cytotoxic, and easy to process. PDMS is transparent and, when assembled into a frame structure of an OC, can be viewed directly outside the chip for imaging, which is a major highlight of PDMS materials [59]. However, PDMS also has shortcomings while manufacturing OCs: PDMS is somewhat hydrophobic, preventing some cells from adhering to growth, and adsorbs small hydrophobic molecules, such as some of the drugs tested, which can affect the results of the experiment [60]. The uncross-linked part of the cured PDMS can leach into the solution [61]. PDMS is prone to solution evaporation, which significantly alters the volume, concentration, and equilibrium on a micro-scale, or even forms bubbles that can block gas–liquid flow or damage cells [56,61,62]. In addition to PDMS, another elastomeric material, POMaC, is used in the construction of vascular scaffolds, forming a network structure with many microchannels that mimic the scaffold structure of a blood vessel [63].

Thermoplastics can retain the visibility, biocompatibility, and chemical stability of PDMS materials while overcoming certain disadvantages of PDMS materials [64]. For example, cyclo-olefin polymer (COP) is transparent in the visible and near-UV regions, has low self-fluorescence for visibility, has no effect on hydrophobic drug distribution, and has ultra-low water vapour permeability, which facilitates cell culture while limiting sample evaporation [64,65]. Polymethyl methacrylate (PMMA) is rigid and transparent, and has very low fluorescence intensity, and is commonly used in the construction of OCs [46,66].

Among inorganic materials, glass is commonly used to prepare OCs. Glass is transparent, suitable for real-time imaging, and does not attract hydrophobic molecules [67]. However, owing to its impermeability, glass is unsuitable for cell culture in an enclosed environment [56].

Table 1. Summary of materials used for organs-on-chips.

Classification				Strengths	Weaknesses
Organ material	Hydrogel	Natural [68]	Collagen	Biocompatible [69]; Biodegradable [21]; Low immunogenicity; Extensive cell adhesive domains [21,23]; Suitable for cell growth and migration; Structure similar to ECM [26]	Weak mechanical properties [70]
			Gelatine		
			Chitosan		
			Alginate		
			Hyaluronic acid		
			Fibrin		
		Synthetic [20]	PEG, PLA, PLGA, PVA, PAAM, PHEMA, PU	Controllable mechanical properties; Stable in batch-to-batch; Controllable degradation properties; Chemical modification	Lack of cell adhesion ligands; Inadequate biocompatibility
		Hybrid	PEGDA/GelMA [35]	Appropriate mechanical properties; More bioactive sites	-
			PEG/fibrinogen [36]	PEG was functionalised to promote cell growth	-
	Cells and tissues	Primary cells [40]		The most phenotypically similar to cells in vivo	Extraction difficulty; Inconstant functionality; Short lifespan; Individual difference
		Immortalised cells [41,42]		Infinite survival; Retention of activity; Repeatable	Low phenotypically similar to cells in vivo
		Embryonic stem cells [44]		Pluripotent; Infinitely proliferative	Ethical restrictions
		Adult stem cells [43]		Easy to extract relatively	Limited differentiation ability

Table 1. Cont.

Classification			Strengths	Weaknesses
		Human induced pluripotent stem cells [43,45].	Retained human relevance; Great differentiation potential; Without ethical restrictions	Individual difference; Low reprogramming output; Genomic instability
		Biopsies [46,47]	More accurate information on the tissue [48]; Maintain the natural extracellular matrices and three-dimensional tissue structures [48]	Cannot survive more than 48 h in ex vivo culture mostly
Chip material	Elastomerics	PDMS [56,57]	Economic; Low cytotoxicity; Ease of processing; Transparent [59]	Hydrophobic; High ability to adsorb small hydrophobic molecules [61]; High gas permeability [56,61,62]
		POMaC [63]	Biodegradable; Biocompatible; Desired mechanical properties	
	Thermoplastics	COP, COC, PC, PS, PMMA	Economic; Transparent; Low absorption; Appropriate gas permeability [64,65]; Low auto-fluorescence [46]	
	Inorganic materials	Glass	Transparent; Stable physical and chemical properties [67]	Diseconomy in fabrication; High gas impermeability [56]

Annotations: PEG, polyethylene glycol; PLA, polylactic acid; PLGA, poly (lactic-co-glycolic acid); PVA, polyvinyl alcohol; PAAM, polyacrylamide; PHEMA, poly (hydroxyethyl methacrylate); PU, polyurethane; PEGDA, poly (ethylene glycol) diacrylate; GelMA, gelatine methacryloyl; PDMS, polydimethylsiloxane; POMaC, poly (octamethylene maleate (anhydride) citrate); COP, cyclo-olefin polymers; COC, cyclic olefin copolymer; PC, polycarbonate; PS, polystyrene; PMMA, polymethyl methacrylate.

2.2. Techniques and Environmental Parameters

Microfabrication technology is used in the fabrication of OC hardware templates or ECM scaffolds [71–73], using photolithography [74] and soft lithography technologies. Photolithography technology focuses on the formation of UV-sensitive materials, where the constructed hardware can be directly applied to OCs or used as a master for soft lithography. Soft lithography technology is a technique for infusing materials such as PDMS into a master plate and removing the template after shaping to obtain a soft and flexible microstructure (Figure 2A). Multi-layered soft lithography utilises 3D stamping techniques for the tight assembly of multi-layered structures [71]. 3D printing enables stereoscopic structure efficiently with high fidelity and wide dimensional pattern ranging from micro- to macroscale without templates or masks [75,76]. The cell and tissue components are mainly printed in 3D, using bioprinting technology to create tissue structures [77,78] or using electrospinning technology to first form a cell growth scaffold [79] and then grow the cells to promote cell growth and distribution.

Microfluidics is a core technology in OC fabrication, which controls the flow of fluid in channels of less than 1 mm, allowing for better simulation of the dynamic cellular and tissue environment [80]. In microchannels, the liquid flows directionally and steadily, without turbulence, and can be used to maintain the stability of chemical gradients over long periods of time [81]. Microfluidics is used to control dynamic changes, such as the flow of the culture fluid delivery and the exchange of gases, simulating the dynamic circulatory changes in the human body's ministries [2,26,73,80,82].

Of course, owing to the flexibility of OC research, various technical supports are required for target OCs under different research objectives, such as the establishment of a liver sinusoidal model with the help of bi-directional electrophoresis techniques and the design of electrodes that enable the radiation electric field to form the hepatocytes into a hexagonal arrangement [83] (Figure 2(B1)).

To better simulate the tissues and organs, designers have replicated many environmental parameters of the body in terms of the microenvironment. In terms of structure, specific tissue morphology and function require different ECM structures for maintenance [84], e.g., the survival of hematopoietic stem cells (HSCs) is closely linked to the bone marrow ecological niche [85]. In terms of biochemical stimulation, specific cytokines and chemokines are delivered to tissues and cells to promote cell survival, proliferation, and migration [86], such as the addition of MCP-1 to GelMA to induce monocyte chemotaxis [87]. In tissue homeostasis, microfluidics provides dynamic nutrients and remove metabolic waste to maintain intracellular homeostasis and control the oxygen gradient between different tissues [88,89] (Figure 2(B2)). In terms of mechanical stimulation, electrical stimulation largely affects cellular morphology and activity, and appropriate electrical stimulation can improve synaptic extension in nerve cells [90] and the assembly of specific morphology in muscle cells [91]. Additionally, appropriate mechanical stimulation can similarly affect cellular alignment and growth trends, such as fluid shear stress [92,93] (Figure 2(B3)).

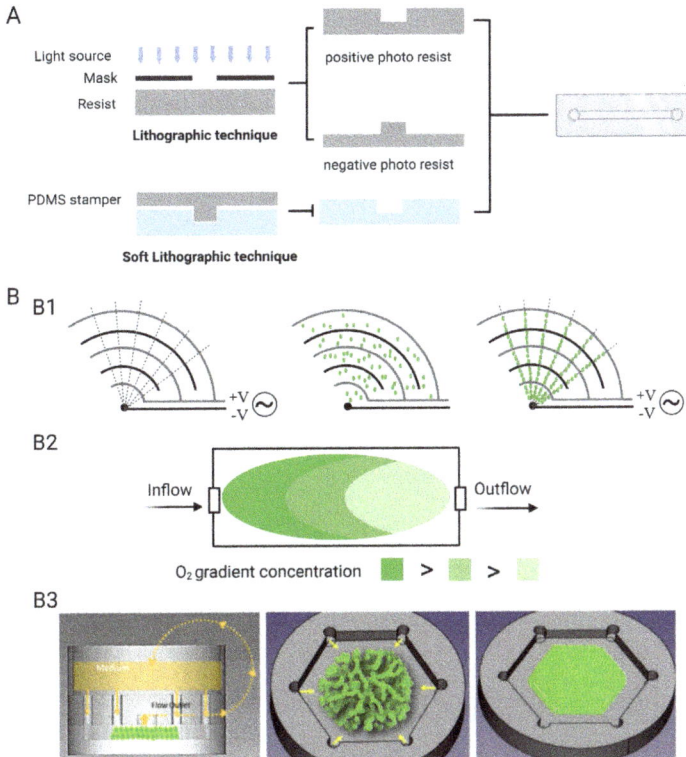

Figure 2. Manufacture of OCs. (**A**) Techniques used in OCs—photolithography technology and soft lithography technology in OCs. (**B**) Environmental parameters influence the tissue formation: (**B1**) The ac DEP voltage distributes liver cells in magnetic direction. (**B2**) Oxygen gradients create tissues with different metabolic levels. (**B3**) Liver cells form hepatic cord along the direction of radial flow. (Reprinted from ref. [93] with permission.)

2.3. Sensors

An important piece of combined equipment for OCs is the sensors. As OCs continue to evolve, developing integrated sensors is vital for monitoring the microenvironment within the chip in real time, continuously and precisely. Sensors can be divided into physical sensors that display pH, temperature, and oxygen, and biosensors that display multiple biomarkers of metabolic processes [94], which can be further divided into optical and electrochemical sensors based on different principles [10].

Optical sensors use light at specific wavelengths to directly detect the absorbance and fluorescence intensity of a substance or indirectly to determine the surface plasmon resonance (SPR) on the probe surface and the binding of the analyte to the probe to determine the analyte concentration [10]. Optical sensors can detect a limited range of substance concentrations; for example, when detecting pH, they require the addition of absorbable phenol red for colour development and, only in the pH range of 6.5–8.0, linearity reflects well and data are accurate [95,96]. However, optical sensors are advantageous in low-oxygen environments because their measurement data are independent of redox reactions [97,98].

Electrochemical sensors are more indirect and flexible, which can be used for more precise quantitative studies. They consist of at least three electrodes for countering, referring, and working. The working electrode has a conductive gel or noble metal containing the reactant (oxidase) attached to it, which reacts with the analyte to produce an exchange of anions and cations. Then, the analyte concentration is calculated by detecting the amperage, potential, and resistance between the working and counter electrodes [10,96]. Electrochemical sensors are designed to be more flexible and to facilitate real-time continuous monitoring [99,100]. Some researchers have used conductive PEDOT:PSS hydrogels wrapped with glucose oxidase (Gox) to prepare working electrodes to create miniature, non-invasive, portable glucose sensors [101]. Researchers have also developed an intestinal barrier chip model to measure transcutaneous resistance within transwell chambers to assess barrier integrity [102,103].

Finally, the construction of an ideal sensor should rely on a combination of optical and electrochemical sensors on demand. In a MOC model, researchers designed an automated monitoring platform with physical sensors and electrochemical biosensors connected in microfluidic channels to reflect micro-environmental parameters (potential of hydrogen, oxygen, and temperature) and biomarkers within the model, respectively. The entire device was placed directly under a microscope to observe the internal morphology of the MOC. MOC also enables in situ and real-time monitoring of the microenvironment, biological components, drug screening, and internal morphology [95].

2.4. Cell Culture Medium

When a single OC, involving only a single cell type, is generated, a culture medium initially formulated for conventional cultures can be used. However, when generating single/multiple OCs involving multiple cell types, the choice of medium becomes more complex because each cell type has specific nutrients and growth factors to sustain growth and function [104]. Therefore, one of the most critical challenges for multi-organ chips is to be able to provide different tissues on the system with a blood-like universal medium to meet the nutritional needs of different cells. So far, there are two ways to solve this problem. One is to improve the properties of the culture medium to expand its application range, and the other way is to utilize the endothelial cell barrier for nutrient separation [16]. For instance, in the connected liver–kidney system, mixing liver-specific medium and kidney-specific medium in a 1:1 manner can come close to meeting the growth needs of both types of cells [105]. In addition, there are multicellular chips that simulate adipose tissue [106] and a multi-organ chip model of liver–fat–skin–lung interaction [107]. However, with an increasing number of organ types in the system, this multiple-mixing approach may result in a less effective medium, as each organ or tissue ends up with a sub-optimal medium, which can greatly affect the functionality and physiological relevance of the system. The connected system can be designed as a single channel or recirculation system, so that the medium can be replenished or replaced at any time, and the barrier formed by the vascular endothelium can also be utilized on the chip platform to segregate the different types of cells, so that they can be cultured with their own optimal medium.

3. Applications

OCs are popular and widely used, including applications in drug absorption, distribution, metabolism, and excretion; in modelling diseases; in building medical resources; and in individualised drug administration. The following is a brief description of the design of OCs for use in these areas.

3.1. Drug Screening

Applications of the intestinal barrier chip model, liver sinusoidal chip model, blood–brain barrier chip model, maternal–foetal barrier chip model, skin-on-a-chip model, and ADME MOC model for drug detection are introduced. The diagrammatic sketch for barriers is shown in Figure 3A.

3.1.1. Intestinal Barrier Chip Model

The intestinal barrier is an important barrier to the absorption of most orally administered drugs, and numerous localised chip models of the intestine have been designed to explore the direction of model design at the end-organ level, such as the colonic crypts-on-a-chip model [48] (Figure 3(B1)). Primary crypts isolated from mice were mixed and cultured in 2D and 3D patterns on a microstructure consisting of PDMS micropores and matrix gel micro pockets to produce continuous millimetre-scale colonic epithelial tissue. This is an effective exploration of the colon-on-a-chip model. It is novel and ingenious to choose targeted tissues and combine 2D and 3D culture methods to better simulate the tissue composition and structure of the crypt.

In contrast, the design of the intestinal barrier-on-a-chip model selected several major cells and chose a Transwell model for its structure (Figure 3(B2)). Caco2-BBE cells and HT29-MTX cells were cultured at a ratio of 9:1 in a mixture of 0.4 µm Transwell chambers to form an intestinal monolayer epithelium, and the basal side of the Transwell was planted with dendritic cells, forming the basic intestinal barrier model [103]. The use of the Transwell chamber was impressive, as it can be used to study cell migration and can also be applied to research the absorption and passage of drugs microscopically; it is the perfect hardware for the intestinal barrier model. In addition, researchers have addressed the problem of quantifying barrier function by measuring the transepithelial electrical resistance (TEER) in the intestinal epithelium. Dendritic cells and HT29-MTX cells respond to exposure to drug components or inflammatory mediators in the culture medium, increasing transmembrane resistance. The absorption of drug breakdown products or the secretion of mucin into vesicles increases transmembrane electrical resistance. The higher the transmembrane resistance, the better the barrier function [16]. Researchers also modified the human Caco2 intestine chip by integrating a micro-oxygen sensor into an in situ oxygen measurement device and placing the chip in an engineered anaerobic chamber to create a physiologically relevant oxygen gradient between the human intestinal epithelium and microvascular endothelial cells, which are cultured in parallel channels separated by a porous matrix-coated membrane within the device. Modified intestinal chip allows stable co-culture of highly complex anaerobic and aerobic intestinal bacterial communities in the same channel as mucus-producing human villous intestinal epithelium, while simultaneously monitoring oxygen levels and intestinal barrier function for at least 5 days in vitro [108].

3.1.2. Blood–Brain Barrier Chip Model

Another barrier to drug delivery is the blood–brain barrier (BBB), which is an important threat to the healing efficacy of nervous system drugs. The BBB is the boundary between the central nervous system and circulatory system that controls transportation between the blood and the brain, limiting the penetration of drugs. It consists mainly of the outer vascular endothelium, middle pericytes, and inner network of astrocytes. The ends of these astrocytes cross pericytes to come into contact with the vasculature and control the inflow of water through aqueous channel 4 (AQP4) [109,110].

Based on this structural basis, researchers produced a simplified BBB-on-a-chip model [111]. The basic structure of the micro-platform was built using PDMS and consisted of an upper layer, polycarbonate porous membrane, lower layer, and a slide (Figure 3C). The upper layer was seeded with 2D human brain microvascular endothelial cells (HB-MECs), and the lower layer was placed with a network of pericytes and 3D astrocytes, between which a porous membrane was placed, significantly reducing the distance between them [18]. Primary cells were selected so that the final microarray replicated the specific markers, membrane transporters, and receptors associated with the BBB to a greater extent.

One of the main mechanisms by which natural HDL is known to pass through the BBB is class B scavenger receptor 1 (SR-B1) [112,113]. Researchers designed mimetic HDL nanoparticles with apolipoprotein A1 (eHNP-A1) and validated this mechanism using a BBB microarray model [18]. The nanoparticle solution was added to the upper medium and compared before and after blocking the SR-B1 channels. The amount of eHNP-A1 in the upper layer, that is, the vascular channel, increased significantly after blocking the SR-B1 channel, whereas there was no significant increase in eHNP-A1 across the semi-permeable membrane nor upon reaching the lower layer, that is, the microenvironmental layer in the brain. In addition, the researchers captured the location of eHNP-A1, demonstrated the distribution of 3D nanoparticles in the microarray model, and elaborated on the different cellular uptakes and receptor-mediated cytokinesis in this model (Figure 3C). The mechanism of HDL penetration of the barrier and the usability of the BBB-on-a-chip model validate each other.

3.1.3. Maternal–Foetal Barrier Chip Model

The placental barrier is also known as the interface between the mother and foetus. This barrier consists of an external trophoblastic layer and an internal foetal endothelial layer. This barrier counts the circulation and communication between the mother and the foetus. The placental barrier-on-a-chip model has provided an excellent tool for studies related to drug and toxicity delivery between the mother and foetus; however, it surpasses this to include breakthroughs in preterm birth induction, hormonal regulation, and maternal–foetal communication. The toxic effects of drugs on the foetus are a major concern when medically administering drugs to pregnant women; however, many in vitro 2D and 3D assay platforms limitedly represent the complex conditions between mother and foetus, and the animal models differ significantly from humans in terms of gestational physiological structure and uterine environment. An excellent placental barrier-on-a-chip model should be created and should be taken a step further for researching the purposeful delivery of drugs from the mother to the foetus.

Researchers used PDMS material to create two microchannels separated by a porous polycarbonate membrane seeded with trophoblastic epithelial cells (BeWo epithelial layer) and foetal vascular endothelial cells (HUVEC layer) to mimic the maternal and foetal environments on either side of the barrier [17,114] (Figure 3D). The researchers verified the gestational deep vein. The inability of heparin, a therapeutic agent for thrombosis and embolism, to penetrate the placental barrier-on-a-chip model is consistent with previous findings. In addition, researchers tested the delivery of glibenclamide, a drug commonly used in gestational diabetes, in this model. The placental barrier microarray model demonstrated the inability of glibenclamide to enter the foetal side under the protection of breast cancer resistance protein (BCRP). Conversely, massive glibenclamide enters the foetal side under the action of BCRP inhibitors [114], validating the physiological protection of BCRP on the foetus. This shows that the placental barrier-on-a-chip model can reconstitute the transport function of the placental barrier and has great potential as a drug screening platform [115].

The above mentioned is a simpler model of the placental barrier, which lacks many important components to reconstruct the maternal–foetal interface [116], such as the lack of many important cellular components, e.g., amnion mesenchymal cells(AMCs) and chorion trophoblast cells(CMCs/CTs) [117]. There are two more well-established placental barrier chip models: one consisting of four parallel chambers culturing amnion epithelial cells (AECs), trophoblast cells, metaphase, and bacteria [118], and the other consisting of four concentric circular channels containing primary AECs, AMCs, CMCs/CTs, and metaphase cells [117]; the latter is superior, in that the four chambers are connected by fine ducts filled with extracellular matrix, which is more realistic than a simple PET membrane (Figure 3D). These designs are more similar in structure and composition to the placental barrier, and, with such models as a cornerstone, future studies on bacterial infections, drug therapy, etc., will be more accessible.

3.1.4. Skin-on-a-Chip Model

The skin barrier is an obstacle that must be examined for all transdermal drugs, such as creams, ointments, solutions, and skin patches, commonly in the form of antibiotic cream for the skin, proprietary Chinese medicine suspensions [119], and pain relief patches for the nervous system [120]. Transdermal drug delivery has many advantages over traditional routes of administration, such as non-invasive administration and avoidance of the first-pass effect of the drug on the digestive system. The drug can act locally or systemically without significant side effects and has a higher safety profile. Animal models are often used in drug experiments to study transdermal drug delivery, but the species variability between animals and humans makes the results lack validity. With increasing restrictions on the use of animals in various countries, we advocate non-animal research methods. The use of skin equivalents is increasingly required for studies of drug penetration, skin irritation, and skin phototoxicity.

Researchers have developed a skin-on-a-chip model that mimics the structure of a Franz-diffusion cell by growing human keratin-forming cells (HaCaT) on a modified electrostatic spun membrane in the middle. The upper layer holds the sample fluid, and the lower layer is filled with type I collagen and connected to a microfluidic channel for easy extraction of the culture fluid and measurement of drug concentration. The lower layer can be removed for tissue staining. This model has been used to study the transdermal transport of caffeine. The maximum concentration of caffeine in the collected cultures was reached at the fifth hour, showing transport kinetics similar to those of human skin samples [121] (Figure 3E). In a full-thickness skin-on-a-chip model, a fibrin-based dermal matrix was used to construct a dermal scaffold and fill the upper surface and interior with keratin-forming cells and fibroblasts, respectively, resulting in a simple full-skin equivalent, which was also shown to be well structured by tissue staining [122] (Figure 3E). Biopsied skin tissue has also been used to replace monolayers of keratin-forming cells [123,124], to establish better models of full-thickness skin-on-a-chip. Other researchers have applied periodic mechanical stimulation to the skin based on a full-thickness skin-on-a-chip model to simulate circadian rhythms, resulting in an aging skin model that can be used for drug development and disease modelling in aging skin [125]. In addition, the subcutaneous vascular component was considered, and skin microarray models containing different vascular channels were created to detect vasodilatation and immune responses to skin stimulation [126,127]. These models are simple and convenient, but they contain only a small number of types of skin cells and lack some important skin accessories, such as nerves and hair follicles, where the hair follicle structure also has an impact on the absorption behaviour of the drug. There are aspects that have not yet been integrated into the skin-on-a-chip model, which is an area where breakthroughs are needed [128].

3.1.5. Liver Sinusoidal Chip Model

The liver is an important site for drug metabolism, and hepatotoxicity is an unavoidable safety indicator in the drug screening process. The liver is the main organ for testing the effectiveness and safety of drugs. The basic liver functional unit is the hepatic sinusoid between the hepatic portal and central vein, consisting of an inner layer of porous endothelial cells, middle layer of hepatic stellate cells, and outer layer of hepatic parenchymal cells. Kupffer cells are also present inside the sinusoid, mediating communication and immune responses [88]. In particular, the partial pressure of oxygen in the hepatic sinusoids gradually decreases during the flow of blood from the periportal to the central vein to regulate the compartment and function of the liver [129].

Accordingly, researchers designed and improved the hepatic sinusoidal-on-a-chip model using glass material instead of PDMS material to create a hollow channel structure that avoids the hydrophobic and oxygen-permeable nature of PDMS. Primary LSECs and stellate cells are grown in the lower layer to form the vascular channels and intrahepatic environment, and primary human hepatocytes and collagen layers are grown in the upper layer, distributing the Kupffer cells within the lower two layers. Primary cells were selected so that the final model contained many specific proteins. In addition, researchers formed different oxygen partitions (oxygen-rich, intermediate, and oxygen-poor) by regulating the flow within the liver and vascular channels through engineering modelling and verified the oxygen partitioning by imaging the ratio of oxygen-sensitive and -insensitive fluorescent beads to form different metabolic gradients [16,88,89] (Figure 3F). The model validity was verified by a bile efflux test and an endothelial cell penetration test, using various imaging modalities. This model was also compared to a PDMS liver sinusoidal-on-a-chip model [130], in which three drugs (Nefazodone, Terfenadine and Acetaminophen) were dissolved and diluted into the vascular channels of the chip, and the effluent was collected daily to determine the remaining drug concentration and calculate the recovery rate. The recovery of acetaminophen, a hydrophilic drug, was 100% in both devices, whereas the recovery of Nefazodone and Terfenadine, hydrophobic drugs, was much greater in the glass device than in the PDMS device. All recoveries were 100% after the addition of drug-loaded LDL. These data demonstrate the drawback of the PDMS material in the fabrication of a chip device, namely, its ability to adsorb hydrophobic molecules [2].

3.1.6. An ADME MOC Model

The MOC model, which is formed by multiple OC, is a more suitable approach for drug development, where drugs undergo absorption, distribution, metabolism, and excretion (ADME) processes in vivo, mainly involving the intestine, liver, kidneys, and organs of action of the target drug, such as the skin, brain, and even bone marrow [16,131–135].

Researchers designed an ADME-on-a-chip model by integrating the gut, liver, kidney, and skin using PDMS and PET membranes to prepare a bilayer of interconnected chambers, with the upper layer serving as the blood circuit and the lower layer as the excretory circuit, with the two layers connected by a proximal tubular culture chamber in the middle of the kidney (Figure 3G). The blood circuit includes an intestinal barrier culture chamber consisting of intestinal epithelium, a liver equivalents culture chamber consisting of liver parenchymal cells and stellate cells, and a skin culture chamber for biopsies and connected microchannels. The excretory circuit consists of a proximal tubular culture chamber and microchannels in the kidney [16,19]. This continuous MOC model was tested for LDH and glucose distribution, and there was a corresponding gap in LDH activity extracted in the different chambers, further suggesting that the four barriers play their respective roles in the passage of LDH [19]. The MOC model can be flexibly designed and adapted for the purpose of the study; for example, heart–liver–lung chip models to study drug effects on each organ [136], liver–kidney chip models, and liver–skin chip models to study drug toxicity [135,137–139].

With the need for constant sampling and testing during experiments, the establishment of a long-term, real-time, continuous testing system is unavoidable. A sensor system for in situ continuous monitoring has been established [95], which is a significant advancement in the development of MOC. MOCs are a flexible and beneficial tool in the drug development process, but their design flexibility also leads to a lack of widely accepted standards for the test tool, which is partly responsible for its limited popularity. Another challenge is the limited survival time of MOCs, which is difficult to match with the time required for drug ADME.

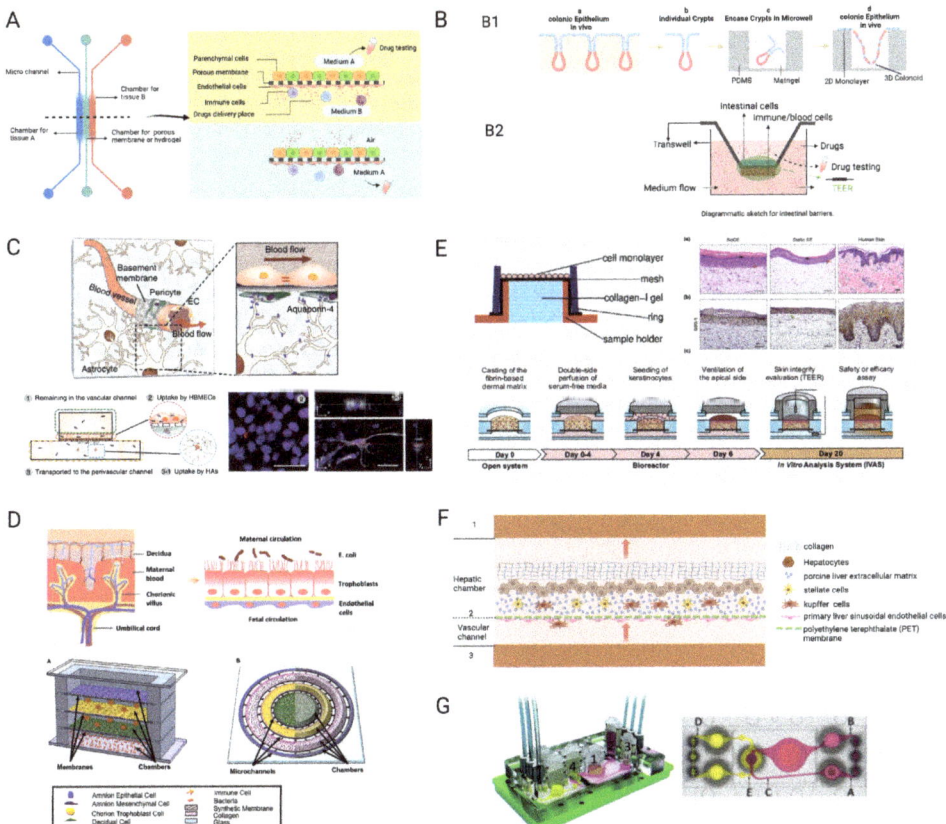

Figure 3. Drug screening by OCs. (**A**) Diagrammatic sketch for barriers. Intestinal barrier, blood–brain barrier, and placental barrier in yellow, airway barrier and skin barrier in green. (**B–G**) The designs of intestinal barrier chip model (**B**), in which B1 is primary colonic crypts-on-a-chip model and B2 is a Transwell modle for intestinal barrier-on-a-chip model. Blood–brain barrier chip model (reprinted from ref. [18] with permission) (**C**), mMaternal–foetal barrier chip model (reprinted from refs. [17,116] with permission) (**D**), in which A was designed to create an infectious preterm birth model to study fetal membranes and B was designed to mimic the feto-maternal interface, including the fetal membranes and maternal decidua. Skin-on-a-chip model [116,121,122] (reprinted from refs. [121,122] with permission) (**E**), Liver sinusoidal chip model (**F**) and ADME MOC model (reprinted from ref. [19] with permission) (**G**), in which pink represents blood flow circuit, yellow represents an excretory flow circuit, numbers represent the four tissue culture compartments for intestine (1), liver (2), skin (3), and kidney (4) tissue. (A, B, C) represent three measuring spots in the surrogate blood circuit and (D, E) represent two spots in the excretory circuit.

3.2. Disease Modelling

The use of OCs models of disease can provide data that are more in accordance with human physiological responses, allowing scholars to gain a deeper understanding of disease characteristics and trends. Their use also reduces animal consumption, as recommended by the "3Rs" principle (replacement, reduction, refinement) in animal ethics.

Here, we focus on an airway-on-a-chip model, simulating disease models for influenza A and COVID-19 infection and using disease models to predict effective drugs for COVID-19 infection [140]; tumour-on-a-chip models, which predict tumour metastasis [141]; and a breast cancer–heart-on-a-chip model to detect chemotherapy toxicity in the heart [142].

3.2.1. Airway-on-a-Chip Model

Researchers grew human bronchial airway epithelial cells and artery endothelial cells in a dual-channel microstructure created by PDMS and PET porous membranes to form an airway-on-a-chip model, combining air and blood channels [15,140] (Figure 4A). This model was infected with influenza A virus, and the infection model was verified by immunofluorescence staining, followed by treatment of the microarray model with an effective therapeutic agent for influenza A, which ultimately showed the effectiveness of the treatment; thus, this proved in reverse that the airway microarray model of viral infection was successful. The researchers then used this chip model to develop a COVID-19 infection airway-on-a-chip model of simulated novel coronavirus infection by pseudotyped syndrome coronavirus type 2 (SARS-CoV-2) and used it to predict effective drugs for novel coronavirus pneumonia in vitro. The predicted drugs were also effective in the prevention and treatment of infection in animal models of COVID-19 infection [140]. The use of this model has demonstrated that OCs models have enormous potential in the treatment of pandemic diseases, alleviating the urgency and burden to develop effective drugs rapidly on occurrence of serious pandemics.

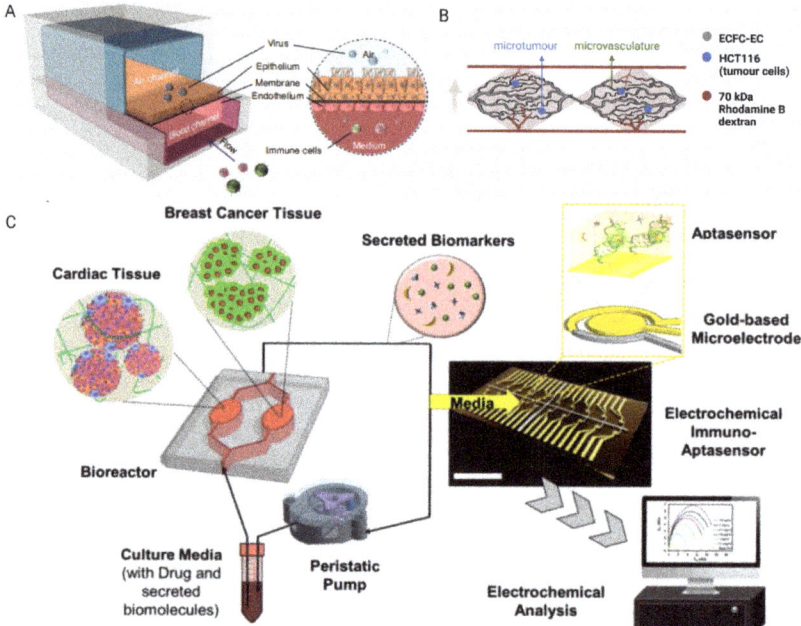

Figure 4. Disease modelling by OCs. (**A–C**) Diagrammatic sketches of an airway-on-a-chip (reprinted from ref. [140] with permission) (**A**), a vascular tumour-on-a-chip (**B**), and a breast cancer–heart-on-a-chip (reprinted from ref. [142] with permission) (**C**).

3.2.2. Tumour-on-a-Chip Models

Researchers have developed vascularised micro-tumour-on-a-chip models for screening effective chemotherapeutic agents [16,141,143,144]. The model was built in PDMS material and bottomless 96-well plates using human vascular endothelial cells in a diamond-shaped culture chamber to self-organise into a 3D microvascular model, growing colorectal tumour cells that differentiated and formed micro-tumours (Figure 4B). This model allows for clear localisation of cell distribution and interactions by histochemical staining. Interestingly, many clinically used chemotherapeutic drugs could be effective in this 3D micro-tumour-on-a-chip model, whereas some of them were not effective when the drugs were also applied to 2D tumour tissue [141]. These findings highlight the superiority of OC models for drug screening compared with 2D cell cultures. It is also possible to build OC models of other tumours to select effective chemotherapeutic drugs [142,145,146].

In addition, many cancer metastases-on-chips have been established to clarify the mechanisms of metastasis in different tumours [147]. Establishing a personalised multi-organ microarray model of a tumour patient can help predict the metastatic activity and trend in that patient's tumour in advance and is a potential area for future study and applications.

3.2.3. Breast Cancer–Heart-on-a-Chip Model

Chemotherapy-induced cardiotoxicity (CIC) is the most likely adverse event in the course of chemotherapy for oncological diseases and is unpredictable, unless irreversible heart failure occurs. Based on clinical experience, researchers chose breast cancer for cardiotoxicity and established the cardiac–breast cancer-on-a-chip model [142]. The researchers co-cultured cardiomyocytes, fibroblasts, and myofibroblasts differentiated from human iPSCs in GelMA hydrogels to form mock heart spheres and similarly cultured breast cancer cells in GelMA, placing them separately in two linked microculture chambers. Addition of TGFβ1 to induce cardiac fibrosis was used to investigate whether a certain degree of myocardial fibrosis promoted the development of CIC (Figure 4C). The chip platform also incorporated an electrochemical multi-array sensor for real-time, continuous detection of multiple biomarkers such as CK-MB, cTnT, and HER-2 [148,149]. Treatment with doxorubicin (DOX) nanoparticles resulted in changes in biomarker indicators, reflecting the suitability of the platform. This microarray model is more of a conceptual model for predicting CIC, but with the concept proposed, a truly practical model is being prepared, and replacing all the cell sources in this model with patient-specific sources may be the way to proceed.

3.3. Treatment

In addition to drug detection and disease modelling, OCs have great potential for use as a flexible medical resource, a development that represents an unexpected breakthrough for both medical treatment and OC itself. Perennial bone marrow-on-a-chip [150], vascular-on-a-chip as a therapeutic scaffold [63], and foreign body corresponding-on-a-chip [87] as an aid for treatment monitoring are currently being investigated.

3.3.1. Bone Marrow-on-a-Chip

The use of OCs as a tool for cultivating resources for disease treatment is a breakthrough in the application of various biomaterials. All types of blood cells originating from HSPCs and their survival are closely linked to the bone marrow cell ecotone, but modelling all aspects of the bone marrow cell ecotone in a more comprehensive way remains unaddressed The bone marrow cell ecotone is structurally complex and consists mainly of cells, such as bone marrow stromal cells and MSCs; it includes a variety of signalling molecules and extracellular matrix components [85,151–153].

The researchers learned from previous superior HSPC culture methods and used 3D ceramic scaffolds of hydroxyapatite-coated zirconium oxide [154], which mimics the porosity and strength of osteochondral stroma; it is filled with MSCs and HSPCs, in which MSCs produce signal molecules and ECM components. It can form a bone marrow model after one week of incubation in vitro. The bone marrow model was placed on a PDMS microchip platform consisting of two independent circular channels [139,150]. In this model,

HSPCs remained in their original state after four weeks, and the ecotone composition remained unchanged, similar to the natural bone marrow ecotone [150]. Establishing this model has helped expand the sources of HSPCs and exploit the potential of an in vitro blood bank of HSPCs that can be used for the treatment of related haematological disorders, which has made them independent of bone marrow donation. This concept was developed to provide inspiration for the treatment of many other systemic diseases (Figure 5A).

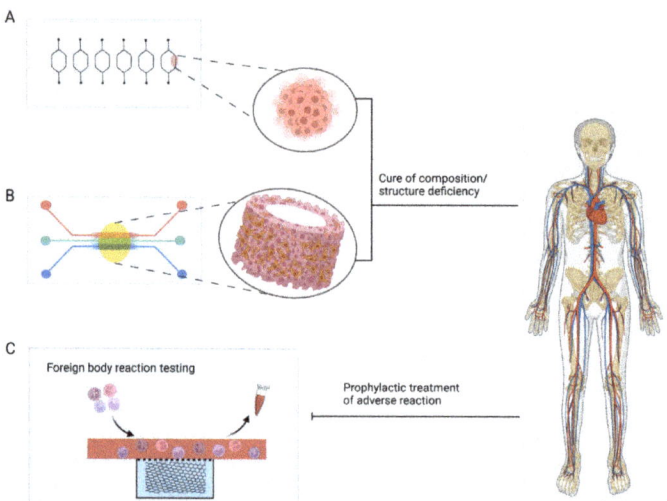

Figure 5. Treatment by OCs. (**A–C**) The treatment concept maps of bone marrow-on-a-chip [150] (**A**), vascular-on-a-chip (**B**), and foreign body corresponding-on-a-chip (**C**).

3.3.2. AngioChip

Some researchers have used OCs to breed a vascular scaffold chip (AngioChip), which is more biocompatible and promotes vascular regeneration (Figure 5B). The POMaC solution was injected into a PDMS porous mould designed by AutoCAD, it was UV-irradiated to form glue, and the PDMS mould was removed to obtain the scaffold structure, which made the final scaffold chip flexible. The scaffold structure was coated with gelatine and placed in a microfluidic PDMS material chip device. HUVECs were infused into the scaffold via a microfluidic system and left to stand until the cells adhered to the scaffold to form a 3D HUVECs vascular scaffold structure [63]. A rat vascular scaffold chip made in the same way was used in Lewis rats in either the artery bypass configuration or the artery-to-vein configuration, which established good blood perfusion and demonstrated excellent biocompatibility. One week after implantation, new angiogenesis was found around the scaffold, which was maintained in vivo for at least five weeks [63,155]. Depending on the requirements, cellular components of different compositions can be infused into the scaffold: HESC-derived hepatocytes with HMSCs for liver-vascular-on-a-chip and HESC-derived cardiomyocytes with HMSCs for heart-vascular-on-a-chip [155]. AngioChip grown using the OC is stable and can be directly anastomosed, allowing analytical exchange inside and outside the vessel and contributing to extensive tissue remodelling. Cells of patient origin can be selected to make the AngioChip a better fit for the patient and better for therapeutic use, but more complete and industrial methods of making the AngioChip are required before this can be performed.

3.3.3. Foreign Body Corresponding-on-a-Chip

In addition to using OCs to cultivate therapeutic resources, researchers have created a monitoring and prevention platform that can detect foreign body responses in vivo [87].

The proposed design further extends the scope of application of OCs platforms. Implantable devices and biomaterials are already widely used in the treatment of diseases, but most implants have an immune cell foreign body response in the host body, which eventually leads to treatment failure or even more serious systemic accidents [156–159].

The foreign body response-on-a-chip is multi-layered and made of PDMS material, consisting of a foreign body (tiny titanium beads wrapped in GelMA) culture chamber at the bottom, a PET semi-permeable membrane in the middle, and a vascular channel containing HUVECs and monocytes in the upper layer [87,95,160]. GelMA gels in the foreign body culture chamber contain MCP-1 factors that mimic the chemokines released by cells exposed to foreign bodies and attract monocytes. Immunofluorescence staining demonstrated the dynamic approach of monocytes to titanium beads under microfluidic conditions and, ultimately, revealed that human monocytes from different donors responded to titanium beads at different levels in this microarray platform and that the phenotype of monocytes near titanium beads does not consistently show M1 or M2, which is consistent with individual variability in immune responses [87]. This suggests that, prior to implantation treatment, time-permitting circulating mononuclear cells from the patient can be extracted for implant-specific immune response assays, which can, to some extent, predict trends in immune levels in that patient post-implantation and can guide prophylactic treatment (Figure 5C).

4. Future Perspectives in Precious Medicine and Wound Healing
4.1. Precision Medicine

Another breakthrough in OCs is individualised medicine, where tissue from clinical patients is used to create OCs, which is similar to the application of disease modelling, but the two are incomparable. Patient-personalised disease models are used to determine disease progression, applicable drugs, and treatments [161,162]. Precision medicine is a thorny path that has been yearned for by the medical industry in recent decades; however, it is still struggling. Perhaps the application of OCs in this area can lead to new concepts and breakthroughs.

Currently, OC is commonly used in precision medicine for tumour drug screening, where patient-derived tumour cells, tissues, or pathological sections are cultured in a microchip, and effective drugs are screened in vitro to guide the patient's clinical treatment plan [163]. It is personalised and has profound implications for subsequent treatment of patients. Although cells cultured in vitro cannot mimic the all-sided composition and characteristics of tumour tissue in vivo, the selection of appropriate tumour sections for microtissue culture allows for long-term and comprehensive drug detection [163,164].

Researchers used tumour tissue from two mesothelioma patients, cultured them in vitro in OCs, and then used the same two chemotherapy combinations for each chip: carboplatin/pemetrexed and cisplatin/pemetrexed. They found that tumour tissues from both patients showed different results for the two chemotherapy regimens. Genomic testing identified one of the mutated loci in patient #1 and no mutation in patient #2 [165]. This study demonstrated the role of OCs in precision medicine for tumours. In addition to the precise selection of drug types, OCs are useful for determining precise drug dosage (Figure 6A). In two patient-derived tumour tissue chip models, the investigators administered each treatment regimen and found that #2 was not dose-dependent for cisplatin; therefore, dosage of cisplatin was appropriately reduced during treatment to mitigate unnecessary toxic effects [165]. Researchers established an OC model containing mouse brain tissue sections and infused the microarray with different doses of STS-simulating chemotherapy drugs, ranging from 10 nM to 6 µM. Tissue staining revealed that the number of apoptotic cells increased with increasing STS concentrations [123]. This suggests that OCs have the potential to test precise drug dosing; however, many factors not included in the microarray model, such as the ratio of drug uptake and metabolism, need to be considered in the process of clinical translation.

In addition, the application of organ chips in precision medicine includes accurate predictions for timely prevention and treatment. For example, many current OCs built using patient tumour tissue predict metastatic trends in tumours [147] or study the toxic effects of chemotherapeutic drugs on other organs. Except for tumour diseases, the foreign body response chip model mentioned above is also a good example of accurate prediction.

OC in precision medicine is widely applicable and not limited to oncological diseases, such as the establishment of airway-on-a-chip for COPD [49], vascular perfusion-on-a-chip [166], and intestinal microbiome-on-a-chip [167,168].

Personalised OC encounters critical challenges from ethical restrictions and access to personalised patient data. The use of patient-derived cells and tissues for research has strict ethical restrictions, and the volume of eligible patients is insufficient for research requirements. The creation of personalised organ chips requires the simulation of multiple environmental parameters from the patient's body which are patient-specific, such as immune levels and the degree of local vascularisation (which affects drug absorption and use). Finally, translating the findings of OC into the patient's body is also a problem that needs to be considered. Determining what proportion of the obtained precise treatment plan should be scaled up to the human body and collecting data on the patients' absorption and metabolism levels are obstacles to the future development of personalised OC. The establishment of a complete patient body-on-a-chip can be a solution.

4.2. Chronic-Wound-on-a-Chip Model

Current models for chronic wound research mainly 2D cellular scratches, 3D skin equivalents, and animal models. It is difficult to heal wounds formed by multiple complex factors acting on the wound surface, mainly complex and long-standing inflammatory reactions. Including multiple skin structures in two dimensions is difficult, and the usability of the study results is limited. Although 3D skin equivalents can present similar skin trauma structures to some extent, they still lack in vivo changes in environmental parameters such as changes in chemical gradients. Researchers have created a trauma microarray model containing blood vessels, immune cells, and dermal structures that allows cell-to-cell interactions to explore the use of anti-inflammatory drugs under inflammatory conditions [169]. We believe that such a chip model is associated with acute trauma, while chronic trauma has more complex cellular components, more difficult-to-control inflammatory conditions, and even specific requirements for blood supply, such as ischaemic chronic trauma and diabetic foot ulcers. Based on this model, by adding multiple cellular components and controlling the proportion of inflammatory cells and the culture fluid composition, we expect to establish a microarray model for chronic wounds.

For example, diabetic foot ulcer (DFU) chip models have not yet been fully established; however, the establishment of in vitro 3D DFU models can be a good inspiration for DFU chip models. Some researchers state that the ideal DFU chip model should embed diseased cells in the scaffold, promote the formation of diseased ECM, and actively elicit immune responses [170]. In the 3D DFU model, patient-derived cells were widely selected for tissue construction and their use slowed down the healing of the model wounds, including fibroblasts, keratin-forming cells, and monocytes. Studies have shown that there is also a large gap in the activity and polarisation of cells extracted in the middle of the wounds, at the edges of the wounds, and in healthy sites [171–174]. These cells are cultured in a high-glucose medium that mimics the high-sugar environment in vivo [171]. By integrating existing 3D models into a microfluidic platform that controls the cell source and culture fluid composition to provide the correct proportion of immune cells, DFU microarray models can be built.

In addition to the existing approach of integrating 3D chronic and acute wound models to form chronic-wound-on-a-chip models, the formation of a chip model of a chronic wound is based on a normal full-layer skin-on-a-chip, which is treated with a drug such as mercaptosuccinic acid (MSA) [175]. The same design can be used for other types of chronic wounds.

4.3. Skin Repair

The establishment of chronic-wound-on-a-chip models helps us study the complex inflammatory situation of chronic wounds, explore active and effective treatment methods, and promote faster healing. However, for difficult-to-heal wounds, the pathological mechanism is very clear, but it is very difficult to complete the healing process, such as in large deep burn wounds.

In the treatment of deep burn wounds, the ultimate goal is to repair the wound; however, patients with deep burns have skin defects and damage to the dermis that prevents spontaneous re-formation of skin to complete healing. Currently, deep burn wounds are often covered with autologous micro-dermis grafts or dECM or hydrogel scaffolds containing mesenchymal stem cells, in the hope of generating good skin coverage. This method is yet to be explored, and autologous skin sources are very limited for patients with large deep burns. We believe that OC can solve this problem by culturing suitable skin tissues in vitro as a therapeutic resource to be transplanted to the wound surface to complete repair. On the one hand, cells of patient origin can be selected for in vitro culture to get rid of the limitation of insufficient resources, and, on the other hand, excellent skin structures can be formed by in vitro 3D bioprinting and cultured for a long-time using microfluidics, which can increase the vascular component and improve the survival rate of the incoming skin tissue in the wound base. As mentioned above, the skin-on a chip model can be cultured on a large scale and transplanted in vivo for surface wound repair.

In addition, missing skin attachments can be repaired to achieve a high level of wound repair. Hair follicles are important accessories that protect the skin, regulate body temperature, and contain sweat glands, erector spinae, blood vessels, nerves, lymphatic vessels, and epithelial and dermal mesenchymal cells [176]. In the widely studied in vitro culture of hair follicles [177], the process of hair follicle formation in the embryo is simulated in vitro, where embryonic-derived epithelial and mesenchymal cells are co-cultured in a collagen scaffold and subsequently transplanted into the skin to form a certain structure and function of hair follicle tissue [178] (Figure 6(B1)). Researchers established a PDMS microwell array with a diameter of 1 mm and depth of 0.5 mm for in vitro large-scale culturing of hair follicle germ, in which mouse embryonic epithelial and mesenchymal cells were co-cultured in microwells, and the surface of the microwell was covered with colloidal material to maintain the cells in a fixed position. Hair follicle structure was formed after 18 days [179] (Figure 6(B2)). We consider this as a preliminary exploration of hair-follicle-on-a-chip, and the integration of microfluidic devices allows a better study of the effect of oxygen content on hair follicle germ development, as found in these studies. A full-layer skin chip model containing hair follicles, blood vessels, and nerves is possible in a large-scale culture chamber, allowing complete wound repair. Although it provides an ideal treatment for patients with large deep burns, there are still difficulties to be eliminated in the process of chip construction.

OCs are currently used in vitro; however, using them in vivo is equally necessary and advantageous. For example, most ischaemic ulcers develop into hard-to-heal wounds when they are treated because of the lack of blood infusion nutrients in the wounds. Inspired by the application of Ocs in vitro, the ulcerated area was closed and connected to a microfluidic and sensor system, allowing the formation of OC devices targeting wound tissue for culture, which can also cultivate cells with the assistance of tissue scaffolds in vivo, such as fibroblasts, epidermal cells, or even hair follicle germ missing from the wounds (Figure 6(B3)). The integrated sensor system can monitor the temperature, pH, cytokines, and other wound factors in real time, and the corresponding treatment can be applied using a micropump at any time. Such a concept has parallels with smart dressings, which have been developing rapidly in recent years. One of the best examples of smart dressings is the real-time monitoring and on-demand treatment of infected wounds, where the temperature of the wound may rise after infection and this information is transmitted through a temperature sensor, which controls the UV light-emitting diode on the dressing, so that the UV-sensitive antibiotic hydrogel dressing starts releasing antibiotics for antimicrobial treatment [180]. A smart dressing can only identify the presence of an infection, and not the degree of infection. It is of single use only and only decides whether to release antibiotics, while dose grasp is not possible with it. In contrast, in vivo OCs allow for a more comprehensive monitoring of wound conditions and more flexible and precise treatment delivery. This study also provides a novel treatment strategy for unhealed wounds.

The concept of in vivo use of organ chips is promising and can be applied not only for skin wound repair but also for tissue treatment in other areas. However, many factors still need to be considered during the implementation process (such as configuration of the culture medium, which promotes the growth of the target cell population without causing tissue hyperplasia), setting the pressure inside the chip system to avoid abnormal bleeding and ischaemia, and, most importantly, making a tight connection between the target site and the chip system, avoiding or eliminating the impact of tissue fluid exudation on the microfluidic system.

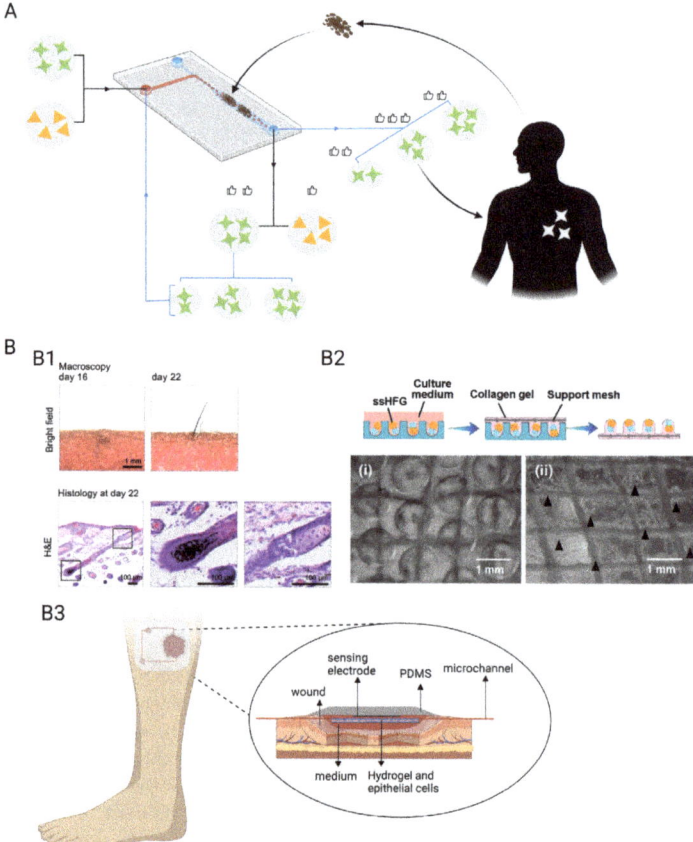

Figure 6. Future perspectives. (**A**) OCs help select the drug types and dosage precisely. The yellow and green shapes represent two different drugs. (**B**) Hair follicle tissue formed in vitro (reprinted from ref. [178] with permission) (**B1**). The boxed areas in the left panels are shown at a higher magnification in the right panels. Hair follicle tissue cultured in mass production in PDMS microwell array (reprinted from ref. [179] with permission) (**B2**). Representative photographs depict HFG appearance prior to (i) and after (ii) the collagen gel was removed from the HFG chip. Arrowheads indicate HFGs. And an assumption for OCs repairing skin in vivo (**B3**).

4.4. Challenges

Many challenges in production of OCs are as follows. First, OCs are difficult to produce and demanding to design. They are designed to mimic the most important aspects and typical features of the tissue, where the nature of problems encounter varies, as do the key aspects and typical features; however, their design is flexible and changeable. Therefore, designers must determine features operating on OCs in consideration during the design phase or when selecting a specific platform, such as channel diameter, angles and input/output ports, bubble traps, biomechanical forces, and the design of biosensors [15]. Most of the cells used in OCs are pluripotent cells and adult stem cells, and many of these cell-derived differentiated cells (e.g., cardiomyocytes) are phenotypically immature, have no standardised protocol for differentiation and maturation, and are difficult to replicate [43]. The choice of extracellular matrix in OCs is also challenging, and no standardised protocol is yet determined for its creation. Decellularized scaffolds or seeded cells in hydrogels can be used to build a suitable environment for cell growth, which is mostly influenced by the composition and arrangement of the scaffold. Therefore, it must be selected and designed carefully to promote appropriate tissue characteristics to form appropriately [181]. The nutrient preferences and aversions of tissues in OCs are different and require associated conservation of many different nutrients. A key challenge for the connected OCs tissue system is, therefore, the provision of this universal cell culture fluid or 'blood mimic'. However, mixed media can solve the problem of a limited number of connected OCs, which is not applicable for connected multiple OCs, and the creation of a single-channel medium that can be added or updated over time is a potential solution that is as-of-yet unexplored [105,141]. OCs cannot replicate certain aspects of the body, and even the most complex MOC may miss some tissues, resulting in a series of OCs missing changes in human metabolism, such as diurnal changes [182], temperature changes [59,183], and changes in drug absorption due to endocrine changes. One solution is to create complex 'micro formulations' to deliver media at particular intervals to compensate for the missing organ [16]; however, this remains a challenge. Finally, the fabrication materials used to fabricate the OCs must be taken into account. Regardless of the material chosen for manufacturing, aspects such as its adsorption properties and biocompatibility should be carefully observed [56,64].

5. Summary

OCs have made drug development faster, economical, and more efficient; they have also enabled a deeper, more detailed understanding of diseases. They have provided novel and interesting approaches for disease treatment and prevention, especially with MOC systems formed by the integration of many OCs, such that their development from one to many can potentially realise body-on-a-chip (BOC) platforms. Although many applications of OCs have been revolutionary, it is believed that there are still more astounding applications to be discovered.

Author Contributions: Conceptualization, Y.L., X.L., M.X. and G.L.; writing—original draft preparation, Y.L. and X.L.; writing—review and editing, Y.L., X.L., Y.Z., W.Z., M.X. and G.L.; supervision, M.X. and G.L.; project administration, M.X. and G.L.; funding acquisition, G.L. All authors have read and agreed to the published version of the manuscript.

Funding: This research was supported by National Key R&D Program of China (2022YFC3006200) and Jiangsu Provincial Department of Science and Technology (BE2018626).

Institutional Review Board Statement: Not applicable.

Informed Consent Statement: Not applicable.

Data Availability Statement: Not applicable.

Conflicts of Interest: The authors declare no conflict of interest.

References

1. Arrowsmith, J.; Miller, P. Trial watch: Phase II and phase III attrition rates 2011-2012. *Nat. Rev. Drug Discov.* **2013**, *12*, 569. [CrossRef]
2. Bhatia, S.N.; Ingber, D.E. Microfluidic organs-on-chips. *Nat. Biotechnol.* **2014**, *32*, 760–772. [CrossRef]
3. Brajsa, K.; Vujasinovic, I.; Jelic, D.; Trzun, M.; Zlatar, I.; Karminski-Zamola, G.; Hranjec, M. Antitumor activity of amidino-substituted benzimidazole and benzimidazo [1,2-a]quinoline derivatives tested in 2D and 3D cell culture systems. *J. Enzyme Inhib. Med. Chem.* **2016**, *31*, 1139–1145. [CrossRef] [PubMed]
4. Van de Stolpe, A.; den Toonder, J. Workshop meeting report Organs-on-Chips: Human disease models. *Lab Chip* **2013**, *13*, 3449–3470. [CrossRef] [PubMed]
5. Rossi, G.; Manfrin, A.; Lutolf, M.P. Progress and potential in organoid research. *Nat. Rev. Genet.* **2018**, *19*, 671–687. [CrossRef]
6. Clevers, H. Modeling Development and Disease with Organoids. *Cell* **2016**, *165*, 1586–1597. [CrossRef]
7. Duval, K.; Grover, H.; Han, L.H.; Mou, Y.; Pegoraro, A.F.; Fredberg, J.; Chen, Z. Modeling Physiological Events in 2D vs. 3D Cell Culture. *Physiology* **2017**, *32*, 266–277. [CrossRef]
8. Ryan, S.L.; Baird, A.M.; Vaz, G.; Urquhart, A.J.; Senge, M.; Richard, D.J.; O'Byrne, K.J.; Davies, A.M. Drug Discovery Approaches Utilizing Three-Dimensional Cell Culture. *Assay Drug Dev. Technol.* **2016**, *14*, 19–28. [CrossRef] [PubMed]
9. Jia, X.; Hua, C.; Yang, F.; Li, X.; Zhao, P.; Zhou, F.; Lu, Y.; Xing, M.; Lu, G. Hydrophobic aerogel-modified hemostatic gauze with thermal management performance. *Bioact. Mater.* **2023**, *26*, 142–158. [CrossRef]
10. Ahadian, S.; Civitarese, R.; Bannerman, D.; Mohammadi, M.H.; Lu, R.; Wang, E.; Davenport-Huyer, L.; Lai, B.; Zhang, B.; Zhao, Y.; et al. Organ-On-A-Chip Platforms: A Convergence of Advanced Materials, Cells, and Microscale Technologies. *Adv. Health Mater.* **2018**, *7*, 1700506. [CrossRef]
11. Huh, D.; Hamilton, G.A.; Ingber, D.E. From 3D cell culture to organs-on-chips. *Trends Cell Biol.* **2011**, *21*, 745–754. [CrossRef] [PubMed]
12. Harink, B.; Le Gac, S.; Truckenmuller, R.; van Blitterswijk, C.; Habibovic, P. Regeneration-on-a-chip? The perspectives on use of microfluidics in regenerative medicine. *Lab Chip* **2013**, *13*, 3512–3528. [CrossRef]
13. Jaalouk, D.E.; Lammerding, J. Mechanotransduction gone awry. *Nat. Rev. Mol. Cell Biol.* **2009**, *10*, 63–73. [CrossRef]
14. Thompson, C.L.; Fu, S.; Knight, M.M.; Thorpe, S.D. Mechanical Stimulation: A Crucial Element of Organ-on-Chip Models. *Front. Bioeng. Biotechnol.* **2020**, *8*, 602646. [CrossRef]
15. Huh, D.; Matthews, B.D.; Mammoto, A.; Montoya-Zavala, M.; Hsin, H.Y.; Ingber, D.E. Reconstituting organ-level lung functions on a chip. *Science* **2010**, *328*, 1662–1668. [CrossRef]
16. Low, L.A.; Mummery, C.; Berridge, B.R.; Austin, C.P.; Tagle, D.A. Organs-on-chips: Into the next decade. *Nat. Rev. Drug Discov.* **2021**, *20*, 345–361. [CrossRef] [PubMed]
17. Zhu, Y.; Yin, F.; Wang, H.; Wang, L.; Yuan, J.; Qin, J. Placental Barrier-on-a-Chip: Modeling Placental Inflammatory Responses to Bacterial Infection. *ACS Biomater. Sci. Eng.* **2018**, *4*, 3356–3363. [CrossRef] [PubMed]
18. Ahn, S.I.; Sei, Y.J.; Park, H.J.; Kim, J.; Ryu, Y.; Choi, J.J.; Sung, H.J.; MacDonald, T.J.; Levey, A.I.; Kim, Y. Microengineered human blood-brain barrier platform for understanding nanoparticle transport mechanisms. *Nat. Commun.* **2020**, *11*, 175. [CrossRef]
19. Maschmeyer, I.; Lorenz, A.K.; Schimek, K.; Hasenberg, T.; Ramme, A.P.; Hubner, J.; Lindner, M.; Drewell, C.; Bauer, S.; Thomas, A.; et al. A four-organ-chip for interconnected long-term co-culture of human intestine, liver, skin and kidney equivalents. *Lab Chip* **2015**, *15*, 2688–2699. [CrossRef]
20. Wieringa, P.A.; Goncalves de Pinho, A.R.; Micera, S.; van Wezel, R.J.A.; Moroni, L. Biomimetic Architectures for Peripheral Nerve Repair: A Review of Biofabrication Strategies. *Adv. Health Mater.* **2018**, *7*, e1701164. [CrossRef] [PubMed]
21. Liaw, C.Y.; Ji, S.; Guvendiren, M. Engineering 3D Hydrogels for Personalized In Vitro Human Tissue Models. *Adv. Health Mater.* **2018**, *7*, 1701165. [CrossRef] [PubMed]
22. Luan, Z.; Liu, S.; Wang, W.; Xu, K.; Ye, S.; Dan, R.; Zhang, H.; Shu, Z.; Wang, T.; Fan, C.; et al. Aligned nanofibrous collagen membranes from fish swim bladder as a tough and acid-resistant suture for pH-regulated stomach perforation and tendon rupture. *Biomater. Res.* **2022**, *26*, 60. [CrossRef]
23. Yang, J.; Zhang, Y.S.; Yue, K.; Khademhosseini, A. Cell-laden hydrogels for osteochondral and cartilage tissue engineering. *Acta Biomater.* **2017**, *57*, 1–25. [CrossRef]
24. Arık, Y.B.; de Sa Vivas, A.; Laarveld, D.; van Laar, N.; Gemser, J.; Visscher, T.; van den Berg, A.; Passier, R.; van der Meer, A.D. Collagen I Based Enzymatically Degradable Membranes for Organ-on-a-Chip Barrier Models. *ACS Biomater. Sci. Eng.* **2021**, *7*, 2998–3005. [CrossRef] [PubMed]
25. Zamprogno, P.; Thoma, G.; Cencen, V.; Ferrari, D.; Putz, B.; Michler, J.; Fantner, G.E.; Guenat, O.T. Mechanical Properties of Soft Biological Membranes for Organ-on-a-Chip Assessed by Bulge Test and AFM. *ACS Biomater. Sci. Eng.* **2021**, *7*, 2990–2997. [CrossRef]
26. Li, W.; Zhang, L.; Ge, X.; Xu, B.; Zhang, W.; Qu, L.; Choi, C.H.; Xu, J.; Zhang, A.; Lee, H.; et al. Microfluidic fabrication of microparticles for biomedical applications. *Chem. Soc. Rev.* **2018**, *47*, 5646–5683. [CrossRef]
27. He, T.; Wang, W.; Chen, B.; Wang, J.; Liang, Q.; Chen, B. 5-Fluorouracil monodispersed chitosan microspheres: Microfluidic chip fabrication with crosslinking, characterization, drug release and anticancer activity. *Carbohydr. Polym.* **2020**, *236*, 116094. [CrossRef]

28. Agarwal, A.; Farouz, Y.; Nesmith, A.P.; Deravi, L.F.; McCain, M.L.; Parker, K.K. Micropatterning Alginate Substrates for in vitro Cardiovascular Muscle on a Chip. *Adv. Funct. Mater.* 2013, *23*, 3738–3746. [CrossRef]
29. Jiang, W.; Li, M.; Chen, Z.; Leong, K.W. Cell-laden microfluidic microgels for tissue regeneration. *Lab Chip* 2016, *16*, 4482–4506. [CrossRef]
30. Lee, K.Y.; Mooney, D.J. Alginate: Properties and biomedical applications. *Prog. Polym. Sci.* 2012, *37*, 106–126. [CrossRef] [PubMed]
31. Yue, K.; Trujillo-de Santiago, G.; Alvarez, M.M.; Tamayol, A.; Annabi, N.; Khademhosseini, A. Synthesis, properties, and biomedical applications of gelatin methacryloyl (GelMA) hydrogels. *Biomaterials* 2015, *73*, 254–271. [CrossRef] [PubMed]
32. Li, X.; Luo, Y.; Yang, F.; Chu, G.; Li, L.; Diao, L.; Jia, X.; Yu, C.; Wu, X.; Zhong, W.; et al. In situ-formed micro silk fibroin composite sutures for pain management and anti-infection. *Compos. Part B Eng.* 2023, *260*, 110729. [CrossRef]
33. Darabi, M.A.; Khosrozadeh, A.; Wang, Y.; Ashammakhi, N.; Alem, H.; Erdem, A.; Chang, Q.; Xu, K.; Liu, Y.; Luo, G.; et al. An Alkaline Based Method for Generating Crystalline, Strong, and Shape Memory Polyvinyl Alcohol Biomaterials. *Adv. Sci.* 2020, *7*, 1902740. [CrossRef]
34. Abdallah, M.; Martin, M.; El Tahchi, M.R.; Balme, S.; Faour, W.H.; Varga, B.; Cloitre, T.; Páll, O.; Cuisinier, F.J.G.; Gergely, C.; et al. Influence of Hydrolyzed Polyacrylamide Hydrogel Stiffness on Podocyte Morphology, Phenotype, and Mechanical Properties. *ACS Appl. Mater. Interfaces* 2019, *11*, 32623–32632. [CrossRef] [PubMed]
35. Wang, Z.; Abdulla, R.; Parker, B.; Samanipour, R.; Ghosh, S.; Kim, K. A simple and high-resolution stereolithography-based 3D bioprinting system using visible light crosslinkable bioinks. *Biofabrication* 2015, *7*, 045009. [CrossRef] [PubMed]
36. Dikovsky, D.; Bianco-Peled, H.; Seliktar, D. The effect of structural alterations of PEG-fibrinogen hydrogel scaffolds on 3-D cellular morphology and cellular migration. *Biomaterials* 2006, *27*, 1496–1506. [CrossRef]
37. Humayun, M.; Chow, C.W.; Young, E.W.K. Microfluidic lung airway-on-a-chip with arrayable suspended gels for studying epithelial and smooth muscle cell interactions. *Lab Chip* 2018, *18*, 1298–1309. [CrossRef]
38. Shim, K.Y.; Lee, D.; Han, J.; Nguyen, N.T.; Park, S.; Sung, J.H. Microfluidic gut-on-a-chip with three-dimensional villi structure. *Biomed. Microdevices* 2017, *19*, 37. [CrossRef]
39. Zhang, X.; Li, L.; Luo, C. Gel integration for microfluidic applications. *Lab Chip* 2016, *16*, 1757–1776. [CrossRef]
40. Wang, Y.I.; Abaci, H.E.; Shuler, M.L. Microfluidic blood-brain barrier model provides in vivo-like barrier properties for drug permeability screening. *Biotechnol. Bioeng.* 2017, *114*, 184–194. [CrossRef]
41. Hare, D.; Collins, S.; Cuddington, B.; Mossman, K. The Importance of Physiologically Relevant Cell Lines for Studying Virus-Host Interactions. *Viruses* 2016, *8*, 297. [CrossRef]
42. Pan, C.; Kumar, C.; Bohl, S.; Klingmueller, U.; Mann, M. Comparative proteomic phenotyping of cell lines and primary cells to assess preservation of cell type-specific functions. *Mol. Cell Proteom.* 2009, *8*, 443–450. [CrossRef]
43. Wnorowski, A.; Yang, H.; Wu, J.C. Progress, obstacles, and limitations in the use of stem cells in organ-on-a-chip models. *Adv. Drug Deliv. Rev.* 2019, *140*, 3–11. [CrossRef] [PubMed]
44. Mummery, C. Stem cell research: Immortality or a healthy old age? *Eur. J. Endocrinol.* 2004, *151* (Suppl. S3), U7-12. [CrossRef]
45. Takahashi, K.; Yamanaka, S. Induction of pluripotent stem cells from mouse embryonic and adult fibroblast cultures by defined factors. *Cell* 2006, *126*, 663–676. [CrossRef]
46. Li, X.; Brooks, J.C.; Hu, J.; Ford, K.I.; Easley, C.J. 3D-templated, fully automated microfluidic input/output multiplexer for endocrine tissue culture and secretion sampling. *Lab Chip* 2017, *17*, 341–349. [CrossRef]
47. Maschmeyer, I.; Hasenberg, T.; Jaenicke, A.; Lindner, M.; Lorenz, A.K.; Zech, J.; Garbe, L.A.; Sonntag, F.; Hayden, P.; Ayehunie, S.; et al. Chip-based human liver-intestine and liver-skin co-cultures--A first step toward systemic repeated dose substance testing in vitro. *Eur. J. Pharm. Biopharm.* 2015, *95*, 77–87. [CrossRef]
48. Wang, Y.; Ahmad, A.A.; Sims, C.E.; Magness, S.T.; Allbritton, N.L. In vitro generation of colonic epithelium from primary cells guided by microstructures. *Lab Chip* 2014, *14*, 1622–1631. [CrossRef]
49. Benam, K.H.; Villenave, R.; Lucchesi, C.; Varone, A.; Hubeau, C.; Lee, H.H.; Alves, S.E.; Salmon, M.; Ferrante, T.C.; Weaver, J.C.; et al. Small airway-on-a-chip enables analysis of human lung inflammation and drug responses in vitro. *Nat. Methods* 2016, *13*, 151–157. [CrossRef] [PubMed]
50. Nawroth, J.; Rogal, J.; Weiss, M.; Brucker, S.Y.; Loskill, P. Organ-on-a-Chip Systems for Women's Health Applications. *Adv. Health Mater.* 2018, *7*, 1700550. [CrossRef] [PubMed]
51. Simoncini, T.; Giannini, A.; Genazzani, A.R. The Long-Term Cardiovascular Risks Associated with Amenorrhea. In *Frontiers in Gynecological Endocrinology*; ISGE Series; Springer: Berlin/Heidelberg, Germany, 2017; pp. 127–132.
52. Werling, D.M.; Geschwind, D.H. Sex differences in autism spectrum disorders. *Curr. Opin. Neurol.* 2013, *26*, 146–153. [CrossRef]
53. Altemus, M.; Sarvaiya, N.; Neill Epperson, C. Sex differences in anxiety and depression clinical perspectives. *Front. Neuroendocrinol.* 2014, *35*, 320–330. [CrossRef]
54. Wenger, N.K.; Ouyang, P.; Miller, V.M.; Bairey Merz, C.N. Strategies and Methods for Clinical Scientists to Study Sex-Specific Cardiovascular Health and Disease in Women. *J. Am. Coll. Cardiol.* 2016, *67*, 2186–2188. [CrossRef]
55. Klein, S.L.; Flanagan, K.L. Sex differences in immune responses. *Nat. Rev. Immunol.* 2016, *16*, 626–638. [CrossRef]
56. Ding, C.; Chen, X.; Kang, Q.; Yan, X. Biomedical Application of Functional Materials in Organ-on-a-Chip. *Front. Bioeng Biotechnol.* 2020, *8*, 823. [CrossRef]
57. McDonald, J.C.; Whitesides, G.M. Poly(dimethylsiloxane) as a material for fabricating microfluidic devices. *Acc. Chem. Res.* 2002, *35*, 491–499. [CrossRef] [PubMed]

58. Liu, Y.; Guan, G.; Li, Y.; Tan, J.; Cheng, P.; Yang, M.; Li, B.; Wang, Q.; Zhong, W.; Mequanint, K.; et al. Gelation of highly entangled hydrophobic macromolecular fluid for ultrastrong underwater in situ fast tissue adhesion. *Sci. Adv.* **2022**, *8*, eabm9744. [CrossRef] [PubMed]
59. Bhattacharjee, N.; Urrios, A.; Kang, S.; Folch, A. The upcoming 3D-printing revolution in microfluidics. *Lab Chip* **2016**, *16*, 1720–1742. [CrossRef]
60. Su, X.; Young, E.W.; Underkofler, H.A.; Kamp, T.J.; January, C.T.; Beebe, D.J. Microfluidic cell culture and its application in high-throughput drug screening: Cardiotoxicity assay for hERG channels. *J. Biomol. Screen* **2011**, *16*, 101–111. [CrossRef]
61. Regehr, K.J.; Domenech, M.; Koepsel, J.T.; Carver, K.C.; Ellison-Zelski, S.J.; Murphy, W.L.; Schuler, L.A.; Alarid, E.T.; Beebe, D.J. Biological implications of polydimethylsiloxane-based microfluidic cell culture. *Lab Chip* **2009**, *9*, 2132–2139. [CrossRef] [PubMed]
62. Paoli, R.; Di Giuseppe, D.; Badiola-Mateos, M.; Martinelli, E.; Lopez-Martinez, M.J.; Samitier, J. Rapid Manufacturing of Multilayered Microfluidic Devices for Organ on a Chip Applications. *Sensors* **2021**, *21*, 1382. [CrossRef] [PubMed]
63. Zhang, B.; Lai, B.F.L.; Xie, R.; Davenport Huyer, L.; Montgomery, M.; Radisic, M. Microfabrication of AngioChip, a biodegradable polymer scaffold with microfluidic vasculature. *Nat. Protoc.* **2018**, *13*, 1793–1813. [CrossRef]
64. Ren, K.; Zhou, J.; Wu, H. Materials for microfluidic chip fabrication. *Acc. Chem. Res.* **2013**, *46*, 2396–2406. [CrossRef]
65. Piruska, A.; Nikcevic, I.; Lee, S.H.; Ahn, C.; Heineman, W.R.; Limbach, P.A.; Seliskar, C.J. The autofluorescence of plastic materials and chips measured under laser irradiation. *Lab Chip* **2005**, *5*, 1348–1354. [CrossRef] [PubMed]
66. Miller, P.G.; Shuler, M.L. Design and demonstration of a pumpless 14 compartment microphysiological system. *Biotechnol. Bioeng.* **2016**, *113*, 2213–2227. [CrossRef]
67. Hirama, H.; Satoh, T.; Sugiura, S.; Shin, K.; Onuki-Nagasaki, R.; Kanamori, T.; Inoue, T. Glass-based organ-on-a-chip device for restricting small molecular absorption. *J. Biosci. Bioeng.* **2019**, *127*, 641–646. [CrossRef]
68. Xu, K.; Wu, X.; Zhang, X.; Xing, M. Bridging wounds: Tissue adhesives' essential mechanisms, synthesis and characterization, bioinspired adhesives and future perspectives. *Burn. Trauma* **2022**, *10*, tkac033. [CrossRef] [PubMed]
69. Huang, Y.; Fan, C.; Liu, Y.; Yang, L.; Hu, W.; Liu, S.; Wang, T.; Shu, Z.; Li, B.; Xing, M.; et al. Nature-Derived Okra Gel as Strong Hemostatic Bioadhesive in Human Blood, Liver, and Heart Trauma of Rabbits and Dogs. *Adv. Health Mater.* **2022**, *11*, e2200939. [CrossRef] [PubMed]
70. Huang, G.; Li, F.; Zhao, X.; Ma, Y.; Li, Y.; Lin, M.; Jin, G.; Lu, T.J.; Genin, G.M.; Xu, F. Functional and Biomimetic Materials for Engineering of the Three-Dimensional Cell Microenvironment. *Chem. Rev.* **2017**, *117*, 12764–12850. [CrossRef]
71. Huang, Y.; Cai, D.; Chen, P. Micro- and nanotechnologies for study of cell secretion. *Anal. Chem.* **2011**, *83*, 4393–4406. [CrossRef]
72. Huh, D.; Leslie, D.C.; Matthews, B.D.; Fraser, J.P.; Jurek, S.; Hamilton, G.A.; Thorneloe, K.S.; McAlexander, M.A.; Ingber, D.E. A human disease model of drug toxicity-induced pulmonary edema in a lung-on-a-chip microdevice. *Sci. Transl. Med.* **2012**, *4*, 159ra147. [CrossRef] [PubMed]
73. Jang, K.J.; Suh, K.Y. A multi-layer microfluidic device for efficient culture and analysis of renal tubular cells. *Lab Chip* **2010**, *10*, 36–42. [CrossRef] [PubMed]
74. Chapanian, R.; Amsden, B.G. Combined and sequential delivery of bioactive VEGF165 and HGF from poly(trimethylene carbonate) based photo-cross-linked elastomers. *J. Control Release* **2010**, *143*, 53–63. [CrossRef] [PubMed]
75. Darabi, M.A.; Khosrozadeh, A.; Mbeleck, R.; Liu, Y.; Chang, Q.; Jiang, J.; Cai, J.; Wang, Q.; Luo, G.; Xing, M. Skin-Inspired Multifunctional Autonomic-Intrinsic Conductive Self-Healing Hydrogels with Pressure Sensitivity, Stretchability, and 3D Printability. *Adv. Mater.* **2017**, *29*, 1700533. [CrossRef]
76. Chang, Q.; He, Y.; Liu, Y.; Zhong, W.; Wang, Q.; Lu, F.; Xing, M. Protein Gel Phase Transition: Toward Superiorly Transparent and Hysteresis-Free Wearable Electronics. *Adv. Funct. Mater.* **2020**, *30*, 1910080. [CrossRef]
77. Matai, I.; Kaur, G.; Seyedsalehi, A.; McClinton, A.; Laurencin, C.T. Progress in 3D bioprinting technology for tissue/organ regenerative engineering. *Biomaterials* **2020**, *226*, 119536. [CrossRef]
78. Mandrycky, C.; Wang, Z.; Kim, K.; Kim, D.H. 3D bioprinting for engineering complex tissues. *Biotechnol. Adv.* **2016**, *34*, 422–434. [CrossRef]
79. Sill, T.J.; von Recum, H.A. Electrospinning: Applications in drug delivery and tissue engineering. *Biomaterials* **2008**, *29*, 1989–2006. [CrossRef]
80. Polte, T.R.; Eichler, G.S.; Wang, N.; Ingber, D.E. Extracellular matrix controls myosin light chain phosphorylation and cell contractility through modulation of cell shape and cytoskeletal prestress. *Am. J. Physiol. Cell Physiol.* **2004**, *286*, C518–C528. [CrossRef] [PubMed]
81. Takayama, S.; Ostuni, E.; LeDuc, P.; Naruse, K.; Ingber, D.E.; Whitesides, G.M. Subcellular positioning of small molecules. *Nature* **2001**, *411*, 1016. [CrossRef]
82. Andersson, H.; van den Berg, A. Microfabrication and microfluidics for tissue engineering: State of the art and future opportunities. *Lab Chip* **2004**, *4*, 98–103. [CrossRef] [PubMed]
83. Ho, C.T.; Lin, R.Z.; Chang, W.Y.; Chang, H.Y.; Liu, C.H. Rapid heterogeneous liver-cell on-chip patterning via the enhanced field-induced dielectrophoresis trap. *Lab Chip* **2006**, *6*, 724–734. [CrossRef]
84. Daley, W.P.; Peters, S.B.; Larsen, M. Extracellular matrix dynamics in development and regenerative medicine. *J. Cell Sci.* **2008**, *121*, 255–264. [CrossRef]
85. Morrison, S.J.; Scadden, D.T. The bone marrow niche for haematopoietic stem cells. *Nature* **2014**, *505*, 327–334. [CrossRef] [PubMed]

86. Lee, K.; Silva, E.A.; Mooney, D.J. Growth factor delivery-based tissue engineering: General approaches and a review of recent developments. *J. R. Soc. Interface* **2011**, *8*, 153–170. [CrossRef] [PubMed]
87. Sharifi, F.; Htwe, S.S.; Righi, M.; Liu, H.; Pietralunga, A.; Yesil-Celiktas, O.; Maharjan, S.; Cha, B.H.; Shin, S.R.; Dokmeci, M.R.; et al. A Foreign Body Response-on-a-Chip Platform. *Adv. Health Mater.* **2019**, *8*, e1801425. [CrossRef] [PubMed]
88. Beckwitt, C.H.; Clark, A.M.; Wheeler, S.; Taylor, D.L.; Stolz, D.B.; Griffith, L.; Wells, A. Liver 'organ on a chip'. *Exp. Cell Res.* **2018**, *363*, 15–25. [CrossRef]
89. Li, X.; George, S.M.; Vernetti, L.; Gough, A.H.; Taylor, D.L. A glass-based, continuously zonated and vascularized human liver acinus microphysiological system (vLAMPS) designed for experimental modeling of diseases and ADME/TOX. *Lab Chip* **2018**, *18*, 2614–2631. [CrossRef]
90. Subramanian, A.; Krishnan, U.M.; Sethuraman, S. Development of biomaterial scaffold for nerve tissue engineering: Biomaterial mediated neural regeneration. *J. Biomed. Sci.* **2009**, *16*, 108. [CrossRef]
91. Nunes, S.S.; Miklas, J.W.; Liu, J.; Aschar-Sobbi, R.; Xiao, Y.; Zhang, B.; Jiang, J.; Masse, S.; Gagliardi, M.; Hsieh, A.; et al. Biowire: A platform for maturation of human pluripotent stem cell-derived cardiomyocytes. *Nat. Methods* **2013**, *10*, 781–787. [CrossRef] [PubMed]
92. Galie, P.A.; Nguyen, D.H.; Choi, C.K.; Cohen, D.M.; Janmey, P.A.; Chen, C.S. Fluid shear stress threshold regulates angiogenic sprouting. *Proc. Natl. Acad. Sci. USA* **2014**, *111*, 7968–7973. [CrossRef]
93. Weng, Y.S.; Chang, S.F.; Shih, M.C.; Tseng, S.H.; Lai, C.H. Scaffold-Free Liver-On-A-Chip with Multiscale Organotypic Cultures. *Adv. Mater.* **2017**, *29*, 1701545. [CrossRef] [PubMed]
94. Rodrigues, R.O.; Sousa, P.C.; Gaspar, J.; Banobre-Lopez, M.; Lima, R.; Minas, G. Organ-on-a-Chip: A Preclinical Microfluidic Platform for the Progress of Nanomedicine. *Small* **2020**, *16*, e2003517. [CrossRef]
95. Zhang, Y.S.; Aleman, J.; Shin, S.R.; Kilic, T.; Kim, D.; Mousavi Shaegh, S.A.; Massa, S.; Riahi, R.; Chae, S.; Hu, N.; et al. Multisensor-integrated organs-on-chips platform for automated and continual in situ monitoring of organoid behaviors. *Proc. Natl. Acad. Sci. USA* **2017**, *114*, E2293–E2302. [CrossRef]
96. Kieninger, J.; Weltin, A.; Flamm, H.; Urban, G.A. Microsensor systems for cell metabolism—From 2D culture to organ-on-chip. *Lab Chip* **2018**, *18*, 1274–1291. [CrossRef]
97. Cohen, Z.J.; Haxha, S.; Aggoun, A. Pulse oximetry optical sensor using oxygen-bound haemoglobin. *Opt. Express* **2016**, *24*, 10115–10131. [CrossRef] [PubMed]
98. Rumpler, M.; Hajnsek, M.; Baumann, P.; Pieber, T.R.; Klimant, I. Monitoring tissue oxygen heterogeneities and their influence on optical glucose measurements in an animal model. *J. Clin. Monit. Comput.* **2018**, *32*, 583–586. [CrossRef]
99. Shin, S.R.; Kilic, T.; Zhang, Y.S.; Avci, H.; Hu, N.; Kim, D.; Branco, C.; Aleman, J.; Massa, S.; Silvestri, A.; et al. Label-Free and Regenerative Electrochemical Microfluidic Biosensors for Continual Monitoring of Cell Secretomes. *Adv. Sci.* **2017**, *4*, 1600522. [CrossRef]
100. Riahi, R.; Shaegh, S.A.; Ghaderi, M.; Zhang, Y.S.; Shin, S.R.; Aleman, J.; Massa, S.; Kim, D.; Dokmeci, M.R.; Khademhosseini, A. Automated microfluidic platform of bead-based electrochemical immunosensor integrated with bioreactor for continual monitoring of cell secreted biomarkers. *Sci. Rep.* **2016**, *6*, 24598. [CrossRef] [PubMed]
101. Xu, C.; Jiang, D.; Ge, Y.; Huang, L.; Xiao, Y.; Ren, X.; Liu, X.; Zhang, Q.; Wang, Y. A PEDOT:PSS conductive hydrogel incorporated with Prussian blue nanoparticles for wearable and noninvasive monitoring of glucose. *Chem. Eng. J.* **2022**, *431*, 134109. [CrossRef]
102. Odijk, M.; van der Meer, A.D.; Levner, D.; Kim, H.J.; van der Helm, M.W.; Segerink, L.I.; Frimat, J.P.; Hamilton, G.A.; Ingber, D.E.; van den Berg, A. Measuring direct current trans-epithelial electrical resistance in organ-on-a-chip microsystems. *Lab Chip* **2015**, *15*, 745–752. [CrossRef] [PubMed]
103. Chen, W.L.K.; Edington, C.; Suter, E.; Yu, J.; Velazquez, J.J.; Velazquez, J.G.; Shockley, M.; Large, E.M.; Venkataramanan, R.; Hughes, D.J.; et al. Integrated gut/liver microphysiological systems elucidates inflammatory inter-tissue crosstalk. *Biotechnol. Bioeng.* **2017**, *114*, 2648–2659. [CrossRef]
104. Cao, U.M.N.; Zhang, Y.; Chen, J.; Sayson, D.; Pillai, S.; Tran, S.D. Microfluidic Organ-on-A-chip: A Guide to Biomaterial Choice and Fabrication. *Int. J. Mol. Sci.* **2023**, *24*, 3232. [CrossRef]
105. Chang, S.Y.; Weber, E.J.; Sidorenko, V.S.; Chapron, A.; Yeung, C.K.; Gao, C.; Mao, Q.; Shen, D.; Wang, J.; Rosenquist, T.A.; et al. Human liver-kidney model elucidates the mechanisms of aristolochic acid nephrotoxicity. *JCI Insight* **2017**, *2*, 95978. [CrossRef] [PubMed]
106. Yang, F.; Cohen, R.N.; Brey, E.M. Optimization of Co-Culture Conditions for a Human Vascularized Adipose Tissue Model. *Bioengineering* **2020**, *7*, 114. [CrossRef]
107. Zhang, C.; Zhao, Z.; Abdul Rahim, N.A.; van Noort, D.; Yu, H. Towards a human-on-chip: Culturing multiple cell types on a chip with compartmentalized microenvironments. *Lab Chip* **2009**, *9*, 3185–3192. [CrossRef] [PubMed]
108. Jalili-Firoozinezhad, S.; Gazzaniga, F.S.; Calamari, E.L.; Camacho, D.M.; Fadel, C.W.; Bein, A.; Swenor, B.; Nestor, B.; Cronce, M.J.; Tovaglieri, A.; et al. A complex human gut microbiome cultured in an anaerobic intestine-on-a-chip. *Nat. Biomed. Eng.* **2019**, *3*, 520–531. [CrossRef]
109. Abbott, N.J.; Patabendige, A.A.; Dolman, D.E.; Yusof, S.R.; Begley, D.J. Structure and function of the blood-brain barrier. *Neurobiol. Dis.* **2010**, *37*, 13–25. [CrossRef]
110. Park, D.; Lee, J.; Chung, J.J.; Jung, Y.; Kim, S.H. Integrating Organs-on-Chips: Multiplexing, Scaling, Vascularization, and Innervation. *Trends Biotechnol.* **2020**, *38*, 99–112. [CrossRef]

111. Staicu, C.E.; Jipa, F.; Axente, E.; Radu, M.; Radu, B.M.; Sima, F. Lab-on-a-Chip Platforms as Tools for Drug Screening in Neuropathologies Associated with Blood-Brain Barrier Alterations. *Biomolecules* **2021**, *11*, 916. [CrossRef]
112. Fung, K.Y.; Wang, C.; Nyegaard, S.; Heit, B.; Fairn, G.D.; Lee, W.L. SR-BI Mediated Transcytosis of HDL in Brain Microvascular Endothelial Cells Is Independent of Caveolin, Clathrin, and PDZK1. *Front. Physiol.* **2017**, *8*, 841. [CrossRef]
113. Wang, H.; Eckel, R.H. What are lipoproteins doing in the brain? *Trends Endocrinol. Metab.* **2014**, *25*, 8–14. [CrossRef] [PubMed]
114. Blundell, C.; Yi, Y.S.; Ma, L.; Tess, E.R.; Farrell, M.J.; Georgescu, A.; Aleksunes, L.M.; Huh, D. Placental Drug Transport-on-a-Chip: A Microengineered In Vitro Model of Transporter-Mediated Drug Efflux in the Human Placental Barrier. *Adv. Health Mater.* **2018**, *7*, 1700786. [CrossRef]
115. Young, R.E.; Huh, D.D. Organ-on-a-chip technology for the study of the female reproductive system. *Adv. Drug Deliv. Rev.* **2021**, *173*, 461–478. [CrossRef]
116. Richardson, L.; Kim, S.; Menon, R.; Han, A. Organ-On-Chip Technology: The Future of Feto-Maternal Interface Research? *Front. Physiol.* **2020**, *11*, 715. [CrossRef] [PubMed]
117. Richardson, L.; Vargas, G.; Brown, T.; Ochoa, L.; Trivedi, J.; Kacerovsky, M.; Lappas, M.; Menon, R. Redefining 3Dimensional placental membrane microarchitecture using multiphoton microscopy and optical clearing. *Placenta* **2017**, *53*, 66–75. [CrossRef] [PubMed]
118. Gnecco, J.S.; Anders, A.P.; Cliffel, D.; Pensabene, V.; Rogers, L.M.; Osteen, K.; Aronoff, D.M. Instrumenting a Fetal Membrane on a Chip as Emerging Technology for Preterm Birth Research. *Curr. Pharm. Des.* **2017**, *23*, 6115–6124. [CrossRef]
119. Arver, S.; Stief, C.; de la Rosette, J.; Jones, T.H.; Neijber, A.; Carrara, D. A new 2% testosterone gel formulation: A comparison with currently available topical preparations. *Andrology* **2018**, *6*, 396–407. [CrossRef]
120. Rasmussen, S.; Horkan, K.H.; Kotler, M. Pharmacokinetic Evaluation of Two Nicotine Patches in Smokers. *Clin. Pharmacol. Drug Dev.* **2018**, *7*, 506–512. [CrossRef]
121. Tarnoki-Zach, J.; Mehes, E.; Varga-Medveczky, Z.; Isai, D.G.; Barany, N.; Bugyik, E.; Revesz, Z.; Paku, S.; Erdo, F.; Czirok, A. Development and Evaluation of a Human Skin Equivalent in a Semiautomatic Microfluidic Diffusion Chamber. *Pharmaceutics* **2021**, *13*, 910. [CrossRef]
122. Sriram, G.; Alberti, M.; Dancik, Y.; Wu, B.; Wu, R.; Feng, Z.; Ramasamy, S.; Bigliardi, P.L.; Bigliardi-Qi, M.; Wang, Z. Full-thickness human skin-on-chip with enhanced epidermal morphogenesis and barrier function. *Mater. Today* **2018**, *21*, 326–340. [CrossRef]
123. Lukacs, B.; Bajza, A.; Kocsis, D.; Csorba, A.; Antal, I.; Ivan, K.; Laki, A.J.; Erdo, F. Skin-on-a-Chip Device for Ex Vivo Monitoring of Transdermal Delivery of Drugs-Design, Fabrication, and Testing. *Pharmaceutics* **2019**, *11*, 445. [CrossRef]
124. Bajza, A.; Kocsis, D.; Berezvai, O.; Laki, A.J.; Lukacs, B.; Imre, T.; Ivan, K.; Szabo, P.; Erdo, F. Verification of P-Glycoprotein Function at the Dermal Barrier in Diffusion Cells and Dynamic "Skin-On-A-Chip" Microfluidic Device. *Pharmaceutics* **2020**, *12*, 804. [CrossRef]
125. Jeong, S.; Kim, J.; Jeon, H.M.; Kim, K.; Sung, G.Y. Development of an Aged Full-Thickness Skin Model Using Flexible Skin-on-a-Chip Subjected to Mechanical Stimulus Reflecting the Circadian Rhythm. *Int. J. Mol. Sci.* **2021**, *22*, 12788. [CrossRef] [PubMed]
126. Jeon, B.; Lee, G.; Wufuer, M.; Huang, Y.; Choi, Y.; Kim, S.; Choi, T.H. Enhanced predictive capacity using dual-parameter chip model that simulates physiological skin irritation. *Toxicol. In Vitro* **2020**, *68*, 104955. [CrossRef] [PubMed]
127. Mori, N.; Morimoto, Y.; Takeuchi, S. Skin integrated with perfusable vascular channels on a chip. *Biomaterials* **2017**, *116*, 48–56. [CrossRef] [PubMed]
128. Zhang, Q.; Sito, L.; Mao, M.; He, J.; Zhang, Y.S.; Zhao, X. Current advances in skin-on-a-chip models for drug testing. *Microphysiol. Syst.* **2018**, *2*. [CrossRef]
129. Jungermann, K.; Kietzmann, T. Oxygen: Modulator of metabolic zonation and disease of the liver. *Hepatology* **2000**, *31*, 255–260. [CrossRef]
130. Lee-Montiel, F.T.; George, S.M.; Gough, A.H.; Sharma, A.D.; Wu, J.; DeBiasio, R.; Vernetti, L.A.; Taylor, D.L. Control of oxygen tension recapitulates zone-specific functions in human liver microphysiology systems. *Exp. Biol. Med.* **2017**, *242*, 1617–1632. [CrossRef]
131. Sung, J.H.; Shuler, M.L. A micro cell culture analog (microCCA) with 3-D hydrogel culture of multiple cell lines to assess metabolism-dependent cytotoxicity of anti-cancer drugs. *Lab Chip* **2009**, *9*, 1385–1394. [CrossRef] [PubMed]
132. Cecen, B.; Karavasili, C.; Nazir, M.; Bhusal, A.; Dogan, E.; Shahriyari, F.; Tamburaci, S.; Buyukoz, M.; Kozaci, L.D.; Miri, A.K. Multi-Organs-on-Chips for Testing Small-Molecule Drugs: Challenges and Perspectives. *Pharmaceutics* **2021**, *13*, 1657. [CrossRef]
133. Esch, E.W.; Bahinski, A.; Huh, D. Organs-on-chips at the frontiers of drug discovery. *Nat. Rev. Drug Discov.* **2015**, *14*, 248–260. [CrossRef]
134. Bhise, N.S.; Ribas, J.; Manoharan, V.; Zhang, Y.S.; Polini, A.; Massa, S.; Dokmeci, M.R.; Khademhosseini, A. Organ-on-a-chip platforms for studying drug delivery systems. *J. Control Release* **2014**, *190*, 82–93. [CrossRef]
135. Herland, A.; Maoz, B.M.; Das, D.; Somayaji, M.R.; Prantil-Baun, R.; Novak, R.; Cronce, M.; Huffstater, T.; Jeanty, S.S.F.; Ingram, M.; et al. Quantitative prediction of human pharmacokinetic responses to drugs via fluidically coupled vascularized organ chips. *Nat. Biomed. Eng.* **2020**, *4*, 421–436. [CrossRef]
136. Skardal, A.; Aleman, J.; Forsythe, S.; Rajan, S.; Murphy, S.; Devarasetty, M.; Pourhabibi Zarandi, N.; Nzou, G.; Wicks, R.; Sadri-Ardekani, H.; et al. Drug compound screening in single and integrated multi-organoid body-on-a-chip systems. *Biofabrication* **2020**, *12*, 025017. [CrossRef]

137. Novak, R.; Ingram, M.; Marquez, S.; Das, D.; Delahanty, A.; Herland, A.; Maoz, B.M.; Jeanty, S.S.F.; Somayaji, M.R.; Burt, M.; et al. Robotic fluidic coupling and interrogation of multiple vascularized organ chips. *Nat. Biomed. Eng.* **2020**, *4*, 407–420. [CrossRef] [PubMed]
138. Leclerc, E.; Hamon, J.; Bois, F.Y. Investigation of ifosfamide and chloroacetaldehyde renal toxicity through integration of in vitro liver-kidney microfluidic data and pharmacokinetic-system biology models. *J. Appl. Toxicol.* **2016**, *36*, 330–339. [CrossRef] [PubMed]
139. Wagner, I.; Materne, E.M.; Brincker, S.; Sussbier, U.; Fradrich, C.; Busek, M.; Sonntag, F.; Sakharov, D.A.; Trushkin, E.V.; Tonevitsky, A.G.; et al. A dynamic multi-organ-chip for long-term cultivation and substance testing proven by 3D human liver and skin tissue co-culture. *Lab Chip* **2013**, *13*, 3538–3547. [CrossRef] [PubMed]
140. Si, L.; Bai, H.; Rodas, M.; Cao, W.; Oh, C.Y.; Jiang, A.; Moller, R.; Hoagland, D.; Oishi, K.; Horiuchi, S.; et al. A human-airway-on-a-chip for the rapid identification of candidate antiviral therapeutics and prophylactics. *Nat. Biomed. Eng.* **2021**, *5*, 815–829. [CrossRef]
141. Phan, D.T.T.; Wang, X.; Craver, B.M.; Sobrino, A.; Zhao, D.; Chen, J.C.; Lee, L.Y.N.; George, S.C.; Lee, A.P.; Hughes, C.C.W. A vascularized and perfused organ-on-a-chip platform for large-scale drug screening applications. *Lab Chip* **2017**, *17*, 511–520. [CrossRef]
142. Lee, J.; Mehrotra, S.; Zare-Eelanjegh, E.; Rodrigues, R.O.; Akbarinejad, A.; Ge, D.; Amato, L.; Kiaee, K.; Fang, Y.; Rosenkranz, A.; et al. A Heart-Breast Cancer-on-a-Chip Platform for Disease Modeling and Monitoring of Cardiotoxicity Induced by Cancer Chemotherapy. *Small* **2021**, *17*, e2004258. [CrossRef]
143. Wang, X.; Phan, D.T.; Sobrino, A.; George, S.C.; Hughes, C.C.; Lee, A.P. Engineering anastomosis between living capillary networks and endothelial cell-lined microfluidic channels. *Lab Chip* **2016**, *16*, 282–290. [CrossRef]
144. Sobrino, A.; Phan, D.T.; Datta, R.; Wang, X.; Hachey, S.J.; Romero-Lopez, M.; Gratton, E.; Lee, A.P.; George, S.C.; Hughes, C.C. 3D microtumors in vitro supported by perfused vascular networks. *Sci. Rep.* **2016**, *6*, 31589. [CrossRef] [PubMed]
145. Hwang, S.H.; Lee, S.; Park, J.Y.; Jeon, J.S.; Cho, Y.J.; Kim, S. Potential of Drug Efficacy Evaluation in Lung and Kidney Cancer Models Using Organ-on-a-Chip Technology. *Micromachines* **2021**, *12*, 215. [CrossRef]
146. Berzina, S.; Harrison, A.; Taly, V.; Xiao, W. Technological Advances in Tumor-On-Chip Technology: From Bench to Bedside. *Cancers* **2021**, *13*, 4192. [CrossRef] [PubMed]
147. Caballero, D.; Kaushik, S.; Correlo, V.M.; Oliveira, J.M.; Reis, R.L.; Kundu, S.C. Organ-on-chip models of cancer metastasis for future personalized medicine: From chip to the patient. *Biomaterials* **2017**, *149*, 98–115. [CrossRef]
148. Kilickap, S.; Barista, I.; Akgul, E.; Aytemir, K.; Aksoyek, S.; Aksoy, S.; Celik, I.; Kes, S.; Tekuzman, G. cTnT can be a useful marker for early detection of anthracycline cardiotoxicity. *Ann. Oncol.* **2005**, *16*, 798–804. [CrossRef] [PubMed]
149. Simoes, R.; Silva, L.M.; Cruz, A.; Fraga, V.G.; de Paula Sabino, A.; Gomes, K.B. Troponin as a cardiotoxicity marker in breast cancer patients receiving anthracycline-based chemotherapy: A narrative review. *Biomed. Pharmacother.* **2018**, *107*, 989–996. [CrossRef]
150. Sieber, S.; Wirth, L.; Cavak, N.; Koenigsmark, M.; Marx, U.; Lauster, R.; Rosowski, M. Bone marrow-on-a-chip: Long-term culture of human haematopoietic stem cells in a three-dimensional microfluidic environment. *J. Tissue Eng. Regen. Med.* **2018**, *12*, 479–489. [CrossRef] [PubMed]
151. Arai, F.; Suda, T. Maintenance of quiescent hematopoietic stem cells in the osteoblastic niche. *Ann. N. Y. Acad. Sci.* **2007**, *1106*, 41–53. [CrossRef]
152. Abdallah, B.M.; Kassem, M. Human mesenchymal stem cells: From basic biology to clinical applications. *Gene Ther.* **2008**, *15*, 109–116. [CrossRef] [PubMed]
153. Lilly, A.J.; Johnson, W.E.; Bunce, C.M. The haematopoietic stem cell niche: New insights into the mechanisms regulating haematopoietic stem cell behaviour. *Stem Cells Int.* **2011**, *2011*, 274564. [CrossRef]
154. Didwania, M.; Didwania, A.; Mehta, G.; Basak, G.W.; Yasukawa, S.; Takayama, S.; de Necochea-Campion, R.; Srivastava, A.; Carrier, E. Artificial hematopoietic stem cell niche: Bioscaffolds to microfluidics to mathematical simulations. *Curr. Top Med. Chem.* **2011**, *11*, 1599–1605. [CrossRef]
155. Zhang, B.; Montgomery, M.; Chamberlain, M.D.; Ogawa, S.; Korolj, A.; Pahnke, A.; Wells, L.A.; Masse, S.; Kim, J.; Reis, L.; et al. Biodegradable scaffold with built-in vasculature for organ-on-a-chip engineering and direct surgical anastomosis. *Nat. Mater.* **2016**, *15*, 669–678. [CrossRef] [PubMed]
156. Langer, R.; Vacanti, J.P. Tissue engineering. *Science* **1993**, *260*, 920–926. [CrossRef]
157. Rafii, S.; Lyden, D. Therapeutic stem and progenitor cell transplantation for organ vascularization and regeneration. *Nat. Med.* **2003**, *9*, 702–712. [CrossRef] [PubMed]
158. Breitbach, M.; Bostani, T.; Roell, W.; Xia, Y.; Dewald, O.; Nygren, J.M.; Fries, J.W.; Tiemann, K.; Bohlen, H.; Hescheler, J.; et al. Potential risks of bone marrow cell transplantation into infarcted hearts. *Blood* **2007**, *110*, 1362–1369. [CrossRef] [PubMed]
159. Badylak, S.F.; Gilbert, T.W. Immune response to biologic scaffold materials. *Semin. Immunol.* **2008**, *20*, 109–116. [CrossRef]
160. Skardal, A.; Murphy, S.V.; Devarasetty, M.; Mead, I.; Kang, H.W.; Seol, Y.J.; Shrike Zhang, Y.; Shin, S.R.; Zhao, L.; Aleman, J.; et al. Multi-tissue interactions in an integrated three-tissue organ-on-a-chip platform. *Sci. Rep.* **2017**, *7*, 8837. [CrossRef]
161. Guenat, O.T.; Geiser, T.; Berthiaume, F. Clinically Relevant Tissue Scale Responses as New Readouts from Organs-on-a-Chip for Precision Medicine. *Annu. Rev. Anal. Chem.* **2020**, *13*, 111–133. [CrossRef]
162. van den Berg, A.; Mummery, C.L.; Passier, R.; van der Meer, A.D. Personalised organs-on-chips: Functional testing for precision medicine. *Lab Chip* **2019**, *19*, 198–205. [CrossRef]

163. Rodriguez, A.D.; Horowitz, L.F.; Castro, K.; Kenerson, H.; Bhattacharjee, N.; Gandhe, G.; Raman, A.; Monnat, R.J.; Yeung, R.; Rostomily, R.C.; et al. A microfluidic platform for functional testing of cancer drugs on intact tumor slices. *Lab Chip* **2020**, *20*, 1658–1675. [CrossRef] [PubMed]
164. Chang, T.C.; Mikheev, A.M.; Huynh, W.; Monnat, R.J.; Rostomily, R.C.; Folch, A. Parallel microfluidic chemosensitivity testing on individual slice cultures. *Lab Chip* **2014**, *14*, 4540–4551. [CrossRef]
165. Mazzocchi, A.R.; Rajan, S.A.P.; Votanopoulos, K.I.; Hall, A.R.; Skardal, A. In vitro patient-derived 3D mesothelioma tumor organoids facilitate patient-centric therapeutic screening. *Sci. Rep.* **2018**, *8*, 2886. [CrossRef]
166. Tsai, M.; Kita, A.; Leach, J.; Rounsevell, R.; Huang, J.N.; Moake, J.; Ware, R.E.; Fletcher, D.A.; Lam, W.A. In vitro modeling of the microvascular occlusion and thrombosis that occur in hematologic diseases using microfluidic technology. *J. Clin. Investig.* **2012**, *122*, 408–418. [CrossRef]
167. Bein, A.; Shin, W.; Jalili-Firoozinezhad, S.; Park, M.H.; Sontheimer-Phelps, A.; Tovaglieri, A.; Chalkiadaki, A.; Kim, H.J.; Ingber, D.E. Microfluidic Organ-on-a-Chip Models of Human Intestine. *Cell Mol. Gastroenterol. Hepatol.* **2018**, *5*, 659–668. [CrossRef]
168. Gumuscu, B.; Albers, H.J.; van den Berg, A.; Eijkel, J.C.T.; van der Meer, A.D. Compartmentalized 3D Tissue Culture Arrays under Controlled Microfluidic Delivery. *Sci. Rep.* **2017**, *7*, 3381. [CrossRef]
169. Biglari, S.; Le, T.Y.L.; Tan, R.P.; Wise, S.G.; Zambon, A.; Codolo, G.; De Bernard, M.; Warkiani, M.; Schindeler, A.; Naficy, S.; et al. Simulating Inflammation in a Wound Microenvironment Using a Dermal Wound-on-a-Chip Model. *Adv. Health Mater.* **2019**, *8*, e1801307. [CrossRef]
170. Ejiugwo, M.; Rochev, Y.; Gethin, G.; O'Connor, G. Toward Developing Immunocompetent Diabetic Foot Ulcer-on-a-Chip Models for Drug Testing. *Tissue Eng. Part C Methods* **2021**, *27*, 77–88. [CrossRef] [PubMed]
171. Ozdogan, C.Y.; Kenar, H.; Davun, K.E.; Yucel, D.; Doger, E.; Alagoz, S. An in vitro 3D diabetic human skin model from diabetic primary cells. *Biomed. Mater.* **2020**, *16*, 015027. [CrossRef] [PubMed]
172. Mascharak, S.; desJardins-Park, H.E.; Longaker, M.T. Fibroblast Heterogeneity in Wound Healing: Hurdles to Clinical Translation. *Trends Mol. Med.* **2020**, *26*, 1101–1106. [CrossRef]
173. Maione, A.G.; Smith, A.; Kashpur, O.; Yanez, V.; Knight, E.; Mooney, D.J.; Veves, A.; Tomic-Canic, M.; Garlick, J.A. Altered ECM deposition by diabetic foot ulcer-derived fibroblasts implicates fibronectin in chronic wound repair. *Wound Repair Regen.* **2016**, *24*, 630–643. [CrossRef]
174. Maione, A.G.; Brudno, Y.; Stojadinovic, O.; Park, L.K.; Smith, A.; Tellechea, A.; Leal, E.C.; Kearney, C.J.; Veves, A.; Tomic-Canic, M.; et al. Three-dimensional human tissue models that incorporate diabetic foot ulcer-derived fibroblasts mimic in vivo features of chronic wounds. *Tissue Eng. Part C Methods* **2015**, *21*, 499–508. [CrossRef]
175. Kim, J.H.; Martins-Green, M. Protocol to Create Chronic Wounds in Diabetic Mice. *J. Vis. Exp.* **2019**, *151*, e57656. [CrossRef]
176. Wang, E.C.E.; Higgins, C.A. Immune cell regulation of the hair cycle. *Exp. Dermatol.* **2020**, *29*, 322–333. [CrossRef] [PubMed]
177. Nilforoushzadeh, M.; Rahimi Jameh, E.; Jaffary, F.; Abolhasani, E.; Keshtmand, G.; Zarkob, H.; Mohammadi, P.; Aghdami, N. Hair Follicle Generation by Injections of Adult Human Follicular Epithelial and Dermal Papilla Cells into Nude Mice. *Cell J.* **2017**, *19*, 259–268. [CrossRef]
178. Asakawa, K.; Toyoshima, K.E.; Ishibashi, N.; Tobe, H.; Iwadate, A.; Kanayama, T.; Hasegawa, T.; Nakao, K.; Toki, H.; Noguchi, S.; et al. Hair organ regeneration via the bioengineered hair follicular unit transplantation. *Sci. Rep.* **2012**, *2*, 424. [CrossRef] [PubMed]
179. Kageyama, T.; Yoshimura, C.; Myasnikova, D.; Kataoka, K.; Nittami, T.; Maruo, S.; Fukuda, J. Spontaneous hair follicle germ (HFG) formation in vitro, enabling the large-scale production of HFGs for regenerative medicine. *Biomaterials* **2018**, *154*, 291–300. [CrossRef] [PubMed]
180. Pang, Q.; Lou, D.; Li, S.; Wang, G.; Qiao, B.; Dong, S.; Ma, L.; Gao, C.; Wu, Z. Smart Flexible Electronics-Integrated Wound Dressing for Real-Time Monitoring and On-Demand Treatment of Infected Wounds. *Adv. Sci.* **2020**, *7*, 1902673. [CrossRef]
181. Liu, H.; Wang, Y.; Cui, K.; Guo, Y.; Zhang, X.; Qin, J. Advances in Hydrogels in Organoids and Organs-on-a-Chip. *Adv. Mater.* **2019**, *31*, e1902042. [CrossRef]
182. Hoyle, N.P.; Seinkmane, E.; Putker, M.; Feeney, K.A.; Krogager, T.P.; Chesham, J.E.; Bray, L.K.; Thomas, J.M.; Dunn, K.; Blaikley, J.; et al. Circadian actin dynamics drive rhythmic fibroblast mobilization during wound healing. *Sci. Transl. Med.* **2017**, *9*, eaal2774. [CrossRef] [PubMed]
183. Gao, X.; Wu, L.; O'Neil, R.G. Temperature-modulated diversity of TRPV4 channel gating: Activation by physical stresses and phorbol ester derivatives through protein kinase C-dependent and -independent pathways. *J. Biol. Chem.* **2003**, *278*, 27129–27137. [CrossRef] [PubMed]

Disclaimer/Publisher's Note: The statements, opinions and data contained in all publications are solely those of the individual author(s) and contributor(s) and not of MDPI and/or the editor(s). MDPI and/or the editor(s) disclaim responsibility for any injury to people or property resulting from any ideas, methods, instructions or products referred to in the content.

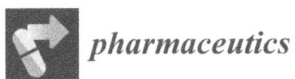

Review

An Overview of the Stability and Delivery Challenges of Commercial Nucleic Acid Therapeutics

Rahul G. Ingle [1,2] and Wei-Jie Fang [1,*]

1. Institute of Drug Metabolism and Pharmaceutical Analysis, College of Pharmaceutical Sciences, Zhejiang University, Hangzhou 310027, China
2. Dr. Rajendra Gode College of Pharmacy, Amravati 444602, India
* Correspondence: wjfang@zju.edu.cn

Abstract: Nucleic acid (NA)-based biopharmaceuticals have emerged as promising therapeutic modalities. NA therapeutics are a diverse class of RNA and DNA and include antisense oligonucleotides, siRNA, miRNA, mRNA, small activating RNA, and gene therapies. Meanwhile, NA therapeutics have posed significant stability and delivery challenges and are expensive. This article discusses the challenges and opportunities for achieving stable formulations of NAs with novel drug delivery systems (DDSs). Here we review the current progress in the stability issues and the significance of novel DDSs associated with NA-based biopharmaceuticals, as well as mRNA vaccines. We also highlight the European Medicines Agency (EMA) and US Food and Drug Administration (FDA)-approved NA-based therapeutics with their formulation profiles. NA therapeutics could impact future markets if the remaining challenges and requirements are addressed. Regardless of the limited information available for NA therapeutics, reviewing and collating the relevant facts and figures generates a precious resource for formulation experts familiar with the NA therapeutics' stability profile, their delivery challenges, and regulatory acceptance.

Keywords: drug delivery; excipient; formulation; mRNA vaccine; nucleic acid therapeutics; stability

1. Introduction

Biopharmaceuticals are at the supreme level of the pharmaceutical market due to their high efficacy, high specificity, and low toxicity profiles [1]. Recently, nucleic acid (NA) therapeutics have emerged as promising candidates for several severe diseases and disorders. NAs are present in all living organisms, including humans, animals, and plants [2]. NAs are naturally occurring chemical compounds; certain small NAs are also synthesized in the laboratory. NAs can be broken down into sugars, phosphoric acid, and a mixture of organic bases (e.g., purines and pyrimidines). NAs have been developed as therapeutic agents and carefully characterized to provide the intended quality, efficacy, and safety profile. NAs are complex and delicate molecules that require sophisticated processes with clever handling during manufacturing, which makes these drugs more expensive. The stability of NAs during manufacturing, handling, shipping, and long-term storage is a major subject of discussion. Excipients play a key role in designing NA therapeutics by improving the manufacturability, stability, quality, and safe delivery of the products [3].

Due to their complex nature, NAs require special attention as active pharmaceutical ingredients (APIs). The alteration in NA quality as a result of physicochemical degradation makes their formulation development challenging. Therefore, several aspects must be considered, including active drug concentration, excipients, delivery routes, and novel drug delivery systems (DDSs). The use of excipients at optimized concentrations aims to maintain the stability of NA therapeutics [4]. However, a key obstacle for the formulation expert is to formulate stable NA therapeutics with the narrow range of excipients usually employed in parenteral settings. Therefore, the launch of novel and ideal excipients to maintain the integrity of significant scientific contribution. Specifically, a critical manufacturing hurdle is precision in the reproducibility of chemical synthesis, the assurance of reproducibility, and the integrity of subsequent batches of the NA therapeutics. For example, the synthesis of thiophosphate derivatives of oligonucleotides results in a mixture of 2^n diastereomers, in which each diastereomer might interact in a slightly different manner. Here, chirality impacts the physical and biological properties of NAs, such as the binding affinity, nuclease stability, etc. [5]. In addition, NA therapeutics are still related with the dilemma of complex drug delivery. This is a fundamental setback preventing the widespread implementation of NA therapeutics. Naked NAs are quickly degraded into physiological fluids and do not accumulate in target tissues [6–8]. Despite these issues, the current NA dosage forms and novel DDSs have enabled the successful launch of NA therapeutics globally. The application of novel DDSs not only improves the long-term storage stability of NAs but also preserves their in vivo efficacy. Therefore, it could be assumed that it is important to conduct an up-to-date survey of the excipients in approved NA therapeutics with novel DDSs. It could serve the biopharmaceutical industry by minimizing the time spent on pre-formulation studies and speeding up the development of stable NA formulations.

Between 2004 and 2021, there have been 23 NA therapeutics approved via the United States Food and Drug Administration (FDA) and/or the European Medicines Agency (EMA) approaches. Among these, fomivirsen (Vitravene) was removed from the European and US markets in 2002 and 2006, respectively, owing to the demand having been undermined. In addition, Macugen (pegaptanib sodium injection), Glybera (alipogene tiparvovec), and Kynamro (mipomersen sodium) were withdrawn from the market in 2019, 2017, and 2022, respectively [9]. Therapeutic NAs formulated in liquid, suspension, and freeze-dried forms, as well as vector-like liposomes/lipids and nanoparticles (NPs), are divided into their functional classes. Antisense oligonucleotides are a major division of approved NA therapeutics. On the other hand, gene therapy has revealed exciting treatment opportunities for numerous severe and rare diseases that have not been cured thus far, although the safety of gene therapy is a major concern. Continuous monitoring is needed to overcome the challenges posed by these new drugs and to increase their contribution as novel therapeutic modalities in the biopharmaceutical industry [10].

To date, one of the major unresolved issues for approved NAs is the high cost of these drugs. For example, nusinersen costs USD $750,000 for the first year and USD $375,000 in subsequent years. Likewise, eteplirsen costs USD $300,000 annually. The expense for high-efficacy, life-saving drugs, such as nusinersen, is likely to be acceptable. In contrast, eteplirsen has a narrow efficacy; therefore, justifying the cost of eteplirsen would be difficult [11,12].

2. Lasting Challenges and Considerations of NA Therapeutics

2.1. NA Therapeutics Stability

NAs could have unique stability issues, similar to protein drugs, due to their complex and fragile nature (Figure 1). Naked or unmodified NAs have extremely short half-lives in circulation due to enzymatic (e.g., nucleases, such as deoxyribonucleases, and RNAse, such as ribonucleases) and chemical (e.g., oxidation, hydrolysis, deamidation, depurination, and strand cleavage) degradation. Therefore, chemical modifications are usually necessary to improve NA stability. Currently, messenger RNA (mRNA) vaccines have become the frontrunners in fighting coronavirus (COVID-19). However, mRNAs alone are prone to nuclease degradation and phosphate backbone hydrolysis through the intramolecular attack of the 2′-hydroxyl group in physiological fluids [13], which is responsible for the short half-life and low efficiency of the mRNA therapeutics due to incompatibility with nuclease, high molecular weight, high negativity, and their hydrophilic and acid-labile nature [14]. Therefore, lipid nanoparticles (LNPs) are employed in COVID-19 mRNA vaccines. A key disadvantage of the approved COVID-19 mRNA-LNP vaccines is the need to be kept under (ultra) cold storage conditions [15], and the stability of mRNA vaccines during storage, handling, and shipping at ambient temperatures is a primary concern [16,17]. As discussed earlier, mRNA could also undergo hydrolytic degradation during storage, handling, and shipping at ambient temperatures. Thus, DDSs, such as LNP, act as a shield for mRNA to prevent degradation and assure its potency.

In the case of antisense oligonucleotides (ASOs), modifications are usually made to the 2′-carbon of the sugar ring or phosphodiester bond. Phosphorothioate modification provides key protection from nucleases and extends the half-life with better stability. A similar phosphonoacetate modification is possible at the ASO backbone, which is totally resistant to nuclease degradation. Another approach to enhance ASO stability is the ribose sugar modification at the 2′-position of the ring, e.g., locked nucleic acids (LNAs) [18,19]. However, in phosphorodiamidate morpholino oligomers (PMOs), ribose sugars are exchanged with phosphodiester bonds and morpholino groups (e.g., casimersen), sometimes referred to as splice switching oligonucleotides (SSOs). For example, nusinersen and eteplirsen are inclusion- and skipping-type SSOs, respectively. In the case of peptide nucleic acids (PNAs), the ribose-phosphate backbone is exchanged with a polyamide backbone [20,21]. In addition, short interfering RNA (siRNA) chemical modifications at various sites, such as phosphate, nucleobases, ribose, poly-2-O-(2,4-dini-trophenyl)-RNA, and oxygen ring replacement with a sulfur group, exhibit enhanced resistance to RNase with better stability. Fluorine, sugar, methoxy, or deoxy modifications at 2′ positions of the ring are other approaches to improve siRNA serum stability [22–24]. On the other hand, targeting the liver is both a major advantage and disadvantage (e.g., immunotoxicity, immunogenesis, degradation of LNP against the harsh GIT conditions) of NA therapeutics [25]. Due to their different particle size and lipid composition, nanocarriers have organ-specific targeting. LNP is likely delivering the drug to the liver. Rizvi et al. [26] measured the organ distribution of protein activity produced by firefly luciferase encoding mRNA-LNP (Luc mRNA-LNP) and found that robust luciferase expression was detected in the liver. Yang et al. [27] used the lipopolyplex (LPP) nanoparticles, formulated by SW-01(a positively charged cationic compound), ionized and non-ionized lipids, carrying with mRNA encoding luciferase which was evaluated for biodistribution pattern. After intramuscular injection (i.m.) into the hind legs of mice, a strong luciferase expression was noticed at the injection site (muscle) but not in the liver.

In addition, the ASOs are modified with PS-linkages (e.g., Kynamro, Tegsedi), and siRNA (e.g., Oxlumo) are well targeted to hepatic delivery. Synthetic therapeutic oligonucleotides (STOs) could control numerous intracellular and extracellular obstacles to interact with their biological RNA targets inside cells. STOs depend on passive exchanges of phosphorothioate (PS) oligonucleotides with cell-surface and plasma proteins to endorse delivery to the kidney and liver. PS-mediated drug delivery was also useful in delivering NA therapeutics (e.g., Spinraza) to CNS tissues [28].

Additionally, gene-based therapies present exclusive challenges due to several factors, including membrane fluidity and permeability and multiple and complex antigen epitopes. Aggregation, oxidation, deamidation, hydrolysis, and adsorption of gene therapies are frequent pathways responsible for degradation. During deamidation, a succinimidyl intermediate is formed due to nucleophilic attack by the adjacent amide over the amide group of asparagine, and the succinimidyl intermediate is hydrolyzed to isoaspartic and aspartic acids [29]. Thus, this causes instabilities in cell-based therapeutics [30], which may lead to the loss of therapeutic efficacy and produce severe immunogenic responses in patients [31]. Therefore, an astute consideration of the degradation processes and triggering factors and the selection of suitable excipients are crucial to protect NA therapeutics against destabilization.

The challenges involved in the successful formulation of NA therapeutics include a variety of physicochemical degradation pathways. The mechanisms of physicochemical degradation with various environmental factors influencing NA stability have been broadly studied. Physical instability is due to exposure to different temperatures, pH, buffer concentrations, presence of oxygen, ultraviolet light, transition metal cations (e.g., copper, ferrous, zinc, magnesium, and nickel), and various stress conditions. For example, uracil is the deamidate product of cytosine, and the process is 100-fold quicker in single-stranded NAs. At higher temperatures and above pH 7, depurination is observed to be sequence-independent. Metal contamination is a significant factor in the degradation of NAs. During the manufacture of NAs, trace amounts of metals present in various raw materials can be established. Transition metal cations have been found to form metal-base pairs by chelation and initiate the breakage of NA strands. Chelation occurs between the NA strands by connecting the cytosines and two adenines, or mixtures thereof [32,33]. Among the transition metals present, copper and ferrous metal ions seem to be strong degradation catalysts. For example, DNA degradation is observed via the intermediate formation of the DNA-copper-hydroperoxide complex by copper ions and ferrous ions, which have been found to be responsible for the degradation of calf thymus DNA due to molecular oxygen [34]. Chemical instability is prevalently caused by hydrolysis, oxidation, depyrimidination, and deamination [35]. In hydrolysis, phosphoester and N-glycosidic bonds are more prone to hydrolytic cleavage. Nucleophilic phosphodiester cleavage is caused by either inter- or intramolecular reactions. Oxidative degradation primarily involves reactive oxygen species (ROS) reactions in which Fenton-type processes are the most frequent origin of ROS. In addition, the formation of covalent intrastrand purine dimers [36] and oxidation through free radicals are considered chief degradative processes for NA therapeutics [37]. Irradiation with NAs was found to generate hydroxyl free radicals that also caused damage [38].

As specified, NA therapeutics are usually formulated as freeze-dried powders, similar to many protein drugs [39,40]. NAs are generally more stable in a freeze-dried (lyophilized) form than in a liquid state. In the freeze-dried form, many of these degradation pathways may be avoided or retarded. Therefore, freeze-drying is advised to be a practical method to sort out stability problems during long-term storage [41]. siRNA has been administered as a dry powder inhalation (DPI) to facilitate the delivery of drugs in lung therapy [42,43]. In addition, Gennova biopharmaceuticals-based mRNA HGCO19 vaccine will be in a lyophilized form. Recently, the approved tozinameran (BNT162b2, Pfizer/BioNTech) and elasomeran (mRNA-1273, Moderna) mRNA vaccines have been considering sucrose as a lyoprotectant [44] due to the surprising loss of mRNA stability and delivery efficiency following the lyophilization of LNP [45,46]. Therefore, it is necessary to optimize freeze-drying parameters and choose a suitable lyoprotectant to achieve a stable product.

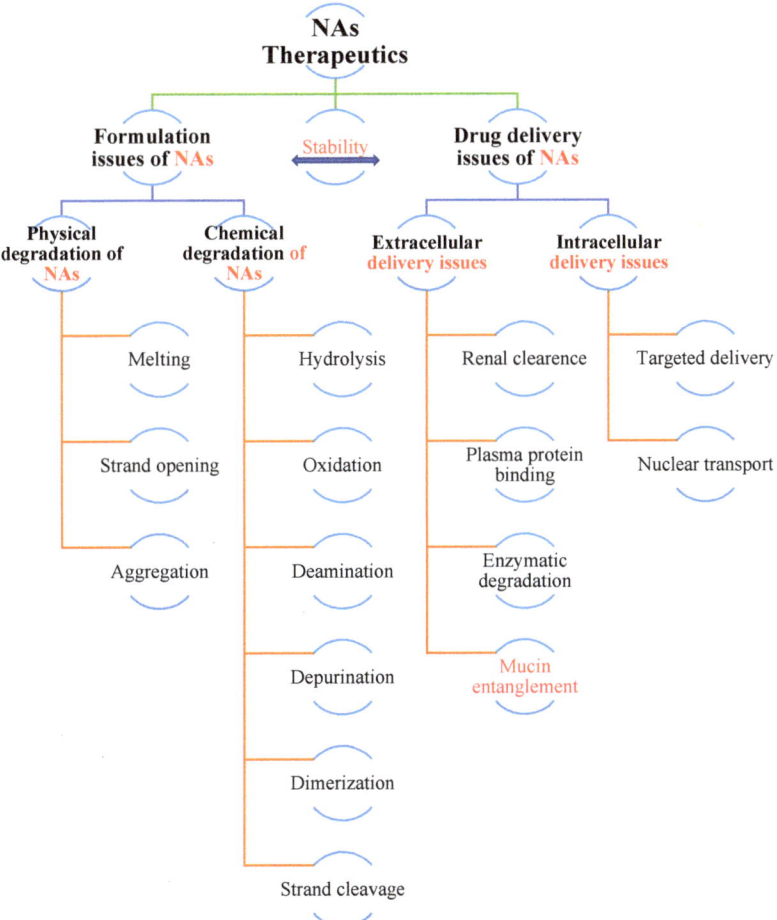

Figure 1. Challenges in the formulation and delivery of NA therapeutics [34].

2.2. NA Therapeutics Delivery

The use of NA therapeutics has climbed significantly in the last decade, but there are still clinical challenges, such as poor pharmacokinetics and pharmacodynamics [47–49]. Incompetent delivery to target organs is a key hurdle preventing the prevalent usage of NA therapeutics (Figure 1). The design of delivery vehicles with particular features renders them stable, efficient, and safe in transfection.

The delivery of NA therapeutics can be influenced by their attributes, such as a negative charge, hydrophilicity, and susceptibility to enzyme degradation [50]. In addition, off-target side effects must be cautiously monitored. Therefore, these issues need to be addressed for the timely development of smart NA formulation. The most commonly engaged strategies to boost NA delivery include chemical, ribose sugar, nucleobases, backbone, and terminal modifications with cell-penetrating moieties. The approaches which have been developed most recently include liposomes, lipoplexes, NPs, DNA cages, DNA nanostructures (framework nucleic acids) [51], microspheres, exosomes [11], gene therapy, spherical NA, red blood cells, biological solids, stimuli-responsive nanotechnology, polyplexes, extracellular vesicles (natural and engineered), micelleplexes, heteroduplex oligonucleotides, niosomes (unilamellar and multilamellar), carbon nanotubes, carbon nanodots, and aptamers [52–63]. Furthermore, Maurer et al. developed magnetic hybrid niosomes (iron-oxide NPs) for siRNA delivery to treat breast cancer [64,65]. All these NA delivery systems have contributed to overcoming several challenges related to NA therapeutics, which include protecting them from degradation and avoiding renal excretion, thereby improving the safety profile.

NP-based drug delivery represents a highly adaptable platform for a variety of therapeutics [66,67]. This includes lipid-based NPs (e.g., liposomes, cubosomes, ionizable, and solid LNPs), polymeric NPs (e.g., natural and synthetic polymers), metal NPs (e.g., gold, silver, and iron), gold NPs (e.g., spherical and nonspherical (such as nanostars, nanorods, and nanocubes)), porous NPs (e.g., porous silicon and mesoporous silica NPs), and metal-organic frameworks (e.g., NU-100) [68–70]. The most frequently employed biodegradable natural polymers are alginate, hyaluronic acids, and chitosan. The current use of synthetic polymers over natural polymers has received noticeably more attention due to their better mechanical and reproducible properties, i.e., dendrimers (e.g., poly-(β-amino ester) (PβAE), poly-(L-lysine) (PLL), and polyamidoamine (PAMAM)), PLGA (polylactic-co-glycolic acid), and PEIs (polyethylene imines) [71,72].

Novel DDSs could enhance the solubility, bioavailability, safety, and PK profiles of systemically administered drugs, leading to enhanced therapeutic efficacy [73]. Therefore, formulation scientists are paying attention to easy and smart DDSs. The current scenario shows rapid commercialization and increasing popularity of nanomedicine dominance over the other DDSs [74–77]. However, liposomes face parallel challenges, including restrictions from the risk of causing immune responses and biodistribution [78]. Due to the suitability of liposomes to both hydrophilic and lipophilic drug candidates, they are used as carriers of choice for various therapeutics [79]. The leading pathway for siRNA therapeutics delivery to the liver was found to be N-acetyl galactosamine (GalNAc), which has proven to be long-acting, therefore, improving the safety profile of the NA therapeutics [80]. In addition, lipid-based carriers (e.g., cationic lipids) [81], polyplexes (many mRNA-based drugs under clinical trials), multivalent cationic non-viral vectors, and polymeric vehicles [82–84] represent the most commonly preferred alternative to viral vectors in gene therapy [85–87]. Viral vectors with antigen-encoding RNA in place of viral genes are prepared by genetic modification of viruses and are effective delivery vehicles. Viral vectors are categorized as replicating and non-replicating vectors [88]. Various RNA viruses, such as adenovirus, picornavirus, flavivirus, and alphavirus, have been used as viral vectors for mRNA delivery. Viral vectors have several limitations, including host genome integration (genotoxicity) and allergic reactions. Therefore, viral vectors have been replaced by non-viral vectors. Non-viral vectors can be classified as hybrid, polymer-based, and lipid-based [36]. They have several benefits over viral vectors, such as ease of production, multi-dosing capabilities, lesser toxicity, and the lack of immunogenicity [89,90]. Therefore, non-viral vectors could be designed with multiple components to overcome physiological barriers [91].

In 1995, the liposome Doxil emerged as the first NP therapeutic. In 2005, human albumin was employed in NP formulations (e.g., Abraxane). Recently, in 2017 [92], the FDA approved the first gene therapies (e.g., Kymriah), which were prepared from the white blood cells of the patients. The great commercial achievement of these DDSs has fascinated many professionals in the field [93]. DDSs play a crucial role in biopharmaceutical formulations, including proteins, monoclonal antibodies, and, recently, NAs. The advanced DDSs promote the high quality and efficacy of the drugs and extend the shelf life of these new molecular entities. Among the approved NA therapeutics, many are delivered as novel DDSs. Patisiran (Onpattro®) is the first commercially available LNP formulation delivered in liposome vesicles. In addition, some gene therapies are associated with adenovirus vectors (e.g., voretigene neparvovecrzyl and onasemnogene abeparvovec-xioi), herpes simplex virus vectors (e.g., talimogene laherparepvec), and gamma retroviral vectors (e.g., strimvelis) [94–96]. Concerning other gene therapies, adeno-associated virus (AAV) has emerged as the principal vector due to the sustainability of the viral genome and its lack of pathogenicity. AAV vectors have special features, such as requiring a helper virus for replication and avoiding pathogenicity. They also have a low tendency for gene integration and, therefore, avoid genotoxicity [97]. The FDA approved Luxturna® as AAV2-based and Zolgensma® as AAV9-based gene therapy, and many more AAV-based gene therapies are under clinical trials [98].

Recently, numerous RNA and DNA vaccines have entered the clinical stages. Among them, mRNA vaccines have become therapeutic targets of interest in many severe diseases and disorders. The safe and efficient delivery of therapeutic mRNAs is one of the key challenges for their wide implementation in humans. mRNAs have concerns such as sensitivity to catalytic hydrolysis, intracellular delivery, and high instability under certain physiological conditions [99]. Recently, developments in mRNA vaccines have been made through their formulation with LNP, which not only provides enhanced delivery and protection but also performs the role of an adjuvant in vaccine reactogenicity [100,101], i.e., the LNP-based delivery of mRNA vaccines against influenza and Zika [102]. In addition, nanoscale delivery platforms (e.g., lipid-derived NPs, polymeric NPs, polymer-lipid hybrid NPs, metal NPs, and peptide complexes) have prolonged the viability of mRNA-based therapeutics, which permit their promising application in protein replacement therapy, genome editing, and cancer immunotherapy [103]. Currently, a major vaccine development platform is advancing with self-assembling drug delivery vehicles, such as cationic monovalent lipids (e.g., N-[1-(2,3-dioleyloxy)propyl]-N,N,N-trimethylammonium chloride (DOTMA), 1,2-dioleoyl-3-tri-methylammonium propane (DOTAP), cationic multivalent lipids (e.g., 2,3-dioleyloxy-N-(2(sperminecarboxaminino)ethyl)-N,N-dimethyl-1-propanaminium trifluoroacetate (DOSPA), dioctadecylamidoglycylspermine (DOGS), neutral lipids (e.g., 1,2-dioleoyl-snglycero-3-phosphoethanolamine (DOPE), dioleoyl phosphatidylcholine (DOPC), and polymeric (e.g., poly(beta-amino esters)), poly(poly-polyesters), poly(colactic glycolic acid), and dioleoyl(DOPC). This involves the use of mRNA-lipid-derived NPs as principal components. In addition to cationic and neutral lipids, anionic lipids have been useful in gene delivery (e.g., dioleoylphosphatidic acid (DOPA), dihexadecyl phosphate (DHPG), dioleoylphosphatidylglycerol (DOPG), and dioleoylphosphatidylserine (DOPS) [104–107].

In particular, LNP-based therapeutics have been proven to be highly biocompatible over polymeric and metal-based delivery systems. It is well-reported that the practice of polymer and metal-based NPs may exert adverse effects [108]. Many vaccine candidates are under clinical trials (e.g., COVAC1, CvnCoV, and LUNAR®-COV-19) [109–112]. Recently, the FDA approved the outstanding vaccine candidate's tozinameran and elasomeran initially under emergency use authorization (EUA) in late 2020 and subsequently granted full approval in mid-2021 for the control of the worldwide COVID-19 pandemic. This has proven to be a breakthrough for the global health emergency of COVID-19. In collaboration with the National Institute of Allergy and Infectious Diseases, Moderna developed the lipid NP-encapsulated mRNA-based vaccine named elasomeran [113]. Simultaneously, Pfizer's mRNA vaccine candidate tozinameran satisfied the entire preliminary efficacy endpoints and was granted the Medicines and Healthcare Products Regulatory Agency (MHRA) approval. The tozinameran vaccine is supplied as a frozen lipid NP suspension. The development of the vaccines was complex, and the Pfizer vaccine (tozinameran) must be stored at -80 to $-60\ °C$, while the Moderna vaccine (elasomeran) must be stored at -25 to $-15\ °C$, making them difficult to handle worldwide, especially in tropical regions.

Therefore, merging NA therapeutics with suitable novel DDSs has become imperative for improving the efficacy with targeted drug delivery and potentially lowering the dose regimens, which may equally reduce the cost.

3. Commercially Approved NA Therapeutics

NA therapeutics can be generally categorized based on the origin and size of the drug. This includes oligonucleotides, ASOs, siRNA, gene therapy, and mRNA vaccines (Table 1) [114]. Oligonucleotides are short DNA or RNA molecules. ASOs are a short single-stranded DNA. The siRNAs are small, double-stranded RNAs with each strand being 20–30 nucleotides. mRNA molecules are composed of thousands of nucleotides with high molecular weights. The modes of action of NAs are different from that of other drugs. NAs are directly delivered to target cells and tissues. Due to their high molecular weight and highly hydrophilic nature, they do not penetrate cells easily and are prone to degradation. Therefore, NAs need high-quality formulations with suitable DDSs to protect them from degradation and to ensure delivery to targeted cells or tissues [115,116]. NA therapeutic formulation development is especially challenging in terms of physical, chemical, and conformational instability. Therefore, an appropriate choice of excipients and drug delivery could lead to high-quality and stable NA therapeutics.

Table 1. Classification of approved nucleic acid (NA) therapeutics.

Biologic Classification	Drug Name (Brand Name)	Subunits	Mol Formula	Target	Indication	Drug Delivery	Approving Agency	Approval Year
Oligonucleotides	Pegaptanib (Macugen)	27	$C_{294}H_{342}F_{13}N_{107}Na_{28}O_{188}P_{28}[C_2H_4O]_2n$	Selectively binds to VEGF165	Neovascular (wet) age-related macular degeneration.	Naked	FDA	2004
	Mipomersen (Kynamro)	20	$C_{230}H_{324}N_{67}O_{122}P_{19}S_{19}$	mRNA of apoB-100	Familial hypercholesterolemia	Naked	FDA	2013
	Defibrotide (Defitelio)	-	$C_{20}H_{21}N_4O_6P$	Adenosine receptors A1, A2a, A2b	Severe hepatic veno-occlusive disease	Naked	FDA	2016
Antisense oligonucleotides	Fomivirsen (Vitravene)	21	$C_{204}H_{243}N_{63}O_{114}P_{20}S_{20}Na_{20}$	30 kDa and 54 kDa immediate-early protein 2	Cytomegalovirus (CMV) retinitis in patients with AIDS	Naked	FDA	1998
	Eteplirsen (Exondys 51)	30	$C_{364}H_{569}N_{177}O_{122}P_{30}$	Forcing the exclusion of exon 51 from the mature DMD mRNA	Duchenne muscular dystrophy	Naked	FDA	2016
	Nusinersen (Spinraza)	18	$C_{234}H_{323}N_{61}O_{128}P_{17}S_{17}Na_{17}$	Survival motor neuron-2 protein	Spinal muscular atrophy	Naked	FDA	2016
	Inotersen (Tegsedi)	20	$C_{230}H_{318}N_{69}O_{121}P_{19}S_{19}$	Transthyretin mRNA	Polyneuropathy	Naked	FDA	2018
	Volanesorsen (Waylivra)	-	$C_{230}H_{320}N_{63}O_{125}P_{19}S_{19}$	Binds to apo C-III mRNA	Familial chylomicronemia syndrome	Naked	EMA	2019
	Golodirsen (Vyondys 53)	25	$C_{305}H_{481}N_{138}O_{112}P_{25}$	Dystrophin	Duchenne muscular dystrophy	Naked	FDA	2019
	Viltolarsen (VILTEPSO)	21	$C_{244}H_{381}N_{113}O_{88}P_{20}$	DMD gene (exon 53 viltolarsen target site)	Duchenne muscular dystrophy	Naked	FDA	2020
	Casimersen (Amondys 45)	20	$C_{268}H_{424}N_{124}O_{95}P_{22}$	DMD gene (exon 45)	Duchenne muscular dystrophy	Naked	FDA	2021
Short interfering RNA (siRNA)	Patisiran (Onpattro)	21	$C_{412}H_{480}N_{148}Na_{40}O_{290}P_{40}$	Transthyretin mRNA	Polyneuropathy	LNP	FDA	2018
	Givosiran (Givlaari)	21	$C_{524}H_{694}F_{16}N_{173}O_{316}P_{43}S_6$	ALAS1 mRNA	Acute hepatic porphyria	N-acetylgalactosamine	FDA	2019
	Lumasiran (Oxlumo)	-	$C_{530}H_{669}F_{10}N_{173}O_{320}P_{43}S_6Na_{43}$	hydroxyacid oxidase-1 (HAO1) mRNA in hepatocytes	Primary hyperoxaluria type 1	N-acetylgalactosamine	FDA	2020
	Inclisiran (Leqvio)	-	$C_{520}H_{679}F_{21}N_{175}O_{309}P_{43}S_6$	Inhibit hepatic translation proprotein convertase subtilisin-Kexin type 9 (PCSK9)	Primary hypercholesterolemia	N-acetylgalactosamine	EMA/FDA	2020/2021
	AMVUTTRA (Vutrisiran)		$C_{530}H_{715}F_9N_{171}O_{323}P_{43}S_6$	Transthyretin mRNA	Amyloidogenic Transthyretin Amyloidosis	Naked	FDA	2022

Table 1. Cont.

Biologic Classification	Drug Name (Brand Name)	Subunits	Mol Formula	Target	Indication	Drug Delivery	Approving Agency	Approval Year
Gene therapy	Voretigene neparvovecrzyl (Luxturna)	-	-	Human retinal pigment epithelial 65 kDa protein (RPE65) encoded gene	Retinal dystrophy	Adeno-associated virus vector	FDA/EMA	2017/2018
	Onasemnogene abeparvovec-xioi (Zolgensma)	-	-	Gene encoding copy delivery to the human SMN protein	Spinal muscular atrophy	Adeno-associated virus	FDA	2019
	Alipogene tiparvovec (Glybera)	-	-	-	Severe pancreatitis	Naked	EMA	2012
	Talimogene laherparepvec (Imlygic)	-	-	For the production of immune response stimulatory protein, human GM-CSF	In recurrent melanoma	Herpes simplex virus 1	FDA/EMA	2015
	Strimvelis	-	-	Activate ADA enzyme	Adenosine deaminase-severe combined immunodeficiency (ADA-SCID)	Gamma retroviral vector	EMA	2016
mRNA vaccines	Tozinameran (Comirnaty) (BNT162b2)	4284	-	SARS-CoV-2S glycoprotein	COVID-19	LNP	FDA/EMA	2021
	Elasomeran (Spikevax) (mRNA-1273)	4284	-	SARS-CoV-2S antigen	COVID-19	LNP	FDA/EMA	2021

Usually, excipients are the key components of a formulation, of which the active drugs comprise only a tiny proportion of the total composition [117]. The key functions of excipients are to improve the safety, stability, and efficacy of therapeutics. A few excipients may be added to formulations to provide tonicity to minimize pain upon injection or to target the easy delivery in the body upon administration (i.e., buffers for pH control, protectants for higher stability, bulking agents for freeze-drying, a surfactant for adsorption control, and salts for osmolality adjustment) [118]. Excipients are comprised of integral components of any formulation. As noted by a model excipient, it is chemically compatible, safe, stable, economical, and multifunctional [119]. In the case of NA formulations, they not only function to regulate shifts in pH but can also stabilize NAs by a variety of mechanisms [92].

The ability of excipients to stabilize therapeutic NAs is notable. The names of excipients used in approved NA therapeutics are shown in Table 2 [120], which summarizes the common excipients included in NA therapeutics for each functional category. The information is briefly tabulated as the commercial name, APIs, dosage form, therapeutic class, excipient compositions, strength, dosage, pH range, administration route, storage condition, and date of approval by the governing authorities (e.g., FDA and EMA).

Table 2. In brief therapeutic information of approved nucleic acid (NA) therapeutics.

API	Dosage Form	Excipients	Strength	Dosage	pH Range	Route of Administration
Pegaptanib (0.3 mg)	Injection/solution	Dibasic sodium phosphate heptahydrate, monobasic sodium phosphate monohydrate, sodium chloride sodium hydroxide, and hydrochloric acid	0.4 mg/mL, 3.47 mg/mL	0.3 mg/90 µL	6.0 to 7.0	IVI
Mipomersen sodium (200 mg)	Injection/solution	Hydrochloric acid and sodium hydroxide	200 mg/mL	200 mg/mL solution	7.5 to 8.5	SC

Table 2. Cont.

API	Dosage Form	Excipients	Strength	Dosage	pH Range	Route of Administration
Eteplirsen (50 mg)	Injection/solution	0.2 mg potassium phosphate monobasic, 0.2 mg potassium chloride, 8 mg sodium chloride, and 1.14 mg sodium phosphate dibasic, anhydrous hydrochloric acid, and sodium hydroxide	50 mg/mL	100 mg/2 mL, 500 mg/10 mL	7.5	IV
Nusinersen (2.4 mg)	Injection/solution	0.16 mg magnesium chloride hexahydrate USP, 0.22 mg potassium chloride USP, 0.21 mg calcium chloride dihydrate USP, 8.77 mg sodium chloride USP, 0.10 mg sodium phosphate dibasic anhydrous USP, 0.05 mg sodium phosphate monobasic dihydrate USP, hydrochloric acid and sodium hydroxide	2.4 mg/mL	12 mg/5 mL	~7.2	IT
Defibrotide sodium (80 mg)	Injection/solution	10 mg sodium citrate USP, hydrochloric acid, and sodium hydroxide	80 mg/mL	200 mg/2.5 mL	6.8–7.8	IV
Inotersen (284 mg)	Injection/solution	Phosphate buffer, hydrochloric acid, and sodium hydroxide	284 mg/1.5 mL	284 mg/1.5 mL	7.5 to 8.5	SC
Patisiran (2.0 mg)	Injection/liposome	13.0 mg (6Z,9Z,28Z,31Z)-heptatriaconta-6,9,28,31 tetraen-19-yl-4-(dimethylamino) butanoate (DLin-MC3-DMA), 3.3 mg 1,2-distearoyl-sn-glycero-3-phosphocholine (DSPC), 6.2 mg cholesterol USP, 1.6 mg α-(3′-[[1,2-di(myristyloxy)propanoxy] carbonylamino]propyl)-ω-methoxy, polyoxyethylene (PEG 2000 C-DMG), 0.2 mg potassium phosphate monobasic anhydrous NF, 2.3 mg sodium phosphate dibasic heptahydrate USP, and 8.8 mg sodium chloride USP	2 mg/mL	10 mg/5 mL	~7.0	IV
Givosiran (189 mg)	Injection/solution	Water for injection	189 mg/mL	189 mg/mL	-	SC
Volanesorsen sodium (200 mg)	Solution	Sodium hydroxide and hydrochloric acid	200 mg of Volanesorsen sodium/mL	285 mg of Volanesorsen/1.5 ml	8.0	SC
Golodirsen (50 mg)	Injection	0.2 mg potassium phosphate monobasic, 0.2 mg potassium chloride, 8 mg sodium chloride, and 1.14 mg sodium phosphate dibasic anhydrous, sodium hydroxide, and hydrochloric acid	50 mg/mL	100 mg/2 mL	7.5	IV
Viltolarsen (50 mg)	Injection/solution	9 mg (0.9%) sodium chloride, sodium hydroxide, and hydrochloric acid	50 mg/mL	250 mg/5 mL	7.0 to 7.5	IV
Casimersen (50 mg)	Injection/solution	0.2 mg potassium chloride, 0.2 mg potassium phosphate monobasic, 8 mg sodium chloride, and 1.14 mg sodium phosphate dibasic	50 mg/mL	100 mg/2 mL	7.5	IV
Voretigene neparvovecrzyl	Solution/suspension	10 mM sodium phosphate, 180 mM sodium chloride, and 0.001% poloxamer 188	5×10^{12} vg/mL	0.3 mL, 0.5 mL in 2 mL	7.3	IOI
Onasemnogene abeparvovec-xioi	Suspension	Onasemnogene abeparvovec (200000000000 1/1 mL) + Onasemnogene abeparvovec (200000000000 1/1 mL) + isopropyl alcohol (0.7 mL/1 mL)	2.0×10^{13} vg/mL	-	-	IV
Talimogene laherparepvec	Injection/suspension	2.44 mg sodium dihydrogen phosphate dihydrate, 15.4 mg disodium hydrogen phosphate dihydrate, 8.5 mg sodium chloride, 40 mg myoinositol, and 20 mg sorbitol	10^6 (PFU)/1 mL	10^6 (PFU)/1 mL (For initial dose), 10^8 (PFU)/1 mL (For subsequent dose)	-	SC/IL

Table 2. Cont.

API	Dosage Form	Excipients	Strength	Dosage	pH Range	Route of Administration
Alipogene tiparvovec	Injection/solution	Potassium dihydrogen phosphate, potassium chloride, sodium chloride, disodium phosphate, and sucrose	3 × 10 12-genome copies/mL	3 × 10 12-genome copies/mL	-	IM
Lumasiran sodium	Solution	Sodium hydroxide and phosphoric acid	94.5 mg/0.5 mL	94.5 mg/0.5 mL	7.0	SC
Inclisiran sodium (284 mg)	Solution	Sodium hydroxide and con. phosphoric acid	189 mg/mL	284 mg/1.5 mL	-	SC
AMVUTTRA (Vutrisiran sodium)	Injection	0.7 mg sodium phosphate dibasic dihydrate, 0.2 mg sodium phosphate monobasic dihydrate, 3.2 mg sodium chloride	26.5 mg/0.5 mL	26.5 mg/0.5 mL	7.0	SC
Tozinameran	Suspension	0.09 mg 1,2-distearoyl-sn-glycero-3-phosphocholine, 0.05 mg 2[(polyethylene glycol)-2000]-N,N-ditetradecylacetamide, 0.43 mg (4-hydroxybutyl)azanediyl)-bis(hexane-6,1-diyl)bis(2-hexyldecanoate), 0.2 mg cholesterol), 0.01 mg potassium chloride, 0.01 mg monobasic potassium phosphate, 0.07 mg dibasic sodium phosphate dihydrate, 6 mg sucrose, and 0.36 mg sodium chloride	30 mcg of mRNA	0.5 mg/1 mL	6.9 to 7.9	IM
Elasomeran	Suspension	Lipids, cholesterol, 1.93 mg (SM-102, polyethylene glycol-2000, 1,2-distearoyl-sn-glycero-3-phosphocholine), 0.31 mg tromethamine, 1.18 mg tromethamine HCl, 0.043 mg acetic acid, 0.12 mg sodium acetate, dimyristoyl glycerol, and 43.5 mg sucrose	100 mcg of mRNA	0.2 mg/1 mL	7.0 to 8.0	IM

(IVI, intravitreal; SC, subcutaneous; IV, intravenous; IM, intramuscular; IL, intralesional; IOI, intraocular injection; IT, intrathecal.).

NA therapeutics are manufactured in different dosage forms (e.g., solution, suspension, freeze-dried, or vector-like liposome/lipids, and NPs). Excipients can play key roles when employed in optimized concentrations [121]. The compositions of approved NA therapeutics are reported, and the relevant information has been gathered from accredited sources, such as DrugBank.com (10 December 2022) and FDA labels (www.fda.gov, 12 December 2022).

The selection of excipients for any formulation requires the verification of some basic factors, such as the API concentration, dosage form (liquid or freeze-dried), administration route, and compatibility. In the case of parenteral formulations, the choice of excipients is fairly limited. Therefore, the proper selection and optimization of excipients are crucial factors for protecting against physicochemical instabilities.

The pH of the formulation has a strong impact on the NA stability. The degradation pathway usually involves a two-step process, such as β-elimination and depurination, which are acid- and base-catalyzed, respectively. A cytosine-deaminated product by sodium bisulfite was detected in acidic buffers (i.e., pH < 6.0) [122]. At an alkaline pH (i.e., pH > 13), the bisulfite adduct is transformed into uracil through bisulfite elimination, whereas an N-glycoside bond cleavage is responsible for the conversion of the pyrimidine-sulfite adduct into a basic site [123]. Therefore, buffers are necessary to maintain the pH at which the specific NA has maximal stability. A pH in a physiological range is more suitable for the easy administration of a drug. It was recommended that a low buffer concentration would minimize the risk of a pH shift [124]. The approved NA therapeutics have specific pH values, i.e., patisiran, viltolarsen, vutrisiran, and lumasiran sodium at pH 7.0; voretigene neparvovecrzyl at pH 7.3; nusinersen at pH 7.2; mipomersen sodium, eteplirsen, inotersen, casimersen, and golodirsen at pH 7.5; volanesorsen sodium at pH 8.0.

The selection of any suitable buffer depends on compatibility with the NA and its formulation excipients. Occasionally, the absence of buffers in NA formulations might negatively impact the quality profile of formulations. In 2015, Garidel et al. tried a successful buffer-free strategy in freeze-dried protein formulations [125]. This might be an important consideration for NA drugs.

The majority of NA therapeutics, including pegaptanib, nusinersen, eteplirsen, vutrisiran, and golodirsen, use monobasic and dibasic sodium phosphate as the buffer. On the other hand, eteplirsen and golodirsen have used monobasic potassium phosphate as the buffering agent to prevent a pH shift. In addition, they also contain sodium chloride, sodium citrate, and/or potassium chloride in optimal concentration ranges as tonicifiers and may protect them from pH oscillations during storage [126].

Primarily, for pH adjustment, mipomersen sodium, inotersen, volanesorsen sodium, defibrotide sodium, inclisiran sodium, casimersen, vutrisiran, and viltolarsen contain sodium hydroxide and hydrochloric acid as excipients. Defibrotide sodium and viltolarsen additionally contain sodium citrate and sodium chloride as tonicifiers, respectively.

In contrast, few NA therapeutics, such as siRNA-based patisiran and both mRNA-based vaccines, are versatile in terms of excipients. All three products are composed of four lipids showing only differences in the storage conditions. For example, patisiran has diverse excipients, such as cholesterol, (6Z, 9Z, 28Z, 31Z)-heptatriaconta-6,9,28,31 tetraen-19-yl-4-(dimethylamino)-butanoate-(DLin-MC3-DMA), functioning as a conjugation for delivery [127], and 1,2-distearoyl-sn-glycero-3-phosphocholine (DSPC) as a helper lipid to protect NPs from aggregation, with diffusible α-(3′-{[1,2-di(myristyloxy)propanoxy]-carbonylamino}propyl)-ω-methoxy, polyoxyethylene (PEG 2000 C-DMG). In addition, all these vaccines play key roles in efficient delivery and enhancing active pharmaceutical ingredients. The carriers may also regulate the safety profile of these drugs to a great extent, which helps to improve the ultimate drug performance and add a valuable contribution to safety, as well as targeted delivery.

In addition, the latest COVID-19 mRNA vaccines contain cholesterol, the helper lipid DSPC, and the diffusible PEG-lipid ((2-[(polyethylene glycol)-2000]-N,N-ditetradecylacetamide, PEG 2000-DMA in tozinameran, or PEG 2000-DMG, 1,2-dimyristoyl-rac-glycero3-methoxypolyethylene glycol-2000 in elasomeran)) [15]. Cholesterol is responsible for lipid membrane fluidity. PEG chain-linked phospholipids function as excipients that furnish a hydrophilic layer and prolong the half-life of mRNA. An optimized concentration of sucrose and sodium phosphate is used to stabilize liposomal NPs during shipping [126]. The ionizable lipids SM-102 and ALC-0315 are employed in the LNP formulations of elasomeran and tozinameran, respectively [15]. Tozinameran and elasomeran contain formulations of ionizable:cholesterol:neutral lipid:PEGylated lipid at molar ratios of 46.3:42.7:9.4:1.6 mol% and 50:38.5:10:1.5 mol%, respectively, along with a lipid:mRNA ratio of 0.05 (w/w). In the mRNA vaccine formulation, sucrose functions as a cryoprotectant during freeze–thaw cycles [128,129]. Similarly, CVnCoV (CureVac/BAYER), currently in phase 2b/3 clinical trials, has molar ratios similar to those of elasomeran [14,130–133]. Currently, several LNP-based mRNA vaccines are in the clinical pipeline to prevent COVID-19, such as ARCT-021 by Arcturus Therapeutics [134], ARCoV by Walvax Biotechnology/Suzhou Abogen Biosciences [135], DS-5670 by Daiichi Sankyo/the University of Tokyo [136], and LNP-nCoV RNA by Imperial College London [137]. In addition, LNP-based mRNA vaccines, such as mRNA-1325 and mRNA-1893 for Zika virus, mRNA-1944 for chikungunya, CV7202 mRNA for rabies, VAL-506440/H10N8 antigen mRNA, and VAL-339851/H7N9 antigen mRNA for influenza are under Phase 1 clinical trial [138]. LNPs composed of biodegradable ionizable lipids could be a promising next-generation delivery system.

A surfactant can stabilize NA by increasing its solubility while minimizing interfacial and nonspecific interactions. The voretigene neparvovecrzyl gene therapy has used poloxamer 188 as a surfactant at optimal concentrations. In addition, patisiran, tozinameran, and elasomeran have PEG 2000 C-DMG, ALC-0159, and PEG-DMG, respectively.

Talimogene laherparepvec contains sorbitol as a stabilizer with sodium dihydrogen and disodium hydrogen phosphate dihydrate as buffering agents. In addition to buffer, nusinersen contains calcium chloride dihydrate with magnesium chloride hexahydrate as complexing agents, which may chelate trace amounts of transition metals present in the buffer to prevent degradation [139]. However, the alipogene tiparvovec injection has used potassium dihydrogen phosphate, disodium phosphate, sucrose, potassium, and sodium chloride as the excipients for formulation. Unfortunately, the sponsor allowed the approval to expire due to the poor commercial absorption of the drug in the market in 2017 [140,141].

In addition to the drug delivery approach, the selection of suitable administration routes is also a significant factor in ensuring efficient and safe drug delivery. Primarily, NA therapeutics are designed for parenteral administration because they are often hard to administer via non-parenteral routes [142]. Therefore, NAs must be formulated as a stable liquid or freeze-dried powder to deliver these drugs safely and efficiently to their target site [143]. To target drug delivery sites, NAs need to be carefully tailored. The novel trends are set to subcutaneous (SC) administration, and the percentage of NA therapeutics approved for SC administration has risen gradually. Among the approved NA therapeutics, 35% of each have been intended for SC and IV administration (Figure 2). Recently, the approved mRNA vaccines for COVID-19 have been administered intramuscularly (IM). NA formulations with a high strength (i.e., >80 mg/mL) are more frequently delivered subcutaneously. Therefore, the NA concentrations in the formulations may depend on the therapeutic effect and the selected administration route for drug delivery. For example, nusinersen (2.4 mg/mL) was administered via the intrathecal route (IT), pegaptanib (0.4 mg/mL) via the intravitreal route (IVI), and mipomersen sodium (200 mg/mL) via the SC route.

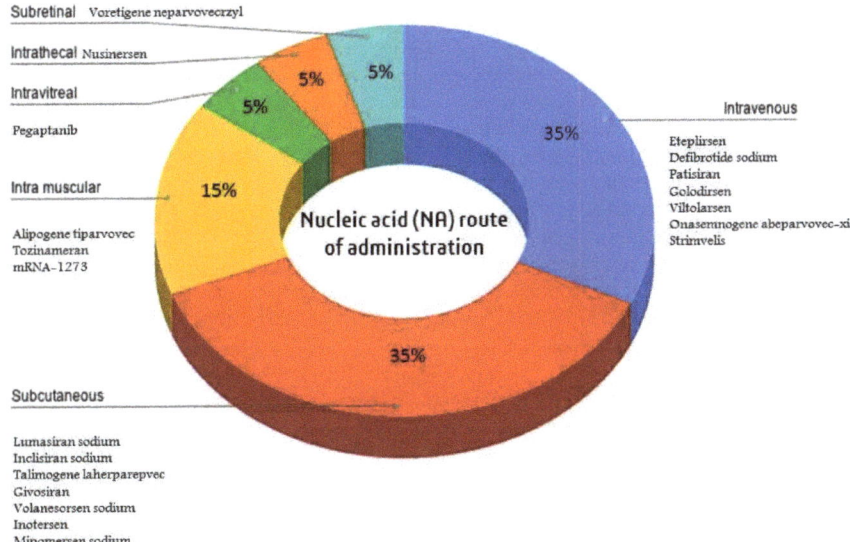

Figure 2. Route of administration allocation for approved NA therapeutics.

It is important to include tonicifiers in NA therapeutics to maintain isotonicity for superior parenteral administration. Most NA therapeutics use potassium chloride and/or sodium chloride as tonicifying agents; however, additional excipients could be added to advance the quality of the therapeutics.

Another crucial aspect is the storage condition. Long-term storage can affect the physicochemical stabilities of NA therapeutics. Sulfur substitutions on the phosphate backbone could easily be exchanged back to dissolved oxygen at elevated temperatures, making the products more prone to nuclease attack. The majority of NA therapeutics are stored at 2–8 °C. The exceptions include voretigene neparvovecrzyl, stored at ≤ -65 °C, alipogene tiparvovec stored at -25 °C to -15 °C, defibrotide sodium stored at 20–25 °C, and givosiran, vutrisiran, and lumasiran stored at 2–25 °C. The new group mRNA vaccines tozinameran (Pfizer-BioNTech) and elasomeran (Moderna) are recommended to be stored at -80 °C to -60 °C and -25 °C to -15 °C, respectively. A recent study concluded that mRNA vaccines are stored at a low temperature to avoid or slow down mRNA degradation by hydrolysis during storage [128].

4. Conclusions and Future Perspectives

Over the past decade, the impact of NA therapeutics has been facilitated by breakthroughs associated with high-end manufacturing and drug delivery in the field of pharmaceuticals. Although excellent growth has been made in NA delivery, including intracellular delivery, several challenges and requirements remain.

This article also discusses the prime considerations pertaining to novel excipients and analyzes their function and rationale in NA therapeutics. To date, 23 NA therapeutics have been approved; however, the publicly accessible awareness of NA therapeutics is extremely limited. Therefore, we recommend that scientists carefully monitor the stability during all stages of NA therapeutics development. Simultaneously, the trend of novel excipients and SC administration is also garnering attention, predominantly in terms of highly concentrated NA therapeutics. In addition, it is important to monitor deficiencies caused by the administration of various NA therapeutics. For example, vutrisiran has caused vitamin-A deficiency in patients. Therefore, the provision of vitamin-A supplementation is a primary concern during the therapeutic application of vutrisiran. In future publications, we aim to discuss the adverse events and the precautionary actions taken during NA therapeutics therapy.

Looking at the current scenario, the development of NAs as therapeutics focuses on long-term stability and the efficiency of DDSs, such as liposomes, NPs, microspheres, or gene therapy. However, there is a need to address several challenges posed by DDSs, such as manufacturing complexity, cost-effectiveness, and safety. In addition, self-amplifying RNA would be a next-generation vaccine platform but requires smart drug delivery vehicles to maintain the long-term stability and efficiency of the drug. In the near future, developing long-acting DDSs to improve the PK and enhance the targeting efficiency at cellular and tissue sites is critical. Formulation scientists could merge advanced techniques, like artificial intelligence and machine learning, with the DDSs to make them more intelligent and potentially more affordable, and easier to use for patients. This continuous advancement presents the hope that remedies for rare or currently untreatable diseases will soon be possible and affordable.

Author Contributions: R.G.I.: Conceptualization, Data curation, Formal analysis, Investigation, Visualization, Software, Methodology, Writing-original draft; W.-J.F.: Conceptualization, Validation, Funding acquisition, Project administration, Supervision, Writing-Review and editing. All authors have read and agreed to the published version of the manuscript.

Funding: This research was funded by the Ministry of Science and Technology of China (Grant No. 2018ZX09J18107-002) and the National Natural Science Foundation of China (Grant No. 81741144).

Acknowledgments: The authors are thankful to the Ministry of Science and Technology of China (Grant No. 2018ZX09J18107-002) and the National Natural Science Foundation of China (Grant No. 81741144) for their financial support.

Conflicts of Interest: The authors declare no conflict of interest.

Abbreviations

AAV: adeno-associated virus; API, active pharmaceutical ingredient; ASOs, antisense oligonucleotides; COVID-19, coronavirus disease-2019; DDSs, drug delivery systems; DSPC, 1,2-distearoyl-sn-glycero-3-phosphocholine; EMA, European Medicines Agency; EUA, emergency use authorization; FDA, United States Food and Drug Administration; IL, intralesional; IM, intramuscular; IOI, intraocular injection; IV, intravenous; IVI, intravitreal; IT, intrathecal; LNP, lipid nanoparticle; mRNA, messenger RNA; NA, nucleic acid; NPs, nanoparticles; PEG-2000C-DMG, α-(3′-{[1,2-di(myristyloxy)propanoxy]-carbonylamino}propyl)-ω-methoxy, polyoxyethylene; PEG2000-DMG, 1,2-dimyristoyl-rac-glycero3-methoxypolyethylene glycol-2000; PS, phosphorothioate; ROS, reactive oxygen species; siRNA, short interfering RNA; SC, subcutaneous; SSO, splice switching oligonucleotide; Synthetic therapeutic oligonucleotides, STOs.

References

1. Bjeloevi, M.; Pobirk, A.; Planinšek, O.; Grabnar, P. Excipients in freeze-dried biopharmaceuticals: Contributions toward formulation stability and lyophilization cycle optimization. *Int. J. Pharm.* **2020**, *576*, 119029. [CrossRef] [PubMed]
2. Rao, V.A.; Kim, J.J.; Patel, D.S.; Rains, K.; Estoll, C.R. A comprehensive scientific Survey of excipients used in currently marketed, therapeutic biological drug products. *Pharm. Res.* **2020**, *37*, 200. [CrossRef]
3. Gervasi, V.; Agnol, R.D.; Cullen, S.; McCoy, T.; Vucen, S.; Crean, A. Parenteral protein formulations: An overview of approved products within the European Union. *Eur. J. Pharm. Biopharm.* **2018**, *131*, 8–24. [CrossRef]
4. Cui, Y.; Cui, P.; Chen, B.; Li, S.; Guan, H. Monoclonal antibodies: Formulations of marketed products and recent advances in novel delivery system. *Drug Dev. Ind. Pharm.* **2017**, *43*, 519–530. [CrossRef]
5. Wan, W.B.; Migawa, M.T.; Vasquez, G.; Murray, H.M.; Nichols, J.G.; Gaus, H.; Berdeja, A.; Lee, S.; Hart, C.E.; Lima, W.F.; et al. Synthesis, biophysical properties and biological activity of second-generation antisense oligonucleotides containing chiral phosphorothioate linkages. *Nucleic Acids Res.* **2014**, *42*, 13456–13468. [CrossRef] [PubMed]
6. Whitehead, K.A.; Langer, R.; Anderson, D.G. Knocking down barriers: Advances in siRNA delivery. *Nat. Rev. Drug Discov.* **2009**, *8*, 129–138. [CrossRef] [PubMed]
7. Cullis, P.R.; Hope, M.J. Lipid nanoparticle systems for enabling gene therapies. *Mol. Ther.* **2017**, *25*, 1467–1475. [CrossRef]
8. Mitragotri, S.; Burke, P.A.; Langer, R. Overcoming the challenges in administering biopharmaceuticals: Formulation and delivery strategies. *Nat. Rev. Drug Discov.* **2014**, *13*, 655–672. [CrossRef]
9. Walsh, G.; Walsh, E. Biopharmaceuticals benchmarks 2022. *Nat. Biotechnol.* **2022**, *40*, 1722–1760. [CrossRef]
10. Cring, M.R.; Sheffield, V.C. Gene therapy and gene correction: Targets, progress, and challenges for treating human diseases. *Gene Ther.* **2020**, *29*, 3–12. [CrossRef]
11. Ke, W.; Afonin, K.A. Exosomes as natural delivery carriers for programmable therapeutic nucleic acid nanoparticles (NANPs). *Adv. Drug Deliv. Rev.* **2021**, *176*, 113835. [CrossRef] [PubMed]
12. Prasad, V. Nusinersen for spinal muscular atrophy: Are we paying too much for too little? *JAMA Pediatr.* **2018**, *172*, 123–125. [CrossRef] [PubMed]
13. Han, X.; Mitchell, M.J.; Nie, G. Nanomaterials for therapeutic RNA delivery. *Matter* **2020**, *3*, 1948–1975. [CrossRef]
14. Weng, Y.; Li, C.; Yang, T.; Hu, B.; Zhang, M.; Guo, S.; Xiao, H.; Liang, X.-J.; Huang, Y. The challenge and prospect of mRNA therapeutics landscape. *Biotechnol. Adv.* **2020**, *40*, 107534. [CrossRef] [PubMed]
15. Schoenmaker, L.; Witzigmann, D.; Kulkarni, J.; Verbeke, R.; Kersten, G.; Jiskoot, W.; Crommelin, D. mRNA-lipid nanoparticle COVID-19 vaccines: Structure and stability. *Int. J. Pharm.* **2021**, *601*, 120586. [CrossRef]
16. Crommelin, D.J.; Anchordoquy, T.J.; Volkin, D.B.; Jiskoot, W.; Mastrobattista, E. Addressing the cold reality of mRNA vaccine stability. *J. Pharm. Sci.* **2021**, *110*, 997–1001. [CrossRef] [PubMed]
17. Verbeke, R.; Lentacker, I.; De Smedt, S.C.; Dewitte, H. The dawn of mRNA vaccines: The COVID-19 case. *J. Control. Release* **2021**, *333*, 511–520. [CrossRef]
18. Morris, G.; O'Brien, D.; Henshall, D.C. Opportunities and challenges for microRNA-targeting therapeutics for epilepsy. *Trends Pharmacol. Sci.* **2021**, *42*, 605–616. [CrossRef]
19. Crooke, S.T.; Liang, X.-H.; Baker, B.F.; Crooke, R.M. Antisense technology: A review. *J. Biol. Chem.* **2021**, *296*, 100416. [CrossRef]
20. Nielsen, P.; Egholm, M.; Berg, R.; Buchardt, O. Sequence-selective recognition of DNA by strand displacement with a thymine-substituted polyamide. *Science* **1991**, *254*, 1497–1500. [CrossRef]
21. Egholm, M.; Buchardt, O.; Christensen, L.; Behrens, C.; Freier, S.M.; Driver, D.A.; Berg, R.H.; Kim, S.K.; Norden, B.; Nielsen, P.E. PNA hybridizes to complementary oligonucleotides obeying the Watson–Crick hydrogen-bonding rules. *Nature* **1993**, *365*, 566–568. [CrossRef] [PubMed]
22. Alshaer, W.; Zureigat, H.; Al Karaki, A.; Al-Kadash, A.; Gharaibeh, L.; Ma'mon, M.H.; Aljabali, A.A.; Awidi, A. siRNA: Mechanism of action, challenges, and therapeutic approaches. *Eur. J. Pharmacol.* **2021**, *905*, 174178. [CrossRef]
23. Parashar, D.; Rajendran, V.; Shukla, R.; Sistla, R. Lipid-based nanocarriers for delivery of small interfering RNA for T therapeutic use. *Eur. J. Pharm. Sci.* **2020**, *142*, 105159. [CrossRef]

24. Bruno, K. Using drug-excipient interactions for siRNA delivery. *Adv. Drug Deliv. Rev.* **2011**, *63*, 1210–1226. [CrossRef]
25. Samaridou, E.; Heyes, J.; Lutwyche, P. Lipid nanoparticles for nucleic acid delivery: Current perspectives. *Adv. Drug Deliv. Rev.* **2020**, *154–155*, 37–63. [CrossRef] [PubMed]
26. Rizvi, F.; Everton, E.; Smith, A.R.; Liu, H.; Osota, E.; Beattie, M.; Tam, Y.; Pardi, N.; Weissman, D.; Gouon-Evans, V. Murine liver repair via transient activation of regenerative pathways in hepatocytes using lipid nanoparticle-complexed nucleoside-modified mRNA. *Nat. Commun.* **2021**, *12*, 613. [CrossRef]
27. Yang, R.; Deng, Y.; Huang, B.; Huang, L.; Lin, A.; Li, Y.; Wang, W.; Liu, J.; Lu, S.; Zhan, Z.; et al. A core-shell structured COVID-19 mRNA vaccine with favorable biodistribution pattern and promising immunity. *Signal Transduct. Target. Ther.* **2021**, *6*, 213. [CrossRef] [PubMed]
28. Gökirmak, T.; Nikan, M.; Wiechmann, S.; Prakash, T.P.; Tanowitz, M.; Seth, P.P. Overcoming the challenges of tissue delivery for oligonucleotide therapeutics. *Trends Pharmacol. Sci.* **2021**, *42*, 588–604. [CrossRef] [PubMed]
29. Mohammad, R. Key considerations in formulation development for gene therapy products. *Drug Discov. Today* **2021**, *27*, 292–303. [CrossRef]
30. Amer, M.H.; White, L.J.; Shakesheff, K.M. The effect of injection using narrow-bore needles on mammalian cells: Administration and formulation considerations for cell therapies. *J. Pharm. Pharmacol.* **2015**, *67*, 640–650. [CrossRef]
31. Falconer, R.J. Advances in liquid formulations of parenteral therapeutic proteins. *Biotechnol. Adv.* **2019**, *37*, 107412. [CrossRef]
32. Medley, C.D.; Muralidhara, B.K.; Chico, S.; Durban, S.; Mehelic, P.; Demarest, C. Quantitation of plasmid DNA deposited on gold particles for particle mediated epidermal delivery using ICP-MS. *Anal. Bioanal. Chem.* **2010**, *398*, 527–535. [CrossRef] [PubMed]
33. Boerner, L.J.; Zaleski, J.M. Metal complex-DNA interactions: From transcription inhibition to photoactivated cleavage. *Curr. Opin. Chem. Biol.* **2005**, *9*, 135–144. [CrossRef] [PubMed]
34. Muralidhara, B.K.; Baid, R.; Bishop, S.M.; Huang, M.; Wang, W.; Nema, S. Critical considerations for developing nucleic acid macromolecule based drug products. *Drug Discov. Today* **2016**, *21*, 430–444. [CrossRef]
35. Daugherty, A.L.; Mrsny, R.J. Formulation and delivery issues for monoclonal B antibody therapeutics. *Adv. Drug Del. Rev.* **2006**, *58*, 686–706. [CrossRef] [PubMed]
36. Pogocki, D.; Schoneich, C. Chemical stability of nucleic acid–derived drugs. *J. Pharm. Sci.* **2000**, *89*, 443–456. [CrossRef]
37. Evans, R.K.; Xu, Z.; Bohannon, K.E.; Wang, B.; Bruner, M.W.; Volkin, D.B. Evaluation of degradation pathways for plasmid DNA in pharmaceutical formulations via accelerated stability studies. *J. Pharm. Sci.* **2000**, *89*, 76–87. [CrossRef]
38. Frelon, S.; Douki, T.; Favier, A.; Cadet, J. Hydroxyl radical is not the main reactive species involved in the degradation of DNA bases by copper in the presence of hydrogen peroxide. *Chem. Res. Toxicol.* **2003**, *16*, 191–197. [CrossRef]
39. Nugraheni, R.; Mulyadi, N.; Yusuf, H. Freeze-dried liposome formulation for small molecules, nucleic acid, and protein delivery. *Sys. Rev. Pharm.* **2020**, *11*, 143–151.
40. Liang, W.; Chan, A.Y.; Chow, M.Y.; Lo, F.F.; Qiu, Y.; Kwok, P.C.L.; Lam, J.K. Spray freeze drying of small nucleic acids as inhaled powder for pulmonary delivery. *Asian J. Pharm. Sci.* **2018**, *13*, 163–172. [CrossRef]
41. Preston, K.B.; Randolph, T.W. Stability of lyophilized and spray dried vaccine formulations. *Adv. Drug Deliv. Rev.* **2021**, *171*, 50–61. [CrossRef] [PubMed]
42. Kubczak, M.; Michlewska, S.; Bryszewska, M.; Aigner, A.; Ionov, M. Nanoparticles for local delivery of siRNA in lung therapy. *Adv. Drug Deliv. Rev.* **2021**, *179*, 114038. [CrossRef] [PubMed]
43. Zoulikha, M.; Xiao, Q.; Boafo, G.F.; Sallam, M.A.; Chen, Z.; He, W. Pulmonary delivery of siRNA against acute lung injury/acute respiratory distress syndrome. *Acta Pharm. Sin. B* **2021**, *12*, 600–620. [CrossRef]
44. Uddin, M.; Roni, M. Challenges of storage and stability of mRNA-based COVID-19 vaccines. *Vaccines* **2021**, *9*, 1033. [CrossRef]
45. Packer, M.; Gyawali, D.; Yerabolu, R.; Schariter, J. White. A novel mechanism for the loss of mRNA activity in lipid nanoparticle delivery systems. *Nat. Commun.* **2021**, *12*, 6777. [CrossRef] [PubMed]
46. Zhao, P.; Hou, X.; Yan, J.; Du, S.; Xue, Y.; Li, W.; Xiang, G.; Dong, Y. Long-term storage of lipid-like nanoparticles for mRNA delivery. *Bioact. Mater.* **2020**, *5*, 358–363. [CrossRef]
47. Yadav, K.; Singh, M.R.; Rai, V.K.; Srivastava, N.; Yadav, N.P. Commercial aspects and market potential of novel delivery systems for bioactives and biological agents. In *Advances and Avenues in the Development of Novel Carriers for Bioactives and Biological Agents*; Academic Press: Cambridge, MA, USA, 2020; pp. 595–620.
48. Megahed, M.; El-Sawy, H.; El-Say, K. The promising expedition of the delivery systems for monoclonal antibodies. In *Advances in the Development of Novel Carriers for Bioactives and Biological Agents*; Academic Press: Cambridge, MA, USA, 2020; pp. 69–103.
49. Herkt, M.; Thum, T. Pharmacokinetics and proceedings in clinical application of nucleic acid therapeutics. *Mol. Ther.* **2021**, *29*, 521–539. [CrossRef]
50. Zhou, S.; Chen, W.; Cole, J.; Zhu, G. Delivery of nucleic acid therapeutics for cancer immunotherapy. *Med. Drug Discov.* **2020**, *6*, 100023. [CrossRef]
51. Chen, L.; Zhang, J.; Lin, Z.; Zhang, Z.; Mao, M.; Wu, J.; Li, Q.; Zhang, Y.; Fan, C. Pharmaceutical applications of framework nucleic acids. *Acta Pharm. Sin. B* **2021**, *12*, 76–91. [CrossRef]
52. Roberts, T.C.; Langer, R.; Wood, M.J.A. Advances in oligonucleotide drug delivery. *Nat. Rev. Drug Discov.* **2020**, *19*, 673–694. [CrossRef]
53. Hu, Q.; Li, H.; Wang, L.; Gu, H.; Fan, C. DNA nanotechnology-enabled drug delivery systems. *Chem. Rev.* **2019**, *119*, 6459–6506. [CrossRef] [PubMed]

54. Scheideler, M.; Vidakovic, I.; Prassl, R. Lipid nanocarriers for microRNA delivery. *Chem. Phys. Lipids* **2020**, *226*, 104837. [CrossRef] [PubMed]
55. Zhang, Y.; Davis, D.A.; AboulFotouh, K.; Wang, J.; Williams, D.; Bhambhani, A.; Zakrewsky, M.; Maniruzzaman, M.; Cui, Z.; Williams, R.O. Williams. Novel formulations and drug delivery systems to administer biological solids. *Adv. Drug Deliv. Rev.* **2021**, *172*, 183–210. [CrossRef] [PubMed]
56. Schulz-Siegmund, M.; Aigner, A. Nucleic acid delivery with extracellular vesicles. *Adv. Drug Deliv. Rev.* **2021**, *173*, 89–111. [CrossRef] [PubMed]
57. Pereira-Silva, M.; Jarak, I.; Alvarez-Lorenzo, C.; Concheiro, A.; Santos, A.C.; Veiga, F.; Figueiras, A. Micelleplexes as nucleic acid delivery systems for cancer-targeted therapies. *J. Control. Release* **2020**, *323*, 442–462. [CrossRef]
58. Asami, Y.; Yoshioka, K.; Nishina, K.; Nagata, T.; Yokota, T. Drug delivery system of therapeutic oligonucleotides. *Drug Discov. Ther.* **2016**, *10*, 256–262. [CrossRef]
59. Gupta, A.; Andresen, J.L.; Manan, R.S.; Langer, R. Nucleic acid delivery for therapeutic applications. *Adv. Drug Deliv. Rev.* **2021**, *178*, 113834. [CrossRef]
60. Fattal, E.; Fay, F. Nanomedicine-based delivery strategies for nucleic acid gene inhibitors in inflammatory diseases. *Adv. Drug Deliv. Rev.* **2021**, *175*, 113809. [CrossRef]
61. Patel, P.; Agrawal, Y. Targeting nanocarriers containing antisense oligonucleotides to cancer cell. *J. Drug Deliv. Sci. Technol.* **2017**, *37*, 97–114. [CrossRef]
62. Zafar, A.; Alruwaili, N.; Imam, S.; Alharbi, K.; Afzal, M.; Alotaibi, N.; Yasir, M.; Elmowafy, M.; Alshehri, S. Novel nanotechnology approaches for diagnosis and therapy of breast, ovarian and cervical cancer in female: A review. *J. Drug Del. Sci. Tech.* **2021**, *61*, 102198. [CrossRef]
63. Subhan, M.; Torchilin, V. siRNA based drug design, quality, delivery and clinical translation. *Nanomed. Nanotech. Bio. Med.* **2020**, *29*, 102239. [CrossRef] [PubMed]
64. Maurer, V.; Altin, S.; Seleci, D.A.; Zarinwall, A.; Temel, B.; Vogt, P.; Strauß, S.; Stahl, F.; Scheper, T.; Bucan, V. In-vitro application of magnetic hybrid niosomes: Targeted siRNA-delivery for enhanced breast cancer therapy. *Pharmaceutics* **2021**, *13*, 394. [CrossRef]
65. Aparajay, P.; Dev, A. Functionalized niosomes as a smart delivery device in cancer and fungal infection. *Eur. J. Pharm. Sci.* **2022**, *168*, 106052. [CrossRef] [PubMed]
66. Johnson, M.B.; Chandler, M.; Afonin, K.A. Nucleic acid nanoparticles (NANPs) as molecular tools to direct desirable and avoid undesirable immunological effects. *Adv. Drug Deliv. Rev.* **2021**, *173*, 427–438. [CrossRef] [PubMed]
67. Zhang, J.; Salaita, K. Smart nucleic acids as future therapeutics. *Trends Biotechnol.* **2021**, *39*, 1289–1307. [CrossRef]
68. He, S.; Wu, L.; Li, X.; Sun, H.; Xiong, T.; Liu, J.; Huang, C.; Xu, H.; Sun, H.; Chen, W.; et al. Metal–organic frameworks for advanced drug delivery. *Acta Pharm. Sin. B* **2021**, *11*, 2362–2395. [CrossRef]
69. Fan, Y.; Marioli, M.; Zhang, K. Analytical characterization of liposomes and other lipid nanoparticles for drug delivery. *J. Pharm. Biomed. Anal.* **2021**, *192*, 113642. [CrossRef]
70. Magar, K.T.; Boafo, G.F.; Li, X.; Chen, Z.; He, W. Liposome-based delivery of biological drugs. *Chin. Chem. Lett.* **2021**, *33*, 587–596. [CrossRef]
71. Wu, L.; Zhou, W.; Lin, L.; Chen, A.; Feng, J.; Qu, X.; Zhang, H.; Yue, J. Delivery of therapeutic oligonucleotides in nanoscale. *Bioact. Mater.* **2022**, *7*, 292–323. [CrossRef]
72. Anwar, M.; Muhammad, F.; Akhtar, B. Biodegradable nanoparticles as drug delivery devices. *Drug Deliv. Sci. Technol.* **2021**, *64*, 1026388. [CrossRef]
73. Subhan, M.; Torchilin, V. Efficient nanocarriers of siRNA therapeutics for cancer treatment. *Transl. Res.* **2019**, *214*, 62–91. [CrossRef] [PubMed]
74. Aminu, N.; Bello, I.; Umar, N.M.; Tanko, N.; Aminu, A.; Audu, M.M. The influence of nanoparticulate drug delivery systems in drug therapy. *J. Drug Deliv. Sci. Technol.* **2020**, *60*, 101961. [CrossRef]
75. Jin, J.-O.; Kim, G.; Hwang, J.; Han, K.H.; Kwak, M.; Lee, P.C. Nucleic acid nanotechnology for cancer treatment. *BBA-Rev. Cancer* **2020**, *1874*, 188377. [CrossRef] [PubMed]
76. Patnaik, S.; Gorain, B.; Padhi, S.; Choudhury, H.; Gabr, G.A.; Shadab; Mishra, D.K.; Kesharwani, P. Recent update of toxicity aspects of nanoparticulate systems for drug delivery. *Eur. J. Pharm. Biopharm.* **2021**, *161*, 100–119. [CrossRef]
77. Barani, M.; Bilal, M.; Sabir, F.; Rahdar, A.; Kyzas, G.Z. Nanotechnology in ovarian cancer: Diagnosis and treatment. *Life Sci.* **2021**, *266*, 118914. [CrossRef]
78. Ickenstein, L.M.; Garidel, P. Lipid-based nanoparticle formulations for small molecules and RNA drugs. *Expert Opin. Drug Deliv.* **2019**, *16*, 1205–1226. [CrossRef]
79. Saraf, S.; Jain, A.; Tiwari, A.; Verma, A.; Panda, P.K.; Jain, S.K. Advances in liposomal drug delivery to cancer: An overview. *J. Drug Deliv. Sci. Technol.* **2020**, *56*, 101549. [CrossRef]
80. Springer, A.; Dowdy, S. GalNAc-siRNA conjugates: Leading the way for delivery of RNAi therapeutics. *Nucleic Acid Ther.* **2018**, *28*, 109–118. [CrossRef]
81. Ponti, F.; Campolungo, M.; Melchiori, C.; Bono, N.; Candiani, G. Cationic lipids for gene delivery: Many players, one goal. *Chem. Phys. Lipids* **2021**, *235*, 105032. [CrossRef]
82. Piotrowski-Daspit, A.S.; Kauffman, A.C.; Bracaglia, L.G.; Saltzman, W.M. Polymeric vehicles for nucleic acid delivery. *Adv. Drug Deliv. Rev.* **2020**, *156*, 119–132. [CrossRef]

83. Blakney, A.K.; McKay, P.F.; Hu, K.; Samnuan, K.; Jain, N.; Brown, A.; Thomas, A.; Rogers, P.; Polra, K.; Sallah, H.; et al. Polymeric and lipid nanoparticles for delivery of self-amplifying RNA vaccines. *J. Control. Release* **2021**, *338*, 201–210. [CrossRef] [PubMed]
84. Shah, A.; Aftab, S.; Nisar, J.; Naeem, M.; Faiza, A.; Iftikhar, J. Nanocarriers for targeted drug delivery. *J. Drug Del. Sci. Tech.* **2021**, *62*, 102426. [CrossRef]
85. Junquera, E.; Aicart, E. Recent progress in gene therapy to deliver nucleic acids with multivalent cationic vectors. *Adv. Colloid Interface Sci.* **2016**, *233*, 161–175. [CrossRef]
86. Hayat, S.M.G.; Farahani, N.; Safdarian, E.; Roointan, A.; Sahebkar, A. Gene delivery using lipoplexes and polyplexes: Principles, limitations and solutions. *Crit. Rev. Eukaryot. Gene Expr.* **2019**, *29*, 29–36. [CrossRef] [PubMed]
87. Tan, X.; Jia, F.; Wang, P.; Zhang, K. Nucleic acid-based drug delivery strategies. *J. Control. Release* **2020**, *323*, 240–252. [CrossRef]
88. Ndwandwe, D.; Wiysonge, C. COVID-19 vaccines. *Curr. Opin. Immunol.* **2021**, *71*, 111–116. [CrossRef]
89. Begum, A.A.; Toth, I.; Hussein, W.M.; Moyle, P.M. Advances in targeted gene delivery. *Curr. Drug Deliv.* **2019**, *16*, 588–608. [CrossRef]
90. Swingle, K.L.; Hamilton, A.G.; Mitchell, M.J. Lipid nanoparticle-mediated delivery of mRNA therapeutics and vaccines. *Trends Mol. Med.* **2021**, *27*, 616–617. [CrossRef]
91. Gupta, V.; Lourenço, S.P.; Hidalgo, I.J. Development of gene therapy vectors: Remaining challenges. *J. Pharm. Sci.* **2021**, *110*, 1915–1920. [CrossRef]
92. Zbacnik, T.J.; Holcomb, R.E.; Katayama, D.S.; Murphy, B.M.; Payne, R.W.; Coccaro, R.C.; Evans, G.J.; Matsuura, J.E.; Henry, C.S.; Manning, M.C. Role of buffers in protein formulations. *J. Pharm. Sci.* **2017**, *106*, 713–733. [CrossRef]
93. Zhong, H.; Chan, G.; Hu, Y.; Hu, H.; Ouyang, D. A comprehensive map of FDA-approved pharmaceutical products. *Pharmaceutics* **2018**, *10*, 263. [CrossRef] [PubMed]
94. Le, T.K.; Paris, C.; Khan, K.S.; Robson, F.; Ng, W.-L.; Rocchi, P. Nucleic acid-based technologies targeting coronaviruses. *Trends Biochem. Sci.* **2021**, *46*, 351–365. [CrossRef] [PubMed]
95. Roncarolo, M.G. Gene Therapy. *N. Eng. J. Med.* **2019**. Available online: https://www.xianjichina.com/news/details_141521.html (accessed on 14 November 2022).
96. van den Berg, A.I.S.; Yun, C.O.; Schiffelers, R.M.; Hennink, W.E. Polymeric delivery systems for nucleic acid therapeutics: Approaching the clinic. *J. Control. Release* **2021**, *331*, 121–141. [CrossRef] [PubMed]
97. Kulkarni, J.A.; Witzigmann, D.; Thomson, S.B.; Chen, S.; Leavitt, B.R.; Cullis, P.R.; van der Meel, R. The current landscape of nucleic acid therapeutics. *Nat. Nanotechnol.* **2021**, *16*, 630–643. [CrossRef]
98. Srivastava, A.; Mallela, K.M.; Deorkar, N.; Brophy, G. Manufacturing challenges and rational formulation development for AAV viral vectors. *J. Pharm. Sci.* **2021**, *110*, 2609–2624. [CrossRef]
99. Reichmuth, A.M.; Oberli, M.A.; Jaklenec, A.; Langer, R.; Blankschtein, D. mRNA vaccine delivery using lipid nanoparticles. *Ther. Deliv.* **2016**, *7*, 319–334. [CrossRef]
100. Pilkington, E.H.; Suys, E.J.; Trevaskis, N.L.; Wheatley, A.K.; Zukancic, D.; Algarni, A.; Al-Wassiti, H.; Davis, T.P.; Pouton, C.W.; Kent, S.J.; et al. From influenza to COVID-19: Lipid nanoparticle mRNA vaccines at the frontiers of infectious diseases. *Acta Biomater.* **2021**, *131*, 16–40. [CrossRef]
101. Buschmann, M.; Carrasco, M.; Alishetty, S.; Paige, M.; Alameh, M.; Weissman, D. Nanomaterial delivery systems for mRNA vaccines. *Vaccines* **2021**, *9*, 65. [CrossRef] [PubMed]
102. Rosa, S.S.; Prazeres, D.M.F.; Azevedo, A.M.; Marques, M.P.C. mRNA vaccines manufacturing: Challenges and bottlenecks. *Vaccine* **2021**, *39*, 2190–2200. [CrossRef]
103. Li, B.; Zhang, X.; Dong, Y. Nanoscale platforms for messenger RNA delivery. *WIREs Nanomed. Nanobiotechnol.* **2019**, *18*, e1530. [CrossRef]
104. Quemener, A.; Bachelot, L.; Forestier, A.; Donnou-Fournet, E.; Gilot, D.; Galibert, M. The powerful world of antisense oligonucleotides: From bench to bedside. *Wiley Interdiscip. Rev. RNA* **2020**, *11*, e1594. [CrossRef] [PubMed]
105. Beg, S.; Almalki, W.H.; Khatoon, F.; Alharbi, K.S.; Alghamdi, S.; Akhter, H.; Khalilullah, H.; Baothman, A.A.; Hafeez, A.; Rahman, M.; et al. Lipid and polymer-based nanocomplexes in nucleic acid delivery as cancer vaccines. *Drug Discov. Today* **2021**, *26*, 1891–1903. [CrossRef] [PubMed]
106. Mukalel, A.; Riley, R.; Zhang, R.; Mitchell, M. Nanoparticles for nucleic acid delivery: Applications in cancer immunotherapy. *Cancer Lett.* **2019**, *458*, 102–112. [CrossRef] [PubMed]
107. Rafael, D.; Andrade, F.; Arranja, A.; Luís, S.; Videira, M. Lipoplexes and polyplexes: Gene therapy. In *Encyclopedia of Biomedical Polymers and Polymeric Biomaterials*; CRC Press: Boca Raton, FL, USA, 2015; pp. 4335–4347.
108. Yang, Y.; Qin, Z.; Zeng, W.; Yang, T.; Cao, Y.; Mei, C.; Kuang, Y. Toxicity assessment of nanoparticles in various systems and organs. *Nanotechnol. Rev.* **2017**, *6*, 279–289. [CrossRef]
109. Kim, J.; Eygeris, Y.; Gupta, M.; Sahay, G. Self-assembled mRNA vaccines. *Adv. Drug Deliv. Rev.* **2021**, *170*, 83–112. [CrossRef] [PubMed]
110. Machhi, J.; Shahjin, F.; Das, S.; Patel, M.; Abdelmoaty, M.; Cohen, J. Nanocarrier vaccines for SARS-CoV-2. *Adv. Drug Deliv. Rev.* **2021**, *171*, 215–239. [CrossRef] [PubMed]
111. Han, H.; Nwagwu, C.; Anyim, O.; Ekweremadu, C.; Kim, S. COVID-19 and cancer: From basic mechanisms to vaccine development using nanotechnology. *Int. Immunopharmacol.* **2021**, *90*, 107247. [CrossRef]

112. Hassett, K.J.; Higgins, J.; Woods, A.; Levy, B.; Xia, Y.; Hsiao, C.J.; Acosta, E.; Almarsson, Ö.; Moore, M.J.; Brito, L.A. Impact of lipid nanoparticle size on mRNA vaccine immunogenicity. *J. Control. Release* **2021**, *335*, 237–246. [CrossRef] [PubMed]
113. Piyush, R.; Rajarshi, K.; Chatterjee, A.; Khan, R.; Ray, S. Nucleic acid-based therapy for coronavirus disease. *Heliyon* **2020**, *6*, e05007. [CrossRef]
114. Available online: https://go.drugbank.com (accessed on 10 December 2022).
115. Yamada, Y. Nucleic acid drugs—Current status, issues, and expectations for exosomes. *Cancers* **2021**, *13*, 5002. [CrossRef]
116. Geary, R.S. Antisense oligonucleotide pharmacokinetics and metabolism. *Expert Opin. Drug Metab. Toxicol.* **2009**, *5*, 381–391. [CrossRef] [PubMed]
117. Nema, S.; Brendel, R.J.; Chan, E.; Maa, Y.-F.; Overcashier, D.; Hsu, C.C. Excipients and their role in approved injectable products: Current usage and future directions. *PDA J. Pharm. Sci. Technol.* **2011**, *65*, 287–332. [CrossRef]
118. Kamerzell, T.; Esfandiary, R.; Joshi, S.; Middaugh, C.; Volkin, D. Protein–excipient interactions: Mechanisms and biophysical characterization applied to protein formulation development. *Adv. Drug Deliv. Rev.* **2011**, *63*, 1118–1159. [CrossRef]
119. Rayaprolu, B.M.; Strawser, J.J.; Anyarambhatla, G. Excipients in parenteral formulations: Selection considerations and effective utilization with small molecules and biologics. *Drug Dev. Ind. Pharm.* **2018**, *44*, 1565–1571. [CrossRef] [PubMed]
120. Available online: https://USFDA.org (accessed on 12 December 2022).
121. Poecheim, J.; Graeser, K.A.; Hoernschemeyer, J.; Becker, G.; Storch, K.; Printz, M. Development of stable liquid formulations for oligonucleotides. *Eur. J. Pharm. Biopharm.* **2018**, *129*, 80–87. [CrossRef] [PubMed]
122. Shapiro, R.; Klein, R.S. The deamination of cytidine and cytosine by acidic buffer solutions-mutagenic implications. *Biochemistry* **1966**, *5*, 2358–2362. [CrossRef] [PubMed]
123. Tanaka, K.; Okamoto, A. Degradation of DNA by bisulfite treatment. *Bioorganic Med. Chem. Lett.* **2007**, *17*, 1912–1915. [CrossRef] [PubMed]
124. Thorat, A.; Munjal, B.; Geders, T.; Suryanarayanan, R. Freezing-induced protein aggregation—Role of pH shift and potential mitigation strategies. *J. Control. Release* **2020**, *323*, 591–599. [CrossRef]
125. Garidel, P.; Pevestorf, B.; Bahrenburg, S. Stability of buffer-free freeze-dried formulations: A feasibility study of a monoclonal antibody at high protein concentrations. *Eur. J. Pharm. Biopharm.* **2015**, *97*, 125–139. [CrossRef]
126. Rosales-Mendoza, S.; Wong-Arce, A.; de Lourdes Betancourt-Mendiola, M. RNA-based vaccines against SARS-CoV-2. In *Biomedical Innovations to Combat COVID-19*; Academic Press: Cambridge, MA, USA, 2022; pp. 129–152.
127. Hovorka, S.; Schoneich, C. Oxidative degradation of pharmaceuticals: Theory, mechanisms and inhibition. *J. Pharm. Sci.* **2001**, *90*, 253–269. [CrossRef]
128. Ball, R.; Bajaj, P.; Whitehead, K. Achieving long-term stability of lipid nano particles: Examining the effect of pH, temperature, and lyophilization. *Int. J. Nanomed.* **2017**, *12*, 305–315. [CrossRef]
129. Suzuki, Y.; Ishihara, H. Difference in the lipid nanoparticle technology employed in three approved siRNA (patisiran) and mRNA (COVID-19 vaccine) drugs. *Drug Metab. Pharmacokinet.* **2021**, *41*, 100424. [CrossRef]
130. Kon, E.; Elia, U.; Peer, D. Principles for designing an optimal mRNA lipid nanoparticle vaccine. *Curr. Opin. Biotechnol.* **2022**, *73*, 329–336. [CrossRef] [PubMed]
131. Jain, S.; Venkataraman, A.; Wechsler, M.E.; Peppas, N.A. Peppas. Messenger RNA-based vaccines: Past, present, and future directions in the context of the COVID-19 pandemic. *Adv. Drug Deliv. Rev.* **2021**, *179*, 114000. [CrossRef]
132. Rauch, S.; Roth, N.; Schwendt, K.; Fotin-Mleczek, M.; Mueller, S.; Petsch, B. mRNA- based SARS-CoV-2 vaccine candidate CVnCoV induces high levels of virus-neutralizing antibodies and mediates protection in rodents. *NPJ Vaccine* **2021**, *6*, 57. [CrossRef] [PubMed]
133. Dolgin, E. CureVac COVID vaccine let-down spotlights mRNA design challenges. *Nature* **2021**, *594*, 483. [CrossRef]
134. de Alwis, R.; Gan, E.; Chen, S.; Leong, Y.; Tan, H.; Zhang, S.; Yau, C.; Low, J.; Kalimuddin, S.; Matsuda, D. A single dose of self-transcribing and replicating RNA-based SARS-CoV-2 vaccine produces protective adaptive immunity in mice. *Mol. Ther.* **2021**, *29*, 1970–1983. [CrossRef]
135. Zhang, N.-N.; Li, X.-F.; Deng, Y.-Q.; Zhao, H.; Huang, Y.-J.; Yang, G.; Huang, W.-J.; Gao, P.; Zhou, C.; Zhang, R.-R.; et al. A thermostable mRNA vaccine against COVID-19. *Cell* **2020**, *182*, 1271–1283.e16. [CrossRef]
136. Kobiyama, K.; Imai, M.; Jounai, N.; Nakayama, M.; Hioki, K.; Iwatsuki-Horimoto, K.; Yamayoshi, S.; Tsuchida, J.; Niwa, T.; Suzuki, T.; et al. Optimization of an LNP-mRNA vaccine candidate targeting SARS-CoV-2 receptor-binding domain. *bioRxiv* **2021**. [CrossRef]
137. McKay, P.F.; Hu, K.; Blakney, A.K.; Samnuan, K.; Brown, J.C.; Penn, R.; Zhou, J.; Bouton, C.R.; Rogers, P.; Polra, K.; et al. Self amplifying RNA SARS-CoV-2 lipid nanoparticle vaccine candidate induces high neutralizing antibody titers in mice. *Nat. Commun.* **2020**, *11*, 3523. [CrossRef] [PubMed]
138. Shuai, Q.; Zhu, F.; Zhao, M.; Yan, Y. mRNA delivery via non-viral carriers for biomedical applications. *Int. J. Pharm.* **2021**, *607*, 121020. [CrossRef] [PubMed]
139. Guzman-Villanueva, D.; El-Sherbiny, I.M.; Herrera-Ruiz, D.; Vlassov, A.V.; Smyth, H.D. Formulation approaches to short interfering RNA and MicroRNA: Challenges and implications. *J. Pharm. Sci.* **2012**, *101*, 4046–4066. [CrossRef] [PubMed]
140. Available online: http://www.xenon-pharma.com/glybera/ (accessed on 15 October 2022).
141. Available online: http://www.drugs.com/uk/glybera.html (accessed on 10 December 2022).

142. Muralidhara, B.K.; Wong, M. Critical considerations in the formulation development of parenteral biologic drugs. *Drug Discov. Today* **2020**, *25*, 574–581. [CrossRef] [PubMed]
143. Mastrobattista, E. Formulation and delivery solutions for the next generation biotherapeutics. *J. Control. Release* **2021**, *336*, 583–597. [CrossRef]

Disclaimer/Publisher's Note: The statements, opinions and data contained in all publications are solely those of the individual author(s) and contributor(s) and not of MDPI and/or the editor(s). MDPI and/or the editor(s) disclaim responsibility for any injury to people or property resulting from any ideas, methods, instructions or products referred to in the content.

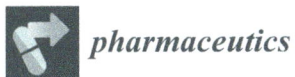

Review

Novel Developments to Enable Treatment of CNS Diseases with Targeted Drug Delivery

Axel H. Meyer [1,*], Thomas M. Feldsien [2], Mario Mezler [1], Christopher Untucht [3], Ramakrishna Venugopalan [2] and Didier R. Lefebvre [2]

1. Quantitative, Translational & ADME Sciences, AbbVie Deutschland GmbH & Co. KG, Knollstraße, 67061 Ludwigshafen, Germany
2. Drug Delivery and Combination Products, Development Sciences, AbbVie Inc., 1 N Waukegan Road, North Chicago, IL 60064, USA
3. Neuroscience Discovery, AbbVie Deutschland GmbH & Co. KG, Knollstraße, 67061 Ludwigshafen, Germany
* Correspondence: axel.meyer@abbvie.com

Abstract: The blood-brain barrier (BBB) is a major hurdle for the development of systemically delivered drugs against diseases of the central nervous system (CNS). Because of this barrier there is still a huge unmet need for the treatment of these diseases, despite years of research efforts across the pharmaceutical industry. Novel therapeutic entities, such as gene therapy and degradomers, have become increasingly popular in recent years, but have not been the focus for CNS indications so far. To unfold their full potential for the treatment of CNS diseases, these therapeutic entities will most likely have to rely on innovative delivery technologies. Here we will describe and assess approaches, both invasive and non-invasive, that can enable, or at least increase, the probability of a successful drug development of such novel therapeutics for CNS indications.

Keywords: central nervous system; blood brain barrier; drug delivery; degradomer; nanoparticles; exosomes; focused ultrasound; convection enhanced delivery; intracerebroventricular delivery

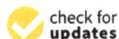

Citation: Meyer, A.H.; Feldsien, T.M.; Mezler, M.; Untucht, C.; Venugopalan, R.; Lefebvre, D.R. Novel Developments to Enable Treatment of CNS Diseases with Targeted Drug Delivery. *Pharmaceutics* 2023, 15, 1100. https://doi.org/10.3390/pharmaceutics15041100

Academic Editors: Vibhuti Agrahari and Prashant Kumar

Received: 21 December 2022
Revised: 7 March 2023
Accepted: 17 March 2023
Published: 29 March 2023

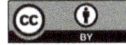

Copyright: © 2023 by the authors. Licensee MDPI, Basel, Switzerland. This article is an open access article distributed under the terms and conditions of the Creative Commons Attribution (CC BY) license (https://creativecommons.org/licenses/by/4.0/).

1. Introduction

A major challenge in the development of treatments against central nervous system (CNS) diseases is ensuring sufficient exposure to target brain tissues to achieve the desired therapeutic effects. A disappointing 98% of small molecule drugs never reach the brain at therapeutic concentrations [1]. The situation is even worse for large-molecule drugs such as antibodies or nucleic-acid based therapeutics. For example, only 0.01–0.1% of a systemically administered dose of antibody will reach the brain, which is often insufficient to elicit a therapeutic effect [2,3]. In the case of naked nucleic acid-based therapeutics such as oligonucleotides, achieving efficient brain tissue exposure would not even be possible without the use of a carrier system [4].

The root cause is the blood-brain barrier (BBB). This complex, multi-cellular and dynamic interface between the blood circulation and the brain tightly preserves brain homeostasis. It enables passage of specific nutrients such as glucose, fatty acids, and amino acids, while at the same time blocking the passage of harmful substances [5]. In doing do, it also acts as a barrier to large therapeutic molecules.

To overcome the BBB, a wide range of delivery technologies, both invasive and non-invasive, have been developed. Receptor-mediated transcytosis (RMT), one of the most advanced, has reached the clinic and holds promise for the delivery of biotherapeutics such as antibodies or enzyme replacement therapies. Since non-invasive approaches to cross the BBB are well covered elsewhere [6], they are not included in this review.

Therapeutic modalities have become more diverse with the advent of gene therapies and degradomers, both of which may require optimized brain delivery systems tailored to their specific needs. The increasing number of gene therapies, both in development and on the market, as well as the ongoing development of degradomers make the challenge of developing efficient delivery technologies for such therapeutic modalities even more pressing.

This realization led us to look at the status of gene therapy and degradomer approaches for CNS indications and to review several delivery technologies for their potential to enable a successful CNS drug development for these types of molecules. The non-invasive approaches include nanoparticles and exosomes. We cover recent medical technology innovations for gene therapy applications and degradomers.

In the final sections, we include a brief survey of medical devices enabling drug delivery, either to the whole brain, or to more localized regions of the brain or the spine: intrathecal (IT), intra-cerebroventricular (ICV), convection-enhanced delivery (CED) and focused ultrasound (FUS).

The central theme that emerges from our review is that delivering a wide range of therapeutics to the brain requires tailored technical solutions, each optimizing the pharmacokinetic profile in brain tissues to achieve therapeutic levels. We show that a convergence between medical technology (MedTech) and pharmacology is increasingly needed to achieve efficacy while reducing side effects associated with off-target exposure.

1.1. Use of Gene Therapy for the Treatment of CNS Indications

Gene therapy aims at modifying a patient's genes for disease treatment by either gene replacement, gene inactivation or by gene introduction. Such approaches can be divided into two categories, viral and non-viral approaches. Historically, approval for gene therapy-based drug products has not been a focus for central nervous system indications. Gene therapy trials have covered a wide range of indications including cancer, monogenic diseases, infectious diseases, and cardiovascular diseases. In 2017 Ginn et al. listed 2597 gene therapy clinical trials for all these indications. Only 47 covered neurological diseases comprising less than 2% of gene therapy trials [7]. This is reflected in the gene therapy products that have reached the market. Even though the first gene therapy product, Gendicíne, was approved in 2003, it took until 2016 for the first gene therapy-based CNS drug, Spinraza, to reach the market. Interestingly, the situation is starting to change. Three more gene therapies for CNS indications have reached the market since 2016, as illustrated in Table 1. Overall, four out of 16 marketed gene or cell therapy products are directed against CNS diseases.

Table 1. Approved gene therapy-based drugs for the treatment of CNS diseases.

Approved	Drug	Indication	Delivery System & Route of Administration	Therapeutic
2016	Spinraza	Spinal Muscular Atrophy	(intrathecal)	Antisense oligonucleotide against SMN2
	Luxturna	Inherited Blind Diseases	Adeno-associated virus Type 2 (subretinal injection)	Retinal pigment epithelium-specific 65 kDa protein
	Brineura	Batten's Disease	(intra-cerebroventricular)	Recombinant TPP1
2019	Zolgensma	Spinal Muscular Atrophy	Adeno-associated Virus Type 9 (intravenous)	SMN1
2021	Delytact	Malignant Glioma	Herpes Simplex Virus Type 1 (intra-tumor)	(oncolytic)

It is worth mention mentioning that these treatments do not rely on systemic application of the gene therapy-based drugs. The commercial approval in 2016 of Spinraza®, an antisense oligonucleotide for the treatment of spinal muscular atrophy (SMA), and subsequent commercial approval in 2017 of Brineura®, a hydrolytic lysosomal N-terminal tripeptidyl peptidase for the treatment of Batten disease, indicates that pharma organizations view the benefits of intrathecal (IT) and intracerebroventricular (ICV) routes of delivery as outweighing limitations (e.g., invasiveness) in the case of niche markets for orphan drugs in the neuroscience space. The commercial approval in 2019 of Zolgensma®, also for the treatment of SMA, represents the first adeno-associated virus (AAV) based drug for a CNS indication [8]. This was followed in 2021 by Delytact which received conditional and time-limited marketing approval for malignant glioma in Japan. To gain more insight into what direction the field is taking we performed a survey in clinicaltrials.gov to identify gene therapy clinical trials specifically for the following neuroscience indications:

Alzheimer's Disease (AD), Parkinson's Disease (PD), Huntington's Disease (HD), Gaucher Disease, Lou Gehrig's Disease (ALS), and Frontotemporal Dementia (FTD). Approximately 3750 results were identified in the search query, and from the query, 16 on-going benchmark trials. The search algorithm at clinicaltrials.gov also searches for synonyms and related terms. The executed search query included the terms 'gene therapy', 'viral vector', 'AAV', 'lentivirus', 'antisense', and 'oligonucleotide'. The query identified approximately 3750 records which included related terms such as 'gene', 'gene transfer', 'DNA therapy', 'therapy', 'treatment', 'therapeutic', 'viral vector', 'viral', 'virus' and 'vector'. The search results then had to be narrowed down using data filtering to identify representative gene therapy studies in the target indications.

A summary of the on-going trials with a clinical phase, associated routes of administration and study duration is given in Table 2. Interestingly, none of the clinical trials utilize systemic delivery or intra-cerebroventricular delivery as a route of administration for gene therapy assets in these indications. Given that viral vectors such as AAV stimulate the immune system after systemic application, a targeted application is a feasible way to reduce/avoid activation of the immune system. Furthermore, only AAV serotypes 8 and 9 have been reported to cross the BBB and enter the brain. Nonetheless, the example of Zolgensma shows that systemic application is possible for a CNS disease.

Table 2. On-going Gene Therapy Trials and Routes of Administration by Disease Indication.

Route of Administration (No. of Studies)	AD	PD	FTD	HD	Gaucher	ALS
Systemic (0)	0	0	0	0	0	0
Intra-Cisterna Magna (5)	NCT03634007 Ph.1/2 2018–2023 (est) NRP	NCT04127578 Ph.1/2 2020–2028 (est) NRP	NCT04747431 Ph.1/2 2021–2027 (est) NRP NCT04408625 Ph.1/2 2020–2027 (est) NRP	0	NCT04411654 Ph.1/2 2021–2028 (est) NRP	0
Intrathecal (4)	NCT03186989 Ph.1/2 2017–2022 NRP	NCT03976349 Ph.1 2019–2023 (est) NRP	0	0	0	NCT04494256 Ph.1/2 2020–2026 (est) NRP NCT04856982 Ph.3 2021–2027 (est) NRP
Intra-Parenchymal (7)	0	NCT01621581 Ph.1 Convection-enhanced delivery 2013–2022 RP [9] NCT04167540 Ph.1 Bilateral image-guided infusion 2020–2027 (est) NRP NCT3720418 Ph.1/2 Neurosurgical delivery 2018–2022 RP [10]	0	NCT04120493 Ph.1/2 MRI-guided infusion 2019–2029 (est) NRP	0	0

Table 2. *Cont.*

Route of Administration (No. of Studies)	AD	PD	FTD	HD	Gaucher	ALS
		NCT01856439 Ph.1/2 Bilateral injection 2011–2022 RP [11] NCT03065192 Ph.1 Neurosurgical infusion 2017–2021 RP [12] NCT03562494 Ph.2 Brain infusion 2018–2023 (est) RP [9]				

NRP = no results posted on www.clinicaltrials.gov (accessed on 16 January 2023); RP = results published; est = estimated study completion date.

1.2. Use of Degradomers for the Treatment of Neurodegenerative Diseases

While gene therapy treatments have made it to the clinics and to the market, even for the treatment of CNS diseases, degradomers are at an earlier stage. Degradomers utilize the intrinsic protein degradation machinery of the cell to remove unwanted, overexpressed, dysfunctional, or dysregulated protein targets [13]. They exist in different forms, which include PROTACs (PROteolysis TArgeting Chimeras), employing the cellular "quality control" machinery to eliminate unwanted proteins [14], AUTACs (AUtophagy-TArgeting Chimera) [15], leading the target into the autophagy mechanism, lysosome targeting chimeras (LYTACs) [16], molecules activating the endoplasmic reticulum-associated degradation (ERAD) pathway, and molecular glues, which transform the target to be structurally modified or tagged as unwanted, and to be destroyed. The degradomers can be differentiated into hetero-bifunctional molecules, including PROTACs, AUTACs, LYTACs and ERAD-pathway targeted molecules, and monofunctional compounds, which are the molecular glues. As the published dataset on PROTACs is currently the largest, we focus on this modality for the hetero-bifunctional molecules. It is expected that the relevance of the AUTACs, LYTACs and ERADs will expand in the future.

Molecular glues mediate their efficacy through proximity-induced degradation [17]. The molecules represent proximity-inducing monofunctional agents, which can have multiple biological effects in the cell. For example, by bringing functional proteins into proximity, or changing the structure of a single protein, they can influence cell signaling, interact with the immune system, remodel chromatin, and also lead to an interaction of the protein of interest (POI) with the ubiquitination system of the cell, which leads to its degradation. For example, Thalidomide and lenalidomide mediate this effect [18], which is described in more detail below in the context of the PROTACs.

As described above, while molecular glues are monofunctional with a relatively low molecular weight, chemical PROTACs are hetero-bifunctional molecules and consist of one binding site for the protein of interest (POI), a linker, and a binding site to the functional cellular protein, which leads the POI towards degradation. Thus, they are generally relatively large, with a molecular weight ranging from 500 to 1000 Da. While they are still comparatively small compared to monoclonal antibodies or peptide or nucleotide drugs, for example, their size causes physicochemical problems, which often leads to low solubility and low permeability across biological membranes. This potentially limits utility for the treatment of CNS diseases, particularly because of the resulting low penetration across the BBB.

Structurally, PROTACs contain a binding site for a specific intracellular ubiquitin ligase or a key autophagy functional protein (LC3), a linker of different lengths and constituents, and a binding site for the POI. PROTACs and AUTACs are, therefore, hetero-bifunctional molecules that bind to the POI and link it to an E3 ubiquitin ligase (PROTAC) through reversible interaction with binding sites on either molecule. By interacting with the E3 ligase the POI is (poly)-ubiquitinated and therefore labeled to undergo intracellular protein degradation in the ubiquitin-proteasome system (UPS; PROTAC).

Current PROTACs bind primarily to Cereblon (CRBN) and von Hippel-Lindau Ligands (VHL) E3 ligases. Current efforts include identifying additional potential ligases, as the CRBL and VHL ligases are expressed ubiquitously, and thus might lead to non-specific and broad-based protein degradation in all tissues. Therefore, more selectively expressed, and more specific ligase binders might lead to a more selective degradation of the POI only in the target tissues [19].

Degradomers have a number of promising advantages over conventional small chemical entities, which include the potential for an effective knock-down of the POI, similar to gene therapy or ribonucleic acid interference (RNAi) approaches, the potential for a catalytical activity, which could alleviate the issue associated with the need to achieve continuously high concentrations of the molecule within the target tissue and cell, and the potential of a selective suppression of certain mutated POIs, which might make it possible for the functional protein allele to take over the activity.

Despite the range of targets and disease states investigated preclinically, the clinical success of hetero-bifunctional degraders is so far limited, and currently described by PROTAC examples only. Nine clinical studies sponsored by Arvinas (NCT03888612, NCT04072952), Celgene (NCT04428788), Kymera (NCT04772885), Nurix (NCT04830137), Haisco Pharmaceutical (NCT04861779), Dialectic Therapeutics (NCT04886622), EnhancedBIO (NCT04669587) and BeiGene (NCT05006716) are currently ongoing. All are in Ph. 1 or Ph. 1/2, mostly for the treatment of cancer and dermatological applications. To date the only clinically relevant study demonstrating efficacy of PROTACs in humans was published in 2020 for the treatment of cancer [20]. The number of PROTAC compounds entering Ph1 clinical trials is rapidly increasing. There are currently over 18 such molecules that are either in dosing or approved for clinical trials, with several more anticipated in 2023. In addition, there have been data releases at conferences and company updates showing data for at least three ongoing programs that have achieved proof of target degradation in humans. Therefore, the degradomer field, spearheaded by PROTACs, is rapidly evolving and sustained publication of clinical efficacy studies is expected. The theoretical potential of degraders for CNS diseases is being investigated in numerous labs. In this context PROTACs have been developed for a range of CNS diseases. Preclinically, they have been described to successfully target tau, α-syn, mutant huntingtin (mHtt), and superoxide dismutase 1 (SOD1) in cellular and animal models. Diseases which are studied in preclinical models include Alzheimer's disease (AD), Parkinson's disease (PD), Huntington's disease (HD), amyotrophic lateral sclerosis (ALS), as well as glioblastoma multiforme (GBM). The advantages of hetero-bifunctional degraders described above also come with challenges for treating CNS diseases. They include the limited penetration across the BBB due to the large size and bulky structure, the non-specific degradation of the POI across the whole CNS, instead of targeted degradation in the affected brain region, the concomitant reduction of proteolytic activity in different neurodegenerative disease states [21], and the transient nature of activity, which requires continuous or multiple treatments throughout the chronic phase of the neurodegenerative disease [22].

The reports describing efficacy of hetero-bifunctional degraders in preclinical in vivo models for CNS diseases are therefore limited. The first published study evaluated peptides with hetero-bifunctional PROTAC activity in in vitro and in vivo models of AD [23]. Compound TH006, a peptide consisting of 32 amino acids, was dosed at 15 mg/kg/day for 10 days in a combination of intranasal and intravenous route of application. The PROTAC reduced cortical Tau levels, as well as Tau in the hippocampus to a lesser extent, in 3xTg-AD mice (B6; 129-Psen1tm1Mpm Tg [APPSwe, Tau P301L] 1Lfa/Mmjax). While the exposure of the compound in the brain was not directly demonstrated in the study, apparently enough TH006 reached the relevant brain structures to modulate Tau levels in the brain of the animals. Arvinas demonstrated the effective penetration of selected PROTAC® degraders through the BBB. As described in a press release, their reference compounds reached brain-to-plasma ratios greater than one. As a result of brain exposure lasting longer than systemic circulation, this ratio rose to 8.9 four hours after dosing. The patent describes efficacy studies with several examples of compounds. Example four reduced total Tau after intra-hippocampal injection in a time-dependent manner in Bl6 mice. Exemplary compounds 82 and 382 demonstrated a 95% reduction of pathological Tau in TG2508 mice after 24 h at doses of 15 and 30 mg/kg, respectively, via parenteral dosing.

While the published results indicate the relevance of hetero-bifunctional degraders for the treatment of CNS disorders, the number of in vivo studies is still limited. There is also not yet a clear understanding of the potential influence of formulations for the penetration of the molecules into the brain. Further studies are required to translate the in vitro results in different cellular models into preclinical in vivo models of neurodegenerative diseases. Translation from rodents to humans is yet another critical step.

Due to their large size, their low permeability across the BBB and complex mode of action, it is not yet fully clear which systemic concentrations are needed to mediate an effect on brain targets. A clear strategy for optimization of the brain availability by rational drug design is not yet available. Therefore, besides serendipitous optimization of the compound structure, the next steps towards functional brain degradomers could be to evaluate methods to increase the systemic exposure of the compound, for example by increasing the circulating drug concentration, or to enhance the systemic half-life through specific slow-release systemic formulations, or to open or circumvent the BBB. Methods for the latter two aspects are exemplified in the present paper.

2. Systemic Delivery

2.1. Nanoparticles

Nanoparticles, such as liposomes, polymeric nanoparticles, and lipid nanoparticles (LNPs), typically have a diameter between 10 and 300 nm. They differ in size, charge, chemical composition and surface properties [24–26]. The first nanoformulations received approval for cancer therapy more than 20 years ago following the discovery of nanoparticles having the potential for increased accumulation in tumor tissue by extravasation through fenestrated blood vessels, a phenomenon termed enhanced permeability and retention (EPR). Several nanoparticle formulations were approved for chemotherapy, for the treatment of fungal infections, hepatitis A and end-stage renal diseases. However, so far only one formulation, Copaxone, has been approved for multiple sclerosis as early as 1996 in the United States and 2001 in the European Union (EU), and to our knowledge is one of the only approved nanoformulation for a CNS disease. Another example is Invega, an intramuscular depot approved by the EU in 2011. However, Invega does not enter the brain directly but increases residence time of the active compound in the blood. Recently, efforts have centered around LNPs, which have found use in COVID vaccinations such as Comirnaty and have proven the therapeutic applicability of these formulations for nucleic acid delivery. To this end Pfizer has entered a four-year research collaboration with Beam Therapeutics utilizing Beam's LNP-based in vivo delivery technology to deliver messenger RNA (mRNA) for gene editing programs for rare diseases in different organs, one being the CNS.

The fact that nanoparticles have only found limited therapeutic uses, especially for the CNS [27], can be attributed to several critical factors such as physicochemical properties, biological interactions with host biofluids and overcoming physiological barriers. Especially the physicochemical properties can give rise to nanoparticle toxicity [28].

Nanoparticles for therapeutic purposes usually contain reagents generally recognized as safe (GRAS). Nevertheless, they can be immunotoxic, eliciting a variety of adverse effects including immunosuppression or immunoenhancement, which in the first case can lead to infections and tumor formation, and in the second case to autoimmunity and hypersensitivity. These effects can be elicited either by the particle itself or by the active pharmaceutical ingredient (API) encapsulated in the particle. Recognition of nanoparticles by the immune system is dependent on their physicochemical properties, their cargo as well as their external milieu such as their protein corona, whose constituents in turn are determined by the nanoparticle's physicochemical properties. In fact, it has been reported that nonviral vectors including lipoplexes have the capability to induce similar or stronger immune reactions than viral vectors [29].

Size determines the ease with which nanoparticles enter their target organ. In general, the smaller they are, the more easily they enter their target organs. However, if nanoparticles are too small (<20 nm) they are cleared from blood via the reticuloendothelial system (RES) and the mononuclear phagocyte system (MPS) [30,31] as well as by filtration via the renal glomeruli, which both lead to a significant reduction in half-life [32,33]. One common strategy to improve half-life apart from size is coating the nanoparticle with polyethylene glycol (PEG) (stealth nanoparticles) that helps avoid recognition by the RES. The upper size limit is mostly defined by the width of the interstitial space of the target organ. If the nanoparticles get too large, diffusion through the interstitial space will be hindered and uptake into target cells inhibited.

A positive charge facilitates interaction with negatively charged cell membranes [34,35] but may trigger toxicity due to easier uptake into cells. Furthermore, positively charged particles are prone to opsonization in body fluids, leading to a corona formation, a coating of the nanoparticle surface by serum proteins, which in turn results in sequestration by the MPS. A promising approach to address the problem of corona formation by coating solid-lipidic-nanoparticles (SLNPs) with a preformulated protein corona was developed within the IMI COMPACT consortium [36,37]. In this approach SLNPs were coated with human serum albumin to which transferrin was conjugated as a targeting ligand for the BBB. This coating is meant to have two effects: First, it should provide protection from binding of serum proteins to the nanoparticles which causes random corona formation. Second, it should keep targeting to the BBB effective. If a targeting ligand is coupled directly to the surface of the nanoparticle, corona formation will mask the ligands, which will block BBB targeting. Since here the targeting ligand is coupled to the corona-mimicking serum albumin, masking of the targeting ligand by the protein corona should be avoided. In vitro studies have demonstrated that this formulation still possessed a strong ability to be taken up by microvascular endothelial cells in the presence of serum in the medium, whereas uptake of nanoparticles without this modified surface were not. In addition, the first in vivo imaging experiments have shown strong signals and long residence time in the brain, indicating an effective targeting of the BBB. Whether this signal is found in the brain or in the vasculature remains to be determined.

Special care must be taken for the release kinetics of the nanoformulation. Many nanoparticulate systems have the problem of a premature burst release of the encapsulated drug. Avoiding this is important for a successful nanoparticle for two reasons [38]. First, encapsulation of a drug can help avoid peripheral side effects. This has been demonstrated, for example with Doxycycline, whose cardiotoxic side effects have been avoided by encapsulation. Second, premature release of the drug can prevent a therapeutic effect by lowering target tissue exposure below the therapeutic threshold. In this regard, it must be kept in mind that nanoparticulate systems will alter the pharmacokinetic (PK) profile of their cargo. While encapsulation of a drug in a nanoparticle may be helpful to avoid systemic side effects elicited by the drug, the pharmacokinetics of the encapsulated drug are driven by the nanoparticle, which may be less favorable than the PK of the original drug.

In addition, nanoparticles need to cross the blood-brain barrier to reach brain tissues. This may require attachment of a targeting moiety to the surface of the particle to promote interaction with the BBB and increase transport into the brain. To this end, several studies in preclinical models of neurodegenerative diseases have shown efficacy of different cargos after packaging into brain-targeted nanoparticles [39–41]. Still, most nanoformulations show a biodistribution profile where most of an applied dose usually ends up in the liver.

Attachment of a surface targeting moiety, in combination with corona mimicry, will increase uptake into the brain to a certain extent but will not prevent most injected nanoparticles from accumulating in the liver.

2.2. Nanoparticles as Potential Brain Bioavailability Enhancers for Payload Carrying Nanoparticles

Recent literature suggests that the biodistribution of nanoformulations can be altered significantly and their clearance by the liver strongly inhibited. An emerging PK-enhancing adjuvant therapy uses payload-free nanoparticles referred to as nanoprimers [42] that have the function of increasing the bioavailability of other nanoparticles, whose function is to carry a therapeutic payload (therapeutic nanoparticles). The PK boosting effect is achieved by administering the nanoprimer prior to the therapeutic nanoparticles, thereby causing a delay in the hepatic clearance of the therapeutic nanoparticles. A secondary benefit is liver toxicity reduction, a common risk with both engineered nanoparticles and viral vectors used to deliver nucleic acid-based therapies.

Preclinical proof-of-concept studies have been conducted to show that payload-free liposomes can be used to increase exposure of nucleic acids in target tissues by temporarily reducing unwanted hepatic clearance [43–45]. In these studies, nanoprimers were engineered to be rapidly phagocytosed by Kupffer Cells (KCs) and Liver Sinusoidal Endothelial Cells (LSECs) after intravenous administration. LSECs are scavenger cells with a diameter of 7–9 µm capable of internalizing particles up to 0.23 µm, while KCs are resident liver macrophages with a diameter of 10–15 µm that can take up larger particles than KCs [46,47].

Germain et al. [43] describe the physicochemical attributes claimed to be optimal for liver accumulation. They argue that nanoprimer particles need to be larger than the fenestration size of the space of Disse to be preferentially cleared by KCs and not by hepatocytes, and smaller than 200 nm to avoid spleen accumulation. They also claim that that the charge should be neither positive, a known source of toxicity, nor too negative, to avoid macrophage internalization. More details on different nanoparticle formulations and liver interactions were recently summarized by Zhang et al. [48].

The study by Germain et al. [43] showed that nanoprimers could enhance the antitumor efficacy of irinotecan-loaded liposomes (with a diameter of 200 nm) for the treatment of colon cancer. Results from this study showed significantly enhanced biodistribution after application of the nanoprimer. Interestingly, an enhanced availability of the liposomes in the blood resulted in a longer liposome persistence in the head as well. In addition to the increased biodistribution to the head, application of nanoprimers showed a long-lasting effect on the biodistribution which was clearly visible even after a 24 h separation between the intravenous injection of the nanoprimer and intravenous infusion of the therapeutic nanoparticles.

Saunders et al. [42] report a preclinical study in mice where LNPs nanoprimers were used to increase levels of two types of LNP-encapsulated nucleic acid in systemic circulation: Human erythropoietin (hEPO) mRNA and Factor VII (FVII) siRNA. Intravenous nanoprimer pre-dosing 1 h prior to the intravenous administration of the loaded LNPs achieved the desired effects, in this case by increasing hEPO expression and by decreasing FVII expression by 49% (blood concentrations). In the same paper a prior liver panel 24 h after the last of three injections of nanoprimers (administered alone) showed no evidence of toxicity as measured by aspartate aminotransferase (AST), alanine aminotransferase (ALT), albumin, and total protein levels. Furthermore, nanoprimer uptake by liver cells was shown to "reduce KC's and LSEC's clearance activity without impacting hepatocyte uptake activity" [Ibid.], thereby suggesting that the vital role of hepatocyte in metabolism, detoxification and protein synthesis had been preserved.

In summary preclinical studies in oncology show that the concept of "nanopriming" is a promising one to enhance the PK of drug-carrying nanoparticles. However, translational implementation is rendered complex by the need to tailor nanoprimer size to organ variations between species. As for viral vectors, it remains unclear to what extent a nanoprimer would be effective at transiently blocking their metabolism. The diameter of Adeno-Associated viruses ranges from 20 to 29 nm [49]. Thus, they may evade the blockading effect of KCs and LSECs by "slipping though" the fenestration of the space of Disse and undergo transcytosis through hepatocytes. Furthermore, AAVs are reported to bind to KCs and LSECs via receptor A and to do so independently of clotting protein Factor X [45]. Whether this binding is sufficient to boost the PK of AAVs remains to be established. Viral vectors would have to bind to KCs and LSEC via receptor A before they slip through the space of Disse. Proof of concept experiments with viral vectors may need to be postponed until pioneers in the nanoprimer field have de-risked the concept. So far biotechnological engineering of the capsid proteins of AAV is another way to obtain enhanced target specificity and less liver clearance, as shown recently [50].

Initial proof-of-concept experiment using nanoprimers should focus on enhancing the PK of large nanoparticles (larger than the space of Disse) to determine if increased brain exposure and half-life can be achieved along with reduced liver toxicity.

2.3. Exosomes

Exosomes are cell-derived vesicles. They are actively secreted by most cell types and have a diameter of 40–100 nm [51]. They are formed in the endolysosomal pathway by inward budding of the membrane of the multivesicular body (MVB). Exosomes are subsequently released from the cell after fusion of the MVB with the cell membrane. Exosomes contain various cargos such as mRNA, non-coding RNAs, microRNA as well as cytoplasmic and membrane proteins [52]. Their physiological and pathophysiological role in CNS diseases has been the subject of intensive studies since their discovery more than 30 years ago. [51]. The fact that exosomes are part of the cell-to-cell communication machinery where they fulfill this function by carrying nucleic acids from one cell to another logically gave rise to the idea of developing exosomes and/or other extracellular vesicle as delivery vectors for RNA- and gene therapies. As a drug delivery system, exosomes are an attractive alternative to viral vectors and other nanoparticles. The fact that they are natural particles provides them with several advantages over AAV as well as synthetic nanoparticles (e.g., LNPs). First, they have a low likelihood of stimulating the immune response as their immunogenicity is lower than that of other delivery vehicles such as viruses or liposomes [53], making them more suitable for repeat dosing. Viral vectors such as AAV have a high propensity to stimulate the immune system resulting in a limited number of doses that can be given to a patient. Similarly, exosomes do not elicit any toxicities due to the natural lipid content of their membranes, a problem often seen with synthetic nanoparticles. Furthermore, the likelihood of being cleared from the circulation by the liver and the reticuloendothelial system (RES) or the immune system is lower. Depending on the therapeutic indication—and thus the target organ that needs to be reached—exosomes can provide a lot of flexibility: As they have an intrinsic targeting ability for different target tissues, exosomes with different targeting profiles can be generated by changing the producing cell line. In addition, exosomes can be genetically engineered to further refine their targeting towards a target organ such as the brain. According to the literature, brain targeting has been accomplished by attachment of peptide-based targeting ligands such as RVG29, g7 or RGD-Dyk. A recent study showed that conjugation of rabies virus glycoprotein-derived peptide (RVG-29) to the exosome surface enhanced brain uptake of the exosomes three-fold [53]. However, none of the peptide-based targeting ligand has been clinically validated yet.

Thus, exosomes have gained much attention as drug delivery vehicles for the treatment of CNS diseases and gene therapy approaches in recent years. Below are just some examples of preclinical studies. Exosomes carrying micro-RNA miR-133b reduced the infarcted area and improved neurological deficits in a middle cerebral aortic occlusion (MCAO) rat model of brain ischemia [54]. A study by Matthew Wood's group showed that conjugation of the rabies virus glycoprotein (RVG-29) peptide to the exosome surface enhanced brain uptake of the exosomes two-fold. BACE1 and Aβ levels were significantly reduced in mouse cortex after intravenous application of RVG-29-coated exosomes loaded with siRNA against BACE1 [55]. The same group confirmed efficient brain delivery of RVG-29-coated exosomes in a Parkinson disease mouse model. A significant reduction in α-synuclein mRNA and protein levels was also observed in several brain regions after injection of RVG-29-coated exosomes loaded with siRNA against α-synuclein [56], but exosome treatments are increasingly finding their way into the clinics as well. The first clinical studies using autologous exosome-based therapies demonstrated good safety and tolerability [57,58]. A recent (January 2022) search in clinicaltrials.gov found 116 clinical studies for "exosomes". While most of these studies use exosomes for diagnostic purposes, 35 studies are pursuing therapeutic interventions using exosomes as delivery vehicles. However, only three of these studies try to treat CNS diseases. The indications mentioned for these studies are stroke (NCT03384433, Ph1/2), depression, anxiety, and dementia (NCT04202770), phase not disclosed) and AD (NCT04388982, Ph1/2). Interestingly, exosomes in study NCT04202770 were applied using focused ultrasound (FUS), thus avoiding BBB transport but relying on transient local opening of the BBB. Currently, another clinical study is investigating the safety and efficacy of allogenic mesenchymal stem cell-derived exosomes in AD patients (NCT04388982).

As a result, various companies (see Table 3) have come into business which develop exosomes as therapeutics for various diseases, some of them already in clinical phases.

Recently the field has moved another step ahead with big pharma companies entering the picture [59]. The first business deals between exosome companies and big pharma companies were announced as early as 2017 when Boehringer Ingelheim and Evox Therapeutics announced a research collaboration on exosome-mediated RNA delivery in Boehringer's therapeutic areas of interest. Over the last two years, additional business deals between small companies developing exosomes as delivery vehicles for therapeutics and big pharma companies have been disclosed, which demonstrate big pharma's increasing interest in this technology. Among the biggest of them are Lilly's deal with Evox Therapeutics on CNS-targeting exosomes for five undisclosed targets which could give up $1.2 billion in milestone payments and Takeda's $900 million deal with Carmine Therapeutics on the development of gene therapies against two undisclosed rare disease targets. This is illustrated in Table 4.

Table 3. Companies Developing Exosome Technologies.

Company	Website (Accessed on 22 March 2023)	Technology	Status
Aegle Therapeutics (Woburn, MA, USA)	www.aegletherapeutics.com	Production of therapeutic-grade extracellular vesicles from bone marrow derived mesenchymal stem cells (MSCs)	Ph1/2a (Imm)
Anjarium Biosciences (Schlieren, Switzerland)	www.anjarium.com	proprietary Hybridosome® delivery technology for non-viral gene therapy	Not disclosed
Aruna Biomedical (Athens, GA, USA)	www.arunabio.com/	Proprietary neural exosomes AB126 (derived from proprietary non-transformed neural stem cells) able to cross the BBB	Preclinical
Capricor Therapeutics (San Diego, CA, USA)	www.capricor.com	Exosomes from proprietary cardiosphere-derived cells and engineered exosomes	Preclinical
Carmine Therapeutics (Cambridge, MA, USA)	www.carminetherapeutics.com	Red blood cell Extracellular Vesicle (RBCEV) Gene Therapy (REGENT®) for the development of next-generation non-viral gene therapies	Not disclosed
Codiak BioScience (Cambridge, MA, USA)	www.codiakbio.com	Proprietary engEx™ platform for designing, engineering, and manufacturing novel exosome therapeutics	Ph1, preclinical for NS
Curexsys (Göttingen, Germany)	www.curexsys.com	Induced mesenchymal stem cells (iMSC) derived exosomes isolated via traceless purification of exosomes (TACS)	Ph2
Evox Therapeutics (Oxford, UK)	www.evoxtherapeutics.com/	Modified exosomes targeting the BBB with the RVG peptide	Preclinical
Exopharm (Melbourne, Australia)	www.exopharm.com	Exosomes as delivery systems for RNA, enzymes, or small molecules, with the possibility of surface modification for specific tissue targeting	Preclinical

Table 3. Cont.

Company	Website (Accessed on 22 March 2023)	Technology	Status
ILIAS Biologics (Daejeon, Republic of Korea)	www.iliasbio.com	Proprietary EXPLOR® platform for intracellular delivery of large-sized protein therapeutics. BBB-targeted exosomes for CNS diseases	Ph1 (inflamm.), preclinical for NS
Kimera Labs (Miramar, FL, USA)	www.kimeralabs.com	Production of MSC-derived exosomes for cosmetic use and scientific and clinical research	Not disclosed
Reneuron (Bridgend, UK)	www.reneuron.com	modified exosomes for brain targeting, according to their website even to specific brain regions	Ph 2b (stroke)
Vesigen Therapeutics (Cambridge, MA, USA)	www.vesigentx.com	Engineered ARrestin-domain 1 Mediated Microvesicles (ARMMs) as a flexible platform for therapeutic delivery	Not disclosed
Mantra Bio (South San Francisco, CA, USA)	www.mantrabio.com	REVEALTM, an exosome engineering platform that to generate targeted exosome vehicles (TEVs) for various therapeutic areas	Not disclosed
Xollent Biotech (Raleigh, NC, USA)	www.xollentbio.com	A variety of applications for exosomes of different origin in oncology, cardiology and cosmetics	Preclinical

Table 4. Business Deals Between Exosome Companies and Big Pharma (from [59], modified).

Companies	Details
Vesigen Therapeutics	Series A round for developing ARRDC1-mediated microvesicles delivering cargos for gene editing, mRNA replacement and RNAi therapeutics ($28.5 million) [60]
Carmine Therapeutics; Takeda	Research agreement using Carmine's proprietary extracellular vesicles (EVs) for the delivery of Takeda's gene therapies against two undisclosed targets (Carmine eligible for milestone payments up to $900 million) [61]
Curexsys GmbH; Evotec	Partnership combining Evotec's proprietary induced pluripotent stem cell (iPSC) platform with Curesys' proprietary exosome isolation technology [62]
Codiak Biosciences; Jazz Pharmaceuticals	Strategic collaboration on the research and development of exosome-based therapies for the treatment of cancer. (Codiak eligible for up to $200 million in milestone payment [63]
Sarepta Therapeutics	Research agreement using Codiak's engineered exosomes for the delivery of Sarepta's gene editing, gene therapy and RNA technologies against neuromuscular diseases (Codiak eligible for up-front and license payments of up to $72.5 million) [64]
Evox Therapeutics; Eli Lilly	Research agreement using Evox's exosomes for the delivery of Lilly's RNAi and antisense oligonucleotide (ASO) therapies against 5 undisclosed targets in neurological disorders (Evox eligible for milestone payments up to $1.2 billion) [65]
Boehringer Ingelheim	Research collaboration on exosome-mediated RNA delivery in Boehringer's therapeutic areas of interest [66]
Takeda	Partnership agreement to develop up to five exosome-based therapeutics for the treatment of rare diseases [67]
ReNeuron; undisclosed partner	Research agreement using ReNeuron's human neural stem cell-derived exosomes to deliver gene-silencing technology of an undisclosed partner [68]

Autologous exosome-based therapies were well tolerated in first clinical cancer studies [58,69]. Still, some issues remain that hinder a broader clinical application of exosomes in CNS disease therapies. First, different functions of exosomes in health and disease have been identified and are not completely understood. These may even be opposing, as exosomes on the one hand mediate tumor prevention, but on the other hand deliver tumor-associated proteins. Selection of the right cell types as starting material for exosome production is important to avoid possible side effects given the varying intrinsic contents of exosomes because of their cellular origin. Mesenchymal stem cells seem to be a suitable source of exosomes, as they have been used in the three clinical studies. In addition, it is still unclear by which mechanism exosomes cross the BBB. Exosomes mostly interact with the cell membrane via membrane fusion, and subsequently deliver their cargo into the cell. Recent studies suggest that exosomes can take different routes through the cell. A routing towards late-endosomes/lysosomes from which they can be released via transcytosis has been described in zebrafish macrophages. Furthermore, they also seem to cross an in vitro BBB via transcellular migration, but only under stroke-like conditions. However, the therapeutic relevance of this route is questionable since disruption of the BBB in stroke occurs after the therapeutic window for treatment initiation [70]. The BBB also is a formidable barrier in other brain diseases such as glioma [71].

A focused optimization of exosomes as delivery systems will only be possible with a deeper knowledge of these processes. In addition to these biological questions, there are technical issues to be solved. Loading exosomes with nucleic acids requires optimization. There are different methods of bringing a cargo into exosomes. Several physical techniques have been reported to enable uptake of cargos into exosomes [72]. Such techniques include sonication, electroporation, and surfactant treatment. However, loading efficiencies of maximally 25% have been reported for most techniques. The loading of nucleic acids can also be achieved by transfecting the producing cells which then overexpress the nucleic acid. The produced exosomes will then contain the expressed nucleic acid. Consequently, a high number of exosomes must be delivered to achieve therapeutic concentration of the drug in the target tissue. Especially for CNS diseases, an improved brain targeting resulting in higher brain uptake would be desired. Although exosomes have an intrinsic propensity to enter the brain, a recent study in mice suggests that only about 0.05% of an injected dose of non-targeted exosomes crosses the BBB [73]. Surface modification of exosomes can increase their brain-targeting efficiency. A recent study showed that conjugation of RVG-29 peptide to the exosome surface enhanced brain uptake of the exosomes, but only by three-fold. The identification of a more efficient targeting ligand will be required to enable a stronger increase in brain uptake. Lastly, production of exosomes in sufficient amounts to support clinical studies is another issue that needs to be solved. Leukapheresis and subsequent ex vivo generation of autologous exosomes has shown to provide sufficient material for clinical studies. Recent technical developments using dynamic 3D cultures suggest a path forward for non-autologous exosomes as delivery systems, as this resulted in a 100-fold increase in yield over the use of 2D cultures. Exosome companies also claim that their proprietary production platforms are scalable and suitable for large scale applications. The fact that some of these are in clinical studies seems to underline this fact.

2.4. Exo-AAVs: Exosomes as Capsid Carriers

Although exosomes move forward slowly towards the market, it is still early days for this technology. Solutions for the issues mentioned are needed for exosomes to progress further as delivery vehicles, especially for CNS therapeutics, but since the field is growing very quickly, additional knowledge to these issues should emerge soon and support the progression of exosomes into the clinic and to the market. Already, first approaches are being developed that broaden the use of exosomes by transporting cargos beyond nucleic acids. An interesting novel application of exosomes developed in recent years is exo-AAVs (also named "vexosomes" or "ev-AAV" (extracellular vesicle-associated AAV), where AAVs associate with exosomes. In this approach, exosomes generated by HEK293T cells transfected with AAV plasmids for AAV1 and AAV2 and isolated from culture medium were found to contain AAVs either associated with the exosomes or even within the exosomes. Approximately 12 and 9% of isolated exosomes contained AAV1 and AAV2 capsids, respectively and the average number of capsids per exosome was 8.2 and 1.2 for AAV1 and AAV2 [74].

In vitro studies transfecting U87 cells, either with AAV1 or AAV1 vexosomes after pre-incubation with an anti-AAV1 neutralizing antibody showed that AAV1 vexosomes yielded a more than four-fold higher transduction efficiency than AAV1. AAV1- and AAV2-vexosomes also showed higher transduction rates compared to free AAV capsids even in the absence of neutralizing antibodies [74]. In vitro studies then showed that ev-AAV containing AAV9 capsids were up to 23 times more resistant to neutralizing antibodies in transducing HeLa cells than AAV9 capsids alone. Furthermore, intravenous injection of a neutralizing dose of immunoglobulin (IVIg) from multiple donors in mice followed by application of either AAV9 or ev-AAV9 showed an increased transduction efficiency in both liver and head as demonstrated by a 5-7-fold higher luciferase signal. This demonstrated that ev-AAV9 are less sensitive to IVIg than free AAV9. Interestingly, decorating the

EVs with RVG as a brain targeting ligand further increased delivery of ev-AAV9 to the brain by 3-4-fold. Interestingly, transduction in liver and heart was strongly reduced with RVG-ev-AAV9 compared to untargeted ev-AAV9 [75]. Another in vivo study showed that intravenous application of exo-AAV9 in mice not only resulted in a similar distribution of the introduced EGFP signal throughout the whole brain compared to free AAV9, but they also showed comparable cellular tropisms in the brain. At the same time, the results showed a significantly higher transduction efficiency of ev-AAV9 compared to free AAV9 in cortex and striatum but not in the hippocampus [76]. However, ev-AAVs show potential beyond the brain. A recent study showed increased efficacy of ev-AAV (here called AAVExo) in a mouse model of lung cancer, where AAVExo demonstrated a significantly higher delivery to the xenografts compared to free AAV [77].

The exo-AAV approach may offer several advantages. Although AAVs are widely used as delivery vehicles for gene therapy approaches, a low likelihood of stimulating an immune response is one of the biggest advantages of exosomes over AAV, especially for repeated dosing. While methods to avoid an immune response after AAV application such as empty capsid decoys [74], balloon catheters and saline flush or removal of neutralizing antibodies from the blood by plasmapheresis [75] have been developed, these methods also have their limitations. Technologies such as plasmapheresis are elaborate technologies which place a heavy burden on the patient and can only be repeated a few times. Protecting the capsids from neutralizing antibodies seems indeed possible with ev-AAVs, as in vitro data suggest. The biodistribution of exosomes shows a majority accumulating in the liver. This is a concern because recent literature [50] highlights the need to keep capsids from entering the liver at a high percentage as this can trigger responses such as liver toxicity. Whether encapsulation of capsids into exosomes can increase safety needs to be demonstrated; at least the data with RVG-ev-AAV9 suggest the possibility to reduce delivery to the liver. This may also be helpful as a large fraction of AAV capsids is sequestered in the liver upon intravenous dosing. On the other hand, the intrinsic targeting property of exosomes may help direct an increased fraction of the ev-AAVs to the target organ, especially the brain, as exosomes possess an intrinsic property to cross the BBB. The in vivo results with RVG-ev-AAV9 suggest that an increased delivery into the brain can be achieved.

While this approach has some intriguing implications, it is still at the early stage. Several points need clarification to objectively assess the full measure of its potential and limitations. Currently, information on exo-AAV in the literature remains limited. Second, only about 10% of the exosomes contain capsids (which is in line with low loading efficiencies for exosomes). Conversely, exosomes can contain up to eight capsids. This means that controls should be put in place to ascertain that the claimed higher transduction of brain cells is indeed based on a higher number of capsids/viruses in the brain. None of the studies so far has confirmed this claim. This is a concern because the mechanism by which exosomes cross the BBB remains unclear. Lastly, optimization of the isolation method to increase the degree exosome loading has not been reported to date.

3. Device-Enabled Drug Delivery

Apart from drug delivery technologies such as receptor-mediated transport (RMT) or intranasal delivery (IN), there are device-enabled drug delivery technologies which allow local delivery to specific regions of brain parenchyma or regions throughout the brain or spinal cord via cerebrospinal fluid (CSF). These technologies are either invasive, such as intracerebroventricular (ICV), intra-cisterna magna (ICM) or intrathecal (IT) injection, or non-invasive such as focused ultrasound (FUS) for BBB disruption. ICM injection is more convenient than ICV application in rodent studies. For safety reasons, however, ICM cannot be used routinely in clinical trials. Both routes of administration provide efficient access to the subarachnoidal space.

3.1. Focused Ultrasound (FUS)

Multiple approaches have been used to disrupt the BBB using focused ultrasound. Disruption of the BBB with focused ultrasound can be accomplished with microbubble injections using implanted transducers or non-invasive phased-array transducers. The biological effects and associated safety profile of the disruption procedure significantly depend on the magnitude of applied ultrasound energy, typically measured as peak negative pressure. The concomitant systemic circulation of injected microbubbles allows a reduction of the peak negative pressure (and ultrasonic energy) needed for BBB disruption. Sizeable peak negative pressure results in irreversible BBB damage while reduced peak negative pressure can avoid irreversible BBB damage. A recent screen in clincialtrials.gov as well as recent literature [78] identified 17 clinical trials using FUS technology. Table 5 provides a summary of the safety assessment period for several clinical trials that utilize microbubbles to disrupt the BBB.

Table 5. Clinical Studies Utilizing FUS with Microbubbles to Disrupt the BBB.

Safety Assessment Period	Date Posted	Microbubble Type	Sponsor	Indication	NCT ID
1 day	August 2019–January 2027	Definity® microbubbles	Neurological Assoc., BrainSonix Corp, Sherman Oaks, CA, USA	Low Grade Glioma	NCT04063514
3 days	October 2019–July 2021	Definity® microbubbles	Elisa Konofagou®, Columbia University, NY, USA	Alzheimer's Disease	NCT04118764
90 days	December 2016–June 2018	Definity® microbubbles	InSightec®, Haifa, Israel	Alzheimer's Disease	NCT02986932
6 months	November 2018–December 2020	Unknown	InSightec®, Haifa, Israel	Alzheimer's Disease	NCT03739905
5 years	September 2018–December 2024	Unknown	InSightec®, Haifa, Israel	Alzheimer's Disease	NCT03671889
6 months	April 2020–December 2020	Definity® microbubbles	InSightec®, Haifa, Israel	Alzheimer's Disease	NCT04526262
1 day	December 2020–December 2021	Definity® microbubbles	InSightec®, Haifa, Israel	Amyotrophic Lateral Sclerosis	NCT03321487
2 weeks	November 2018–December 2021	Luminity® microbubbles	InSightec®, Haifa, Israel	Parkinson's Disease	NCT03608553
1 day [1]	January 2015–July 2021	Definity® microbubbles	InSightec®, Haifa, Israel	Brain tumors	NCT02343991
~26 weeks	October 2018–December 2021	Definity® microbubbles	InSightec®, Haifa, Israel	Glioblastoma	NCT03712293
~52 weeks	August 2018–December 2024	Definity® microbubbles	InSightec®, Haifa, Israel	Glioblastoma	NCT03616860
~52 weeks	June 2018–December 2024	Definity® microbubbles	InSightec®, Haifa, Israel	Glioblastoma	NCT03551249
~42 weeks	October 2018–Mar 2022	Definity® microbubbles	InSightec®, Haifa, Israel	Breast cancer/Brain metastases	NCT03714243
45 days [2] (2 weeks)	August 2018–June 2019	Sonovue®	NaviFUS®, Tapei City, Taiwan	Recurrent Glioblastoma	NCT03626896
38 weeks	June 2020–December 2022	Sonovue®	NaviFUS®, Tapei City, Taiwan	Recurrent Glioblastoma	NCT04446416
52 weeks	October 2014–July 2018	Sonovue®	Carthera®, Paris, France	Recurrent Glioblastoma	NCT02253212
~39 weeks	April 2017–October 2020	Sonovue®	Carthera®, Paris, France	Alzheimer's Disease	NCT03119961

[1] The area that was sonicated by FUS was surgically resected 24 h after sonication. [2] The area that was sonicated by FUS was surgically resected 2 weeks after sonication.

The safety of disrupting the BBB using microbubbles has been controversial [5,79,80]. Vikram Patel, former deputy director of the Division of Applied Regulatory Science at the Center for Drug Evaluation and Research at United States Food and Drug Administration (FDA) commented specifically on the safety aspects of closing the BBB "as soon as possible to limit exposure of the brain to chemicals or toxins other than the intended therapeutic compounds". Kovacs et al. [81] provided evidence that even relatively low ultrasonic energies used with Optison® microbubbles induced immediate expression of damage associated molecular patterns (DAMP), heat shock protein 70 and other cytokines associated with a sterile inflammatory response. These patterns are also found in traumatic brain injury. Recently Schregel et al. [82] delivered an Optison® microbubble dose in combination with the same peak negative pressure used in the experiment by Kovacs et al. [83] to intentionally induce focal lesions resulting in experimental autoimmune encephalomyelitis (EAE) as a disease model of multiple sclerosis in mice.

Accumulation of blood factors in the brain has been implicated in neuroinflammation and neurodegeneration in the CNS. Thrombin activates NF-κB signaling in microglia to promote oxidative stress and activates pro-inflammatory response in microglia, contributing to neuronal cell death [83]. Fibrinogen regulates inflammation in the CNS and contributes to neurodegenerative progression [84]. Fibrinogen accumulation in oligodendrites leads to myelin loss and axon degeneration, leading to cell death [85]. Complement system acts as a key regulator in glial phagocytosis and contributes to cytokine production and inflammatory response in the brain [86,87]. This means that FUS parameters would need to be tightly controlled to avoid the crossing of the BBB by blood coagulation factors.

FUS technology, as currently designed, cannot be used to increase BBB permeability efficiently and transiently over wide areas of the brain. Accordingly, there have been no clinical studies that evaluate disruption of large volumes of the brain while co-administering a therapeutic drug yet. Due to the limited focal area of the ultrasound beams, disruption of a large area of the brain would either require a highly multiplexed disruption algorithm to target multiple cortical volumes at once or a steerable ultrasound beam to achieve widespread coverage (or both). The largest volume of disruption evaluated to date is approximately 24 cm^3 [88], which would require nearly 60 "large volume" treatment sessions of considerable duration to treat the entire brain volume. As such, the approach would not be practical.

Furthermore, co-localization and synchronization of the ultrasound field, microbubbles and therapeutic agents are a particularly challenging obstacle to optimizing drug exposure at the target tissue of interest. The timing of delivery for optimal concentration of the microbubble and therapeutic agent with the ultrasound field at the small target site is critical to achieve consistent passage of the therapeutic agent to the target tissue when BBB disruption is minimally transient. Microbubbles travel through the lungs before entering the arteries within the brain, and a loss in the concentration of microbubbles in the lungs is to be expected [89]. Since the degree of BBB disruption is dependent on the concentration of microbubbles [90], the magnitude of disruption during a single pulse sequence is necessarily very dynamic.

In addition, infrastructure costs and requirements to properly perform the BBB disruption procedure are high [80] and limit access for patient treatments. The cost for a single InSightec Exablate® 4000 system is estimated at $2,000,000 [91] and a single ablation treatment for essential tremor is estimated at $23,500 [92]. If these costs are similar for a MRgFUS system for BBB disruption, there will be significant reimbursement hurdles utilizing this technology to enhance drug distribution.

Another important point to consider is the fact that microbubbles are currently classified as drugs for use as contrast agents to be used in conjunction with diagnostic ultrasound equipment. A different intended use of microbubbles to mechanically disrupt the blood brain barrier is likely to fit the definition of a medical device, which would require a change in classification from drug to device.

Even in the best-case scenario, i.e., "one time" drug delivery to limited regions of the brain (a few cubic millimeters), several technical challenges remain to be solved. This is compounded by safety concerns, commercially available microbubbles originally approved as contrasting agents (i.e., a different intended use) and complex regulatory hurdles on which experts in the field have yet to provide clear pathway to approval.

Despite years of feasibility experimentation reported in numerous publications and conference presentations, FUS applications for widely disrupting the BBB cannot be counted as a scalable platform for commercial development in the foreseeable future. In this context, when we consider more challenging scenarios, e.g., large neuroscience markets where drug exposure is required over large cortical volumes, or even more daunting, where repeated doses are required over large cortical volumes, the prospects for a breakthrough with current FUS technology are very low. However, several promising innovations, such as the use of Rapid Short Pulse (RaSP) ultrasound, may become more viable technologies for future clinical studies.

3.2. Intra CSF Delivery

In a recent review paper [93], we highlighted that there are two schools of thought on the delivery of large proteins to deep brain tissues via the cerebrospinal fluid (CSF). The early school posits that the rate-limiting role of molecular size on protein diffusion through the interstitial space limits the utility of intra-CSF delivery to the treatment of brain tissues that are either located within, or in contact with, the CSF ventricular/ meningeal system as in the case of leptomeningeal metastases. A more recent school has gained recognition following advances in ex vivo and in vivo imaging that revealed the existence of a CSF "microcirculation" system within brain tissues, at times, referred to as the "glymphatic system" [94] As a result, the CSF circulation that was first thought to be useful only to reach tissues in the immediate vicinity of the CSF circulatory system, is increasingly viewed as a pathway for a more rapid intake of therapeutics into deep brain tissues.

Under this new paradigm, deep penetration of the brain by large molecules is achievable via perivascular pathways as demonstrated in primates [95]. The existence of deep penetrating perivascular pathways also has far-reaching implications on cross-species translation and on the effect of molecular weight of CSF solutes on rate of transport within the parenchyma. Such pathways allow micro-convective transport that scales with brain size. Under the intra-parenchymal CSF diffusion paradigm, CSF enabled-drug transport was widely regarded not to be scalable to higher order species. Diffusion was seen as limiting penetration distance and as presenting a major hindrance to the penetration of therapeutics with high molecular weight. However, over the past two decades there have been multiple clinical studies employing ICV injection. First indications for efficacy have been seen in these studies [96,97] suggesting therapeutic concentrations of the drug in the parenchyma.

The implications for drug delivery via CSF microcirculation are far reaching, as shown in a widely cited paper by Yadav et al. [95]. They observed widespread distribution of an anti-BACE1 antibody and of a control IgG antibody after 6 weeks of ICV infusion in primates. Continuous ICV delivery of an anti-BACE1 antibody achieved a steady-state concentration in the CSF within 4 days. Antibody distribution was near uniform across the brain parenchyma after 6 weeks, ranging from 20 to 40 nM, which led to a robust and sustained reduction (~70%) of CSF amyloid-βx-40 peptides. A rat study by Kouzehgarani et al. [98] also demonstrated the suitability of CSF microcirculation for drug delivery. They showed that an antibody penetrates the brain parenchyma starting approximately 30 min after a single intra Cisterna Magna (ICM) injection and continues to do so even 4 h after injection. Even after 24 h the antibody is still present in the tissue.

In contrast, no tissue penetration was observed 4 h after intravenous injection, even with a 30-fold higher dose than in the ICM study. The penetration extended into subcortical regions including the hippocampus. Similarly, two studies performed in Tg2576 mice demonstrated a therapeutic effect of chronically ICV-infused antibodies after 5 and 2 weeks of infusion, respectively [99,100]. This pioneering research has shown that the intra-CSF delivery of large protein therapeutics can achieve widespread distribution and target engagement in deep brain tissues. This indicates that intra-CSF administration can be an attractive option to reach and engage targets in brain tissues when (a) the BBB is poorly permeable to the therapeutic such as in the case of vectorized nucleic acid therapeutics, degradomers or biopharmaceuticals, (b) widespread areas of the brain need to be treated which is not achievable with local delivery with modalities such as FUS or intra-parenchymal injections/infusions, (c) systemic delivery would either lead to unacceptable off-target toxicity, or (d) lead to the degradation or rapid clearance of the therapeutic, and (e) there is no evidence of brain toxicity. Finally, the severity of the condition and treatment benefits may justify an invasive route of administration in the patient. In such cases, intra-CSF administration can provide a convenient short cut to collect proof of concept data on the efficacy of a therapeutic.

Several studies have been published showing that maintaining a steady-state drug concentration in the SAS is a necessary condition to reach deep areas of the brain [95,101,102]. This is to counteract the dilutive effect of rapid CSF turnover (ranging from 13 times a day in mice to 4 times a day in humans). Thus, determining a suitable intra-CSF dosing regimen requires modeling, CSF sampling studies or a combination of the two.

The above concept is well illustrated in a study by Fleischhack et al. [103] comparing bolus ICV administration with continuous intravenous (CIV) administration of chemotherapy agent Etoposide in patients with metastatic medulloblastoma. Five daily ICV bolus doses (0.5 mg per day) via an indwelling subcutaneous reservoir achieved more than a 100-fold peak exposure compared to intravenous infusion. CSF clearance caused each peak to be followed by a steep trough, however. Repeated intraventricular etoposide administration was only minimally toxic, was well tolerated, and steady state ICV exposure exceeding that achieved with continuous intravenous infusion was suggested as a follow-up study.

Route of Intra-CSF Administration for Deep Brain Penetration

Intra CSF administration for delivery to the brain can be achieved via intrathecal (IT), intra-cerebroventricular (ICV) or intra-cisterna magna (ICM) infusion. As seen in Table 1 all ongoing clinical studies in the indications that we screened for used the IT or the ICM route for drug application. However, one clinical trial is currently in Ph2a/b (NCT04153175) in which sodium valproate is administered intra-cerebroventricularly to treat refractory epilepsy [104].

Until recently, the IT route was preferred over ICV route whenever possible due to the risk of infection from long-term use of ICV. For the treatment of deep regions of the brain, excluding ICV delivery comes at a cost. With CSF "near stagnant" in the lumbar area, IT delivery requires pumping a higher initial dose to reach the subarachnoid space (SAS) at therapeutic levels, a precondition to sustained penetration via the microcirculation system. In contrast, ICV leverages brain physiology by infusing the drug in proximity to the site of CSF production, thereby allowing the drug to go with the outward flow of the CSF in the direction of the SAS. This is illustrated by a study published by Vuillemenot et al. [105] describing TPP1 enzyme replacement therapy to treat CLN2, an ultra-rare and rapidly progressing brain disorder that affects an estimated 20 children born in the United States each year. When comparing IT and ICV delivery of TPP1 in primates treated with a single infusion, they found that although CSF and plasma PK profiles were equivalent between ICV or IT infusion, ICV infusion achieved increased TTP1 exposure in all areas of the brain, particularly in the striatum and the thalamus.

The above case studies in both rodents and primates confirm the scalability of ICV delivery and, more generally, the viability of harnessing CSF microcirculation across species with major difference in brain size, a notion that continues to be met with skepticism in some neuroscience circles. However, the pharmaceutical industry is beginning to take note of the promise of ICV for intra-CSF delivery, as exemplified by Genentech in the aforementioned anti-BACE-1 study, which was conducted in collaboration with Medtronic.

IT delivery is well suited for the delivery of lipophilic drugs to the spinal cord area, with diminishing utility for reaching the cerebral SAS due to their rapid absorption in the spinal cord SAS. Moreover, the low rate of CSF circulation in the lumbar area further increases therapeutic concentrations within the confined of the spinal SAS. The situation is less clear cut in the case of therapeutic proteins. While therapeutic proteins do not readily bind to spinal tissues, their distribution beyond spinal CSF remains hindered by the slow CSF circulation in the lumbar area. This hurdle can be overcome by infusing the drug with an implanted pump to steadily replace the drug fraction that is cleared from the cervical area. In fact, IT application of morphine for pain relief was described as early as 1979 [106]. More recently Prialt® has been added to that list, which is the only FDA-approved non-opioid medication for the treatment of chronic pain [107]. Furthermore, intrathecal baclofen is approved by the FDA for the treatment of spasticity [108].

To better understand the role of intra-CSF delivery in the treatment of spinal cord injury (SCI) a search of ongoing clinical trials was conducted on the "SCI clinical trial" website [109]. The first screening excluded non-pharmaceutical modalities as well as chronic management of co-morbidities. The search results revealed that four of nine SCI studies utilized IT delivery as shown in Table 6. When focusing on those SCI trials where the mode of action for neural regeneration was either repulsive guidance molecule receptor A (RGMA) pathway inhibition (AbbVie's ABT-555 and Mitsubishi's MT-3921) or NGR-1 pathway inhibition (ReNetX Bio's AXER-204 and Novartis's NG-101-ATI355), two of these studies utilized intravenous delivery. Published literature indicated that intravenous delivery for MT-3139 (anti-RGMA from Mitsubishi) was chosen out of clinical convenience after successful POC in primates using IT delivery [110–114]. In contrast, AXER-204 and NG-101-ATI355 were dosed in humans via the IT route after successful preclinical studies in primates.

Table 6. SCI benchmarking results: preferred routes of administration for the treatment of SCI.

Drug	Company/Partner	Indication	Clinical Phase	Modality	Target	Route of Administration
ABT-555 (ELEZANUMAB)	AbbVie	Acute cervical SCI	Phase 2	Antibody to inhibit the Neogenin and BMP pathways	RGMa (N-terminal)	Intravenous infusion
AXER-204	ReNetX Bio	Chronic cervical SCI	Phase 1/2	Fusion protein to Inhibit the NgR pathway	Nogo-A, MAG, and OMgp	Intrathecal Infusion
MT-3921	Mitsubishi Tanabe	Acute cervical SCI	Phase 2	Antibody to inhibit the BMP pathway	RGMa (C-terminal)	Intravenous infusion
NG-101/ATI-355	Novartis	Acute cervical SCI	Phase 2	Fc antibody fragment to inhibit the NgR pathway	Nogo-A	Intrathecal Injection

3.3. Convection Enhanced Delivery

The Blood-Brain-Tumor Barrier (BBTB) in GBM tumors can be highly heterogeneous, with permeability to protein therapeutics ranging from high at the tumor core of high grade GBM to low, or extremely low, in unresectable regions such as tumor margins or sparsely infiltrated areas distal from the core. Furthermore, there is mounting evidence from preclinical and clinical studies that BBTB heterogeneity significantly limits efficacy following systemic delivery [115].

To evaluate this hypothesis, a preclinical study in mice was conducted to explore the benefits of administering two antibody-drug conjugates, Depatuxizumab mafodin (ABT-414) and Serclutamab talirine (ABBV-321), via convection enhanced delivery (CED) as an alternative to systemic delivery [116]. Efficacy was evaluated by using an intracranially implanted EGFRviii-amplified patient-derived xenograft (PDX) refractory to treatment via intraperitoneal (IP) delivery (implying BBB impermeability). Four consecutive doses of ABT-414 administered with CED led to a 5-fold increase in mouse longevity compared to weekly systemic administration. It was concluded that ABT-414 is well tolerated as infusion was only associated with modest elevation in glial fibrillary acidic protein (GFAP) without loss of NeuN staining or increased infiltration of CD68-positive cells and resulted in extended survival in orthotopic GBM PDXs. Similarly, a single dose of ABBV-321 administered with CED led to a significant increase in mouse longevity compared to weekly systemic administration. With intra-tumoral administration, two out of three mice were still alive after 300 days vs. a median survival of <60 days with the systemically dosed negative controls. However, ABBV-321 had a much narrower therapeutic window when delivered by CED. More importantly, this study showed that CED is a promising method to enhance delivery across the BBTB.

Publications by Hadaczek et al. [117] and Johnston et al. [118] also describe CED protocols to deliver AAV2-GDNF, AAV2-TK in the striatum and putamen regions of monkeys, resulting in prolonged increases in dopaminergic neural activity and associated locomotor activity.

A necessary condition for CED to be an option is when the regions of the brain requiring drug exposure are precisely located and of relatively small size. Examples of conditions meeting these criteria are clinical study NCT04120493 for early-stage HD, clinical study NCT04167540 for early or late-stage PD, or clinical study NCT01621581 for advanced PD.

4. Conclusions and Outlook

Brain delivery technologies, non-invasive, invasive, and device-mediated, are in different states of maturity. Each of these has specific properties that may be useful for different indications, e.g., local vs global delivery. Table 7 summarizes the properties of delivery technologies sharing the function of enhancing the brain biodistribution of therapeutics ranging from small molecules, degraders, biologics to nucleic acids. The null hypothesis assumes that a technology works as intended until proven otherwise.

Exosomes are currently a hot topic, and various companies have started to invest heavily into this technology. However, despite considerable progress made over the last 10 years, there are still many unresolved issues. Still, exo-AAVs represent an exciting novel development. Although this approach is in an even earlier stage it may present an intriguing opportunity to broaden the use of AAVs in indications that require repeated dosing. To our knowledge nanoprimers are the first technology that tries to concomitantly modulate both the biodistribution and the PK of nanoparticles. While this improves the chances for a successful development for peripheral indications, it does not resolve the issue of opsonization (corona formation) and the resulting loss of brain targeting efficacy. Although the first published results look quite promising, the available literature on nanoprimers remains scarce. Future studies will show if this technology can live up to its promise. In addition, the field is currently lacking a clinically validated targeting ligand.

Focused ultrasound (FUS) technologies have limited preclinical utility in niche areas. A review performed on FUS shows that the technology does not fully live up to the expectations set by its advocates in academic circles as a scalable drug delivery technology. The current embodiments of the technology are not suited to treat large areas of the brain and suffer from safety and regulatory issues that make it difficult to implement beyond phase 1.

Device-based methods to circumvent the BBB, such as convection enhanced delivery (CED) or intra-cerebroventricular delivery (ICV), show more promise preclinically and clinically. There are scalable solutions from the clinic and to commercial launch. The Renishaw NeuroInfuse® system is suitable for both acute (single delivery) and chronic repeat delivery paradigms, whereas other CED equipment suppliers only have delivery solutions for acute delivery paradigms. Cerebral Therapeutic's ICVRx® Infusion System is a fully implanted delivery system that consists of a dual lumen port and ICV catheter, enabling ICV infusion as well as aspiration of ventricular CSF for biomarker analysis. The ICVRx® is attached to either a port or refillable pump to allow intermittent or continuous delivery, respectively. The fully implanted design improves the safety profile over designs requiring an external pump interface.

A recent study in rodents has shown that a humanized antibody administered via CSF penetrated the entire brain at a rate and depth that has surprised many subject matter experts. The circulatory pathway leading to this rapid tissue exposure is described in a 2021 review paper [93]. Benchmarking shows that some companies use device-based modalities for the delivery of nucleic acid in clinical studies. While device-based modalities currently would clearly be impractical for large primary indications, the authors of this paper recommend considering implantable ICV to achieve rapid results in niche markets, particularly those involving acute morbidities with rapid progression. ICV delivery should also be considered for target validation studies, even if the eventual preferred mode of delivery is systemic. To this end, it would be interesting to validate the corona mimicry approach for its ability to maintain the brain targeting capability of nanoparticles.

Table 7. Maturity and Potential Impact of "Brain-Biodistribution Enhancing" Technologies Surveyed.

Category	Sub-Category	Exo-Somes	Exo-AAVs	Nano-Primers	FUS (Focused Ultrasound)	CED (Convection Enhanced Delivery)	ICV (Intra-Cerebro-Ventricular)	IT (Intra-Thecal)
Potential medical impact (Null Hypothesis)	Preclinically enabling	y	y	y	y	y	y	y
	Medically enabling	y	y	TBD	y	y	y	y
	Medically transformative	TBD	n	n	n	TBD	y	n
Extent of brain tissue exposure		All brain tissues	All brain tissues	n/a	Inherently limited	Limited to targeted area	All brain tissues	Spinal tissues
Technology maturity	Readiness for Phase 1/2	y	n	n	Phase I only	y	y	y
	Safety (Chronic)	TBD	TBD	Potential secondary tox	TBD	Y as implant	Y as implant	Y as implant
	Safety (Short term)	y	TBD	Potential secondary tox	y	y	y	y
	Regulatory pathway	y	TBD	Nanoparticle predicate	n	y	y	y
	Invasiveness/medical benefit ratio (Chronic treatment)	n/a	n/a	Non-invasive	Non-invasive FUS, micro-bubbles are invasive (n)	y	y	y
	Invasiveness/medical benefit ratio[x] (Short-term treatment)	n/a	n/a	Non-invasive	Non-invasive FUS, micro-bubbles are invasive (n)	y	y	y
	Adoption prospect by patient & care givers & payers	No foreseeable issue	No foreseeable issue	No foreseeable issue	n	y with design modification	y	y
Business impact (Null hypothesis)	Large markets/Primary indications	Stroke, potentially others	Too early to tell	Too early to tell	n	n	n	y
	Niche markets/Secondary indications	Others	Too early to tell	Too early to tell	y	y	y	y
	R&D productivity/Preclinical studies	y	y	y	y	y	y	y
Potential threat in Neuro-science	Rate of evolution	Rapidly advancing clinical stage	Very early, slow progress	Rapidly advancing POC stage	Low	Steady advancement	Significant recent advances	Low
	Competitive risk	High	Low	Low	Low	Medium	High in niche areas	High
Neuroscience assets that may benefit		Biologics, degraders	AAV-delivered therapeutics	Payload-carrying nanoparticles	All therapeutics	All therapeutics	All therapeutics	Treatment of SCI

Author Contributions: Conceptualization, A.H.M., T.M.F., M.M., C.U., R.V. and D.R.L.; writing—original draft preparation, A.H.M., T.M.F., M.M., C.U. and D.R.L.; writing—review and editing, A.H.M., T.M.F., M.M., C.U., R.V. and D.R.L. All authors have read and agreed to the published version of the manuscript.

Funding: This research received no external funding.

Institutional Review Board Statement: Not applicable.

Informed Consent Statement: Not applicable.

Data Availability Statement: Not applicable.

Conflicts of Interest: All authors are employees of AbbVie and may own AbbVie stock. AbbVie participated in the interpretation of data, review, and approval of the publication. AbbVie did not provide any additional funding.

References

1. Pardridge, W.M. CNS drug design based on principles of blood–brain barrier transport. *J. Neurochem.* **1998**, *70*, 1781–1792. [CrossRef]
2. Abbott, N.J.; Patabendige, A.A.K.; Dolman, D.E.M.; Yusof, S.R.; Begley, D.J. Structure and function of the blood-brain barrier. *Neurobiol. Dis.* **2010**, *37*, 13–25. [CrossRef]
3. St-Amour, I.; Paré, I.; Alata, W.; Coulombe, K.; Ringuette-Goulet, C.; Drouin-Ouelet, J.; Vandal, M.; Soulet, D.; Bazin, R.; Calon, F. Brain bioavailability of human intravenous immunoglobulin and its transport through the murine blood-brain barrier. *J. Cereb. Blood Flow Metab.* **2013**, *33*, 1983–1992. [CrossRef]
4. Tan, J.-K.Y.; Sellers, D.L.; Pham, B.; Pun, S.H.; Horner, P.J. Non-viral nucleic acid delivery strategies to the central nervous system. *Front. Mol. Neurosci.* **2016**, *9*, 108. [CrossRef]
5. Banks, W.A. From blood–brain barrier to blood–brain interface: New opportunities for CNS drug delivery. *Nat. Rev. Drug Discov.* **2016**, *15*, 275–292. [CrossRef]
6. Terstappen, G.C.; Meyer, A.H.; Bell, R.D.; Zhang, W. Strategies for delivering therapeutics across the blood-brain barrier. *Nat. Rev. Drug Discov.* **2021**, *20*, 362–383. [CrossRef]
7. Ginn, S.L.; Amaya, A.K.; Alexander, I.E.; Edelstein, M.; Abedie, M.R. Gene therapy clinical trials worldwide to 2017: An update. *J. Gene Med.* **2018**, *20*, e3015. [CrossRef]
8. He, X.; Urip, B.A.; Zhang, Z.; Ngan, C.C.; Feng, B. Evolving AAV-delivered therapeutics towards ultimate cures. *J. Mol. Med.* **2021**, *99*, 593–617. [CrossRef]
9. McFarthing, K.; Prakash, N.; Simuni, T. Clinical Trial Highlights: 1. Gene Therapy for Parkinson's, 2. Phase 3 study in focus—Intec Pharma's Accordion pill, 3. Clinical trial resources. *J. Park. Dis.* **2019**, *9*, 251–264. [CrossRef]
10. Beyer, M.; Truehart, T. Axovant Announces Clinical Updates from AXO-AAV-GM2 and Axo-Lenti-PD Studies. Available online: https://investors.siogtx.com/news-releases/news-release-details/axovant-announces-clinical-updates-axo-aav-gm2-and-axo-lenti-pd (accessed on 24 March 2023).
11. Palfi, S.; Gurruchaga, J.S.; Ralph, G.S.; Lepetit, H.; Lavisse, S.; Buttery, P.C.; Watts, C.; Miskin, J.; Kelleher, M.; Deeley, S.; et al. Long-term safety and tolerability of ProSavin, a lentiviral vector-based gene therapy for Parkinson's disease: A dose escalation, open-label, phase $\frac{1}{2}$ trial. *Lancet* **2014**, *383*, 1138–1146. [CrossRef]
12. Christine, C.W.; Bankiewicz, K.S.; Van Laar, A.D.; Richardson, R.M.; Ravina, B.; Kells, A.P.; Boot, B.; Martin, A.J.; Nutt, J.; Thompson, M.E.; et al. Magnetic resonance imaging-guided phase 1 trial of putaminal AADC gene therapy for Parkinson's disease. *Ann. Neurol.* **2019**, *85*, 704–714. [CrossRef]
13. Delport, A.; Hewer, R. Inducing the degradation of Disease-related proteins using heterobifunctional molecules. *Molecules* **2019**, *24*, 3272. [CrossRef]
14. Sakamoto, K.M.; Kim, K.B.; Kumagai, A.; Mercurio, F.; Crews, C.M.; Deshaies, R.J. Protacs: Chimeric molecules that target proteins to the Skp1-Cullin-F box complex for ubiquitination and degradation. *Proc. Natl. Acad. Sci. USA* **2001**, *98*, 8554–8559. [CrossRef]
15. Takahashi, D.; Moriyama, J.; Nakamura, T.; Miki, E.; Takahashi, E.; Sato, A.; Akaike, T.; Itto-Nakama, K.; Arimoto, H. AUTACs: Cargo-Specific Degraders Using Selective Autophagy. *Mol. Cell* **2019**, *76*, 797–810. [CrossRef]
16. Banik, S.M.; Pedram, K.; Wisnovsky, S.; Ahn, G.; Riley, N.M.; Bertozzi, C.R.R. Lysosome-targeting chimaeras for degradation of extracellular proteins. *Nature* **2020**, *584*, 291–297. [CrossRef]
17. Dong, G.; Ding, Y.; He, S.; Sheng, C. Molecular Glues for Targeted Protein Degradation: From Serendipity to Rational Discovery. *J. Med. Chem.* **2021**, *64*, 10606–10620. [CrossRef]
18. Schreiber, S.L. The rise of molecular glues. *Cell* **2021**, *184*, 3–9. [CrossRef]
19. Ishida, T.; Ciulli, A. E3 ligase ligands for PROTACs: How they were found and how to discover new ones. *SLAS Discov.* **2021**, *26*, 484–502. [CrossRef]

20. Petrylak, D.P.; Gao, X.; Vogelzang, N.J.; Garfield, M.H.; Taylor, I.; Moore, M.D.; Peck, R.A.; Burris, H.A., III. First-in-Human Phase I Study of ARV-110, an Androgen Receptor (AR) PROTAC Degrader in Patients (pts) with Metastatic Castrate-Resistant Prostate Cancer. *J. Clin. Oncol.* **2020**, *38*, 3500. [CrossRef]
21. Thibaudeau, T.A.; Anderson, R.T.; Smith, D.M. A common mechanism of proteasome impairment by neurodegenerative disease-associated oligomers. *Nat. Commun.* **2018**, *9*, 1097. [CrossRef]
22. Farrell, K.; Jarome, T.J. Is PROTAC technology really a game changer for central nervous system drug discovery? *Expert Opin. Drug Discov.* **2021**, *16*, 833–840. [CrossRef]
23. Chu, T.-T.; Gao, N.; Li, Q.-Q.; Chen, P.-G.; Yang, X.-F.; Chen, Y.-X.; Zhao, Y.-F.; Li, Y.-M. Specific Knockdown of Endogenous Tau Protein by Peptide-Directed Ubiquitin-Proteasome Degradation. *Cell Chem. Biol.* **2016**, *23*, 453–461. [CrossRef]
24. Kamaly, N.; Yameen, B.; Wu, J.; Farokhzad, O.C. Degradable controlled-release polymers and polymeric nanoparticles: Mechanisms of controlling drug release. *Chem. Rev.* **2016**, *116*, 2602–2663. [CrossRef]
25. DeMarino, C.; Schwab, A.; Pleet, M.; Mathiesen, A.; Friedman, J.; El-Hage, N.; Kashanchi, F. Biodegradable Nanoparticles for Delivery of Therapeutics in CNS Infection. *J. Neuroimmune Pharmacol.* **2017**, *12*, 31–50. [CrossRef]
26. Fonseca-Santos, B.; Gremiao, M.P.; Chorilli, M. Nanotechnology-based drug delivery systems for the treatment of Alzheimer's disease. *Int. J. Nanomed.* **2015**, *10*, 4981–5003. [CrossRef]
27. Anselmo, A.C.; Mitragotri, S. Nanoparticles in the clinic: An update. *Bioeng. Transl. Med.* **2016**, *1*, 10–29. [CrossRef]
28. Sukhanova, A.; Bozrova, S.; Sokolov, P.; Berestovoy, M.; Karaulov, A.; Nabiev, I. Dependence of Nanoparticle Toxicity on their Physical and Chemical Properties. *Nanoscale Res. Lett.* **2018**, *13*, 44. [CrossRef]
29. Sakurai, H.; Kawabata, K.; Sakurai, F.; Nagakawa, S.; Mizuguchi, H. Innate Immune Response Induced by Gene Delivery Vectors. *Int. J. Pharm.* **2008**, *354*, 9–15. [CrossRef]
30. Albanese, A.; Tang, P.S.; Chan, W.C.W. The effect of nanoparticle size, shape, and surface chemistry on biological systems. *Ann. Rev. Biomed. Eng.* **2012**, *14*, 1–16. [CrossRef]
31. Liu, X.; Huang, N.; Li, H.; Jin, Q.; Ji, J. Surface and size effects on cell interaction of gold nanoparticles with both phagocytic and nonphagocytic cells. *Langmuir* **2013**, *29*, 9138–9148. [CrossRef]
32. Dreaden, E.C.; Austin, L.A.; Mackey, M.A.; El-Sayed, M.A. Size matters: Gold nanoparticles in targeted cancer drug delivery. *Therapeut. Deliv.* **2012**, *3*, 457–478. [CrossRef]
33. Zuckerman, J.E.; Choi, C.H.J.; Han, H.; Davis, M.E. Polycation-siRNA nanoparticles can disassemble at the kidney glomerular basement membrane. *Proc. Natl Acad. Sci. USA* **2012**, *109*, 3137–3142. [CrossRef]
34. Hühn, D.; Kantner, K.; Geidel, C.; Brandholt, S.; De Cock, I.; Soenen, S.J.H.; Rivera Gil, P.; Montenegro, J.-M.; Braeckmans, K.; Müllen, K.; et al. Polymer-coated nanoparticles interacting with proteins and cells: Focusing on the sign of the net charge. *ACS Nano* **2013**, *7*, 3253–3263. [CrossRef]
35. Chen, L.; Mccrate, J.M.; Lee, J.C.-M.; Li, H. The role of surface charge on the uptake and biocompatibility of hydroxyapatite nanoparticles with osteoblast cells. *Nanotechnology* **2011**, *22*, 105708. [CrossRef]
36. Available online: https://www.imi.europa.eu/sites/default/files/uploads/documents/projects/COMPACT_summary_final_report.pdf (accessed on 25 October 2022).
37. Kaleta, L.; Meyer, A.; Ried, C.; Rohe, M.; Schäker-Theobald, C.; Talmon, S.; Untucht, C.; Zimmermann, T. Albumin-Modified Nanoparticles Carrying a Targeting Ligand. International Patent WO2019048531A1, 14 March 2019.
38. Bhattacharjee, S. Understanding the burst release phenomenon: Towards designing effective nanoparticulate drug-delivery systems. *Ther. Deliv.* **2021**, *12*, 21–36. [CrossRef]
39. Liu, Z.; Gao, X.; Kang, T.; Jiang, M.; Miao, D.; Gu, G.; Hu, Q.; Song, Q.; Yao, L.; Tu, Y.; et al. B6 peptide-modified PEG-PLA nanoparticles for enhanced brain delivery of neuroprotective peptide. *Bioconjugate Chem.* **2013**, *24*, 997–1007. [CrossRef]
40. Liu, Y.; An, S.; Li, J.; Kuang, Y.; He, X.; Guo, Y.; Ma, H.; Zhang, Y.; Ji, B.; Jiang, C. Brain-targeted co-delivery of therapeutic gene and peptide by multifunctional nanoparticles in Alzheimer's disease mice. *Biomaterials* **2016**, *80*, 33–45. [CrossRef]
41. Vilella, A.; Belletti, D.; Sauer, A.K.; Hagmeyer, S.; Sarowar, T.; Masoni, M.; Stasiak, N.; Mulvihill, J.J.E.; Rouzi, B.; Forni, F.; et al. Reduced plaque size and inflammation in the APP23 mous emodel for Alzheimer's disease after chronic application of polymeric nanoparticles for CNS targeted zinc delivery. *J. Trace Elem. Med. Biol.* **2018**, *49*, 210–221. [CrossRef]
42. Saunders, N.R.M.; Paolini, M.S.; Fenton, O.S.; Poul, L.; Devalliere, J.; Mpabani, F.; Damon, A.; Bergère, M.; Jibault, O.; Germain, M.; et al. A Nanoprimer to improve the systemic delivery of siRNA and mRNA. *Nano Lett.* **2020**, *20*, 4264–4269. [CrossRef]
43. Germain, M.; Meyre, M.-E.; Poul, L.; Paolini, M.; Berjaud, C.; Mpabani, F.; Bergère, M.; Levy, L.; Pottier, A. Priming the body to receive the therapeutic agent to redefine treatment benefit/risk profile. *Sci. Rep.* **2018**, *8*, 4797. [CrossRef]
44. Liu, T.; Choi, H.; Zhou, R.; Chen, I.-W. RES blockade: A strategy for boosting efficiency of nanoparticle drug. *Nano Today* **2015**, *10*, 11–21. [CrossRef]
45. Jacobs, F.; Wisse, E.; De Geest, B. The role of Liver Sinusoidal Cells in Hepatocyte-Directed Gene Transfer. *Am. J. Pathol.* **2010**, *176*, 14–21. [CrossRef]
46. Van Dijk, R.; Montenegro-Miranda, P.S.; Riviere, C.; Schilderink, R.; ten Bloemendaal, L.; van Gorp, J.; Duijst, S.; de Waarrt, D.R.; Beuers, U.; Haiisma, H.J.; et al. Polyinosinic Acid Blocks Adeno-Associated Virus Macrophage Endocytosis In Vitro and Enhances Adeno-Associated Virus Liver-Directed Gene Therapy In Vivo. *Hum. Gene Ther.* **2013**, *24*, 807–813. [CrossRef]

47. Germain, M.; Meyer, M.-E.; Pottier, A.; Laurent, L. Pharmaceutical Composition, Preparation and Uses Thereof. International Patent WO 2016/083333 A1, 2 June 2016.
48. Zhang, Y.N.; Poon, W.; Tavares, A.J.; McGilvray, I.; Chan, W.C.W. Nanoparticle-liver interactions: Cellular uptake and Hepatobiliary elimination. *J. Control. Release* **2016**, *240*, 332–348. [CrossRef]
49. Berns, K.I.; Giraud, C. Biology of Adeno-Associated Virus. In *Adeno-Associated Virus (AAV) Vectors in Gene Therapy. Current Topics in Microbiology and Immunology*; Berns, K.I., Giraud, C., Eds.; Springer: Berlin/Heidelberg, Germany, 1996; Volume 218. [CrossRef]
50. Goertsen, D.; Flytzanis, N.C.; Goeden, N.; Chuapoco, M.R.; Cummins, A.; Chen, Y.; Fan, Y.; Zhang, Q.; Sharma, J.; Duan, Y.; et al. AAV capsid variants with brain-wide transgene expression and decreased liver targeting after intravenous delivery in mouse and marmoset. *Nat. Neurosci.* **2021**, *25*, 106–115. [CrossRef]
51. Simons, M.; Raposo, G. Exosomes-vesicular carriers for intercellular communication. *Curr. Opin. Cell Biol.* **2009**, *21*, 575–581. [CrossRef]
52. ElAndaloussi, S.; Mäger, I.; Breakefield, X.O.; Wood, M.J.A. Extracellular vesicles: Biology and emerging therapeutic opportunities. *Nat. Rev. Drug Discov.* **2013**, *12*, 3347–3357.
53. Yang, J.; Zhang, X.; Chen, X.; Wang, L.; Yang, Y. Exosome mediated delivery of miR-124 promotes neurogenesis after ischemia. *Mol. Ther. Nucleic Acids* **2017**, *7*, 278–287. [CrossRef]
54. Xin, H.; Wang, F.; Li, Y.; Lu, Q.-E.; Cheung, W.L.; Zhang, Y.; Zhang, Z.G.; Chopp, M. Secondary release of exosomes from astrocytes contributes to the increase in neural plasticity and improvement of functional recovery after stroke in rats treated with exosomes harvested from microRNA133b- overexpressed multipotent mesenchymal stromal cells. *Cell Transplant.* **2017**, *26*, 243–257.
55. Alvarez-Erviti, L.; Seow, Y.; Yin, H.; Betts, C.; Lakhal, S.; Wood, M.J.A. Delivery of siRNA to the mouse brain by systemic injection of targeted exosomes. *Nat. Biotechnol.* **2011**, *29*, 341–345. [CrossRef]
56. Cooper, J.M.; Wiklander, P.B.O.; Nordin, J.Z.; Al-Shawi, R.; Wood, M.J.A.; Vithlani, M.; Schapira, A.H.V.; Simons, J.P.; El-Andaloussi, S.; Alvarez-Erviti, L. Systemic exosomal siRNA delivery reduced alpha-synuclein aggregates in brains of transgenic mice. *Mov. Disord.* **2014**, *29*, 1476–1485. [CrossRef] [PubMed]
57. Dai, S.; Wei, D.; Wu, Z.; Zhou, X.; Wei, X.; Huang, H.; Li, G. Phase 1 clinical trial of autologous ascites-derived exosomes combined with GM-CSF for colorectal cancer. *Mol. Ther.* **2008**, *16*, 782–790. [CrossRef] [PubMed]
58. Morse, M.A.; Garst, J.; Osada, T.; Khan, S.; Hobeika, A.; Clay, T.M.; Valente, N.; Shreeniwas, R.; Sutton, M.A.; Delcayre, A.; et al. A phase 1 study of dexosome immunotherapy in patients with advanced non-small cell lung cancer. *J. Transl. Med.* **2005**, *3*, 9. [CrossRef] [PubMed]
59. Zipkin, M. Big Pharma buys into exosomes for drug delivery. *Nat. Biotechnol.* **2020**, *38*, 1226–1228. [CrossRef] [PubMed]
60. Available online: https://www.vesigentx.com/about/news/vesigen-therapeutics-launches-with-usd-28-5-million-series-a-investment-led-by-leaps-by-bayer-and-morningside-ventures/ (accessed on 6 October 2022).
61. Available online: https://www.carminetherapeutics.com/post/carmine-therapeutics-takeda-collaborate-to-develop-novel-non-viral-gene-therapies (accessed on 6 October 2022).
62. Available online: https://www.curexsys.com/evotec-und-sartorius-finance-cirexsys/ (accessed on 6 October 2022).
63. Available online: https://ir.codiakbio.com/news-releases/news-release-details/jazz-pharmaceuticals-and-codiak-biosciences-announce-strategic (accessed on 6 October 2022).
64. Available online: https://ir.codiakbio.com/news-releases/news-release-details/sarepta-therapeutics-and-codiak-biosciences-collaborate-research (accessed on 6 October 2022).
65. Available online: https://www.evoxtherapeutics.com/News/Jun-2020/Evox-Therapeutics-Enters-Into-Lilly-Collaboration (accessed on 6 October 2022).
66. Available online: https://www.fiercebiotech.com/biotech/boehringer-forges-alliance-uk-exosome-specialist-evox (accessed on 6 October 2022).
67. Available online: https://www.evoxtherapeutics.com/News/March-2020/Evox-Therapeutics-and-Takeda-collaboration (accessed on 6 October 2022).
68. Available online: http://tools.euroland.com/tools/PressReleases/GetPressRelease/?ID=3554419&lang=en-GB&companycode=services (accessed on 6 October 2022).
69. Escudier, B.; Dorval, T.; Chaput, N.; André, F.; Caby, M.P.; Novault, S.; Flament, C.; Leboulaire, C.; Borg, C.; Amigorena, S.; et al. Vaccination of metastatic melanoma patients with autologous dendritic cell (DC) derived exosomes: Results of the first phase I clinical trial. *J. Transl. Med.* **2005**, *3*, 10. [CrossRef]
70. Li, C.; Sun, T.; Jiang, C. Recent advances in nanomedicine for the treatment of ischemic stroke. *Acta Pharm. Sin. B* **2021**, *11*, 1767–1788. [CrossRef]
71. Ruan, C.; Liu, L.; Zhang, Y.; He, X.; Chen, X.; Zhang, Y.; Chen, Q.; Guo, Q.; Sun, T.; Jiang, C. Substance P-modified human serum albumin nanoparticles loaded with paclitaxel for targeted therapy of glioma. *Acta Pharm. Sin. B* **2018**, *8*, 85–96. [CrossRef]
72. Fu, S.; Wang, Y.; Xia, X.; Zheng, J.C. Exosome engineering: Current progress in cargo loading and targeted delivery. *NanoImpact* **2020**, *20*, 100261. [CrossRef]
73. Chen, C.C.; Liu, L.; Ma, F.; Wong, C.W.; Guo, X.E.; Chacko, J.V.; Farhoodi, H.P.; Zhang, S.X.; Zimak, J.; Ségaliny, A.; et al. Elucidation of exosome migration across the Blood-Brain Barrier model in vitro. *Cell. Mol. Bioeng.* **2016**, *9*, 509–529. [CrossRef]

74. Maguire, C.A.; Balaj, L.; Sivaraman, S.; Crommentuijn, M.H.W.; Ericsson, M.; Mincheva-Nilsson, L.; Baranov, V.; Gianni, D.; Tannous, B.A.; Sena-Esteves, M.; et al. Microvesicle-associated AAV Vector as a novel gene delivery system. *Mol. Ther.* **2012**, *20*, 960–971. [CrossRef]
75. Gyorgy, B.; Fitzpatrick, Z.; Crommentuijn, M.H.W.; Mu, D.; Maguire, C.A. Naturally enveloped AAV vectors for shielding neutralizing antibodies and robust gene delivery in vivo. *Biomaterials* **2014**, *35*, 7598–7606. [CrossRef]
76. Hudry, E.; Martin, C.; Gandhi, S.; Gyorgy, B.; Maguire, C.A. Exosome-associated AAV vector as a robust and convenient neuroscience tool. *Gene Ther.* **2016**, *23*, 380–392. [CrossRef]
77. Liu, B.; Li, Z.; Huang, S.; He, S.; Chen, F.; Liang, Y. AAV-containing exosomes as a novel vector for improved gene delivery to lung cancer cells. *Front. Cell Dev. Biol.* **2021**, *13*, 707607. [CrossRef]
78. Chen, K.-T.; Wei, K.-C.; Liu, H.-L. Theranostic Strategy of Focused Ultrasound Induced Blood Brain Barrier Opening for CNS Disease Treatment. *Front. Pharmacol.* **2019**, *10*, 86. [CrossRef]
79. Lipsman, N.; Meng, Y.; Bethune, A.J.; Huang, Y.; Lam, B.; Masellis, M.; Herrmann, N.; Heyn, C.; Aubert, I.; Boutet, A.; et al. Blood Brain Barrier Opening in Alzheimer's Disease using MR-guided Focused Ultrasound. *Nat. Commun.* **2018**, *9*, 2336. [CrossRef]
80. National Academies of Sciences, Engineering, and Medicine; Health and Medicine Division; Board on Health Sciences Policy; Forum on Neuroscience and Nervous System Disorders. *Enabling Novel Treatments for Nervous System Disorders by Improving Methods for Traversing the Blood-Brain Barrier: Proceedings from a Workshop*; National Academies Press: Washington, DC, USA, 2018.
81. Kovacs, Z.I.; Kim, S.; Jikaria, N.; Frank, J.A. Disrupting the Blood Brain Barrier by Focused Ultrasound Induces Sterile Inflammation. *Proc. Nat. Acad. Sci. USA* **2016**, *114*, E75–E84. [CrossRef]
82. Schregel, K.; Baufeld, C.; Palotai, M.; Meroni, R.; Fiorina, P.; Wuerfel, J.; Sinkus, R.; Zhang, Y.-Z.; McDannold, N.; White, J.P.; et al. Targeted Blood Brain Barrier Opening with Focused Ultrasound Induces Focal Macrophage/Microglial Activation in Experimental Autoimmune Encephalomyelitis. *Front. Neurosci.* **2021**, *15*, 665722. [CrossRef]
83. Jeon, M.T.; Kim, K.-S.; Kim, E.S.; Lee, S.; Kim, J.; Hoe, H.-S.; Kim, D.-G. Emerging Pathogenic Role of Peripheral Blood Factors following BBB Disruption in Neurodegenerative Disease. *Ageing Res. Rev.* **2021**, *68*, 101333. [CrossRef]
84. Adams, R.A.; Schachtrup, C.; Davalos, D.; Tsigelny, I.; Akassoglou, K. Fibrinogen Signal Transduction as a Mediator and Therapeutic Target in Inflammation: Lessons from Multiple Sclerosis. *Curr. Med. Chem.* **2007**, *14*, 2925–2936. [CrossRef]
85. Montagne, A.; Nikolakopoulou, A.M.; Zhao, Z.; Sagare, A.P.; Si, G.; Lazic, D.; Barnes, S.R.; Daianu, M.; Ramanathan, A.; Go, A.; et al. Pericyte Degeneration Causes White Matter Dysfunction in the Mouse Central Nervous System. *Nat. Med.* **2018**, *24*, 326–337. [CrossRef]
86. Bohlson, S.S.; O'Conner, S.D.; Hulsebus, H.J.; Ho, M.-M.; Fraser, D.A. Complement C1q and C1q-Related Molecules Regulate Macrophage Polarization. *Front. Immunol.* **2014**, *5*, 402. [CrossRef]
87. Fraser, D.A.; Pisalyaput, K.; Tenner, A.J. C1q Enhances Microglial Clearance of Apoptotic Neurons and Neuronal Blebs and Modulates Subsequent Inflammatory Cytokine Production. *J. Neurochem.* **2010**, *112*, 733–743. [CrossRef]
88. Park, S.H.; Baik, K.; Jeon, S.; Chang, W.S.; Ye, B.S.; Chang, J.W. Extensive Frontal Focused Ultrasound Mediated Blood-Brain Barrier Opening for the Treatment of Alzheimer's Disease: A Proof of Concept Study. *Transl. Neurodegener.* **2021**, *10*, 44. [CrossRef] [PubMed]
89. Definity® (Perflutren Lipid Microsphere) Injectable Suspension Prescribing Information, RefID: 4649217 Revised 07/2020. Available online: https://www.accessdata.fda.gov/drugsatfda_docs/label/2020/021064s023lbl.pdf (accessed on 24 March 2023).
90. Zhao, B.; Chen, Y.; Liu, J.; Zhang, L.; Wang, J.; Yang, Y.; Lv, Q.; Xie, M. Blood Brain Barrier Disruption Induced by Diagnostic Ultrasound Combined with Microbubbles in Mice. *Oncotarget* **2018**, *9*, 4897–4914. [CrossRef] [PubMed]
91. Truong, K. InSightec Wants to Usher in a New Era of Incisionless Surgery. MedCity News. 2019. Available online: https://medcitynews.com/2019/07/insightec-wants-to-usher-in-a-new-era-of-incisionless-surgery/ (accessed on 25 October 2022).
92. Health Quality Ontario. Magnetic Resonance-Guided Focused Ultrasound Neurosurgery for Essential Tremor: A Health Technology Assessment. *Ont. Health Technol. Assess. Ser.* **2018**, *18*, 1–141.
93. Kouzehgarani, G.N.; Feldsien, T.; Engelhard, H.H.; Mirakhur, K.K.; Phipps, C.; Nimmrich, V.; Clausznitzer, D.; Lefebvre, D.R. Harnessing Cerebrospinal Fluid Circulation for Drug Delivery to Brain Tissues. *Adv. Drug Deliv. Rev.* **2021**, *173*, 20–59. [CrossRef] [PubMed]
94. Jessen, N.A.; Finmann Munk, A.S.; Lundgaard, I.; Nedergaard, M. The glymphatic system—A beginner's guide. *Neurochem. Res.* **2015**, *40*, 2583–2599. [CrossRef]
95. Yadav, D.B.; Maloney, J.A.; Wildsmith, K.R.; Fuji, R.N.; Meilandt, W.J.; Solanoy, H.; Lu, Y.; Peng, K.; Wilson, B.; Chan, P.; et al. Widespread brain distribution and activity following i.c.v. infusion of anti-beta-secretase (BACE1) in nonhuman primates. *Br. J. Pharmacol.* **2017**, *174*, 4173–4185. [CrossRef]
96. Paul, G.; Zaghrisson, O.; Varrone, A.; Almqvist, P.; Jerling, M.; Rehncrona, S.; Linderoth, B.; Bjarmarz, H.; Shafer, L.L.; Coffey, R.; et al. Safety and tolerability of intracerebroventricular PDGF-BB in Parkinson's diesease patients. *J. Clin. Investig.* **2015**, *125*, 1339–1346. [CrossRef]
97. Van Damme, P.; Tilkin, P.; Mercer, K.J.; Terryn, J.; D'Hondt, A.; Herne, N.; Tousseyn, T.; Claeys, K.G.; Thal, D.R.; Zachrisson, O.; et al. Intracerebroventricular delivery of vascular endothelial growth factor in patients with amyotrophic lateral sclerosis, a phase I study. *Brain Commun.* **2020**, *2*, fcaa160. [CrossRef]

98. Kouzehgarani, G.N.; Kumar, P.; Bolin, S.; Reilly, E.; Lefebvre, D.R. Biodistribution Analysis of an Anti-EGFR Antibody in the Rat Brain: Validation of CSF Microcirculation as a Viable Pathway to Circumvent the Blood-Brain Barrier for Drug Delivery. *Pharmaceutics* **2022**, *14*, 1441. [CrossRef]
99. Thakker, D.; Weatherspoon, M.R.; Harrison, J.; Keene, T.E.; Lane, D.S.; Kaemmerer, W.F.; Stewart, G.R.; Shafer, L.L. Intracerebroventricular amyloid-beta antibodies reduce cerebral amyloid angiopathy and associated micro-hemorrhages in aged Tg2576 mice. *Proc. Natl. Acad. Sci. USA* **2009**, *106*, 4501–4506. [CrossRef]
100. Ishii, T.; Muranaka, R.; Tashiro, O.; Nishimura, M. Chronic intracerebroventricular administration of anti-neuropeptide Y antibody stimulates starvation-induced feeding via compensatory responses in the hypothalamus. *Brain Res.* **2007**, *1144*, 91–100. [CrossRef]
101. Tangen, K.; Nestorov, I.; Verma, A.; Sullivan, J.; Holt, R.W.; Linninger, A.A. In Vivo Intrathecal Tracer Dispersion in Cynomolgus Monkey Validates Wide Biodistribution Along Neuraxis. *IEEE Trans. Biomed. Eng.* **2020**, *67*, 1122–1132. [CrossRef]
102. Thakker, D.R.; Adams, E.; Stewart, G.R.; Shafer, L. *Distribution of Molecules through the Cerebral Spinal Fluid (CSF) of Non-Human Primates: Influence of Delivery Site, Flow Rate, and MOLECULAR mass of the Test Agent*; Society for Neuroscience: Washington, DC, USA, 2011.
103. Fleischhack, G.; Reif, S.; Hasan, C.; Jaehde, U.; Hettmer, S.; Bode, U. Feasibility of intraventricular administration of etoposide in patients with metastatic brain tumours. *Br. J. Cancer* **2001**, *84*, 1453–1459. [CrossRef]
104. Cook, M.; Murphy, M.; Bulluss, K.; D'Souza, W.; Plummer, C.; Priest, E.; Williams, C.; Sharan, A.; Fisher, R.; Pincus, S.; et al. Anti-seizure therapy with a long-term, implanted intra-cerebroventricular delivery system for drug-resistant epilepsy: A first-in-man study. *eClinicalMedicine* **2020**, *22*, 100326. [CrossRef]
105. Vuillemenot, B.R.; Kennedy, D.; Reed, R.P.; Boyd, R.B.; Butt, M.T.; Musson, D.G.; Keve, S.; Cahayag, R.; Tsuruda, L.S.; O'Neill, C.A. Recombinant human tripeptidyl peptidase-1 infusion to the monkey CNS: Safety, pharmacokinetics, and distribution. *Toxicol. Appl. Pharmacol.* **2014**, *277*, 49–57. [CrossRef]
106. Wang, J.K.; Nauss, L.A.; Thomas, J.E. Pain relief by intrathecally applied morphine in man. *Anesthesiology* **1979**, *50*, 149–151. [CrossRef]
107. De Andres, J.; Hayek, S.; Perruchoud, C.; Lawrence, M.M.; Reina, M.A.; De Andres-Serrano, C.; Rubio-Haro, R.; Hunt, M.; Yaksh, T.L. Intrathecal drug delivery: Advances and applications in the management of chronic pain patient. *Front. Pain Res.* **2022**, *3*, 900566. [CrossRef]
108. Penn, R.D. Intrathecal baclofen for severe spasticity. *Ann. N. Y. Acad. Sci.* **1988**, *531*, 157–166. [CrossRef]
109. SCI Clinical Trial Website. Available online: https://scitrials.org/triallist (accessed on 19 October 2022).
110. Available online: https://clinicaltrials.gov/ct2/show/NCT04295538 (accessed on 19 October 2022).
111. Available online: https://clinicaltrials.gov/ct2/show/NCT04096950 (accessed on 19 October 2022).
112. Available online: https://ichgcp.net/clinical-trials-registry/NCT04096950 (accessed on 19 October 2022).
113. Available online: https://clinicaltrials.gov/ct2/show/record/NCT03989440 (accessed on 19 October 2022).
114. Available online: https://clinicaltrials.gov/ct2/show/NCT03935321 (accessed on 19 October 2022).
115. Marin, B.M.; Porath, K.A.; Jain, S.; Kim, M.; Conage-Pough, J.E.; Oh, J.-H.; Miller, C.L.; Talele, S.; Kitange, G.J.; Tian, S.; et al. Heterogeneous delivery across the blood-brain barrier Limits the efficacy of an EGFR-targeting antibody drug conjugate in GBM. *Neuro-Oncol.* **2021**, *23*, 20423–22053. [CrossRef] [PubMed]
116. Porath, K.; Regan, M.; Griffith, J.; Jain, S.; Stopka, S.; Burgenske, D.; Bakken, K.; Carlson, B.; Decker, P.; Vaubel, R.; et al. Convection enhanced delivery of EGFR targeting antibody-drug conjugates Serclutamab talirine and Depatux-M in glioblastoma patient derived xenografts. *Neurooncol. Adv.* **2022**, *4*, vdac130. [CrossRef] [PubMed]
117. Hadaczek, P.; Kohutnicka, M.; Krauze, M.T.; Bringas, J.; Pivirotto, P.; Cunningham, J.; Bankiewicz, K. CED of Adeno-Associated Virus Type 2 (AAV2) into the striatum and transport of AAV2 within monkey brain. *Hum. Gene Ther.* **2006**, *17*, 291–302. [CrossRef] [PubMed]
118. Johnston, L.C.; Eberling, J.; Pivirotto, P.; Hadaczek, P.; Federoff, H.J.; Forsayeth, J.; Bankiewicz, K.S. Clinically Relevant Effects of CED od AAV2-GDNF on the dopamine Nigrostriatal Pathway in aged Rhesus monkeys. *Hum. Gene Ther.* **2009**, *20*, 497–510. [CrossRef]

Disclaimer/Publisher's Note: The statements, opinions and data contained in all publications are solely those of the individual author(s) and contributor(s) and not of MDPI and/or the editor(s). MDPI and/or the editor(s) disclaim responsibility for any injury to people or property resulting from any ideas, methods, instructions or products referred to in the content.

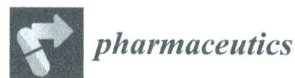

Article

A Single Injection with Sustained-Release Microspheres and a Prime-Boost Injection of Bovine Serum Albumin Elicit the Same IgG Antibody Response in Mice

Renée S. van der Kooij [1], Martin Beukema [2], Anke L. W. Huckriede [2], Johan Zuidema [3], Rob Steendam [3], Henderik W. Frijlink [1] and Wouter L. J. Hinrichs [1,*]

[1] Groningen Research Institute of Pharmacy, Department of Pharmaceutical Technology and Biopharmacy, University of Groningen, Antonius Deusinglaan 1, 9713 AV Groningen, The Netherlands
[2] Department of Medical Microbiology and Infection Prevention, University Medical Center Groningen, University of Groningen, Antonius Deusinglaan 1, 9713 AV Groningen, The Netherlands
[3] InnoCore Pharmaceuticals, L.J. Zielstraweg 1, 9713 GX Groningen, The Netherlands
* Correspondence: w.l.j.hinrichs@rug.nl; Tel.: +31-(0)50-36-32398

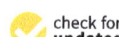

Citation: van der Kooij, R.S.; Beukema, M.; Huckriede, A.L.W.; Zuidema, J.; Steendam, R.; Frijlink, H.W.; Hinrichs, W.L.J. A Single Injection with Sustained-Release Microspheres and a Prime-Boost Injection of Bovine Serum Albumin Elicit the Same IgG Antibody Response in Mice. *Pharmaceutics* **2023**, *15*, 676. https://doi.org/10.3390/pharmaceutics15020676

Academic Editors: Vibhuti Agrahari and Prashant Kumar

Received: 20 January 2023
Revised: 6 February 2023
Accepted: 10 February 2023
Published: 16 February 2023

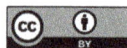

Copyright: © 2023 by the authors. Licensee MDPI, Basel, Switzerland. This article is an open access article distributed under the terms and conditions of the Creative Commons Attribution (CC BY) license (https://creativecommons.org/licenses/by/4.0/).

Abstract: Although vaccination is still considered to be the cornerstone of public health care, the increase in vaccination coverage has stagnated for many diseases. Most of these vaccines require two or three doses to be administered across several months or years. Single-injection vaccine formulations are an effective method to overcome the logistical barrier to immunization that is posed by these multiple-injection schedules. Here, we developed subcutaneously (s.c.) injectable microspheres with a sustained release of the model antigen bovine serum albumin (BSA). The microspheres were composed of blends of two novel biodegradable multi-block copolymers consisting of amorphous, hydrophilic poly(ε-caprolactone)-poly(ethylene glycol)-poly(ε-caprolactone) (PCL-PEG-PCL) blocks and semi-crystalline poly(dioxanone) (PDO) blocks of different block sizes. In vitro studies demonstrated that the release of BSA could be tailored over a period of approximately four to nine weeks by changing the blend ratio of both polymers. Moreover, it was found that BSA remained structurally intact during release. Microspheres exhibiting sustained release of BSA for six weeks were selected for the in vivo study in mice. The induced BSA-specific IgG antibody titers increased up to four weeks after administration and were of the same magnitude as found in mice that received a priming and a booster dose of BSA in phosphate-buffered saline (PBS). Determination of the BSA concentration in plasma showed that in vivo release probably took place up to at least four weeks, although plasma concentrations peaked already one week after administration. The sustained-release microspheres might be a viable alternative to the conventional prime-boost immunization schedule, but a clinically relevant antigen should be incorporated to assess the full potential of these microspheres in practice.

Keywords: bovine serum albumin; immune response; monolithic microspheres; multi-block copolymer; single-injection vaccine; sustained release

1. Introduction

Although vaccination is one of the most successful medical interventions in history, coverage has not improved over the last decade for several diseases. In 2021, 18.2 million infants worldwide remained unvaccinated with the three-dose diphtheria-tetanus-pertussis (DTP3) vaccine and an additional 6.8 million only received an initial dose. This highlights a lack of access to immunization services, which is especially a problem in low- and middle-income countries [1,2]. To improve global vaccination coverage, the World Health Organization set up the Immunization Agenda 2030, with one of the objectives being the development of new vaccines, technologies, and improved products [3]. An example of an improved vaccine product is a single-injection vaccine formulation, such as a microsphere-based formulation, for vaccines that normally require multiple doses [4,5]. With this technology, the problem of the 6.8 million infants that were only partially vaccinated with the DTP3 vaccine could, for instance, be solved.

In a previous study, we developed polymeric core-shell microspheres that released the model antigen bovine serum albumin (BSA) after a lag time of three to seven weeks [6]. By co-injecting these microspheres together with a solution of BSA, a pulsatile release profile could potentially be obtained that mimics the current prime-boost immunization schedule with multiple doses at specific time intervals. Incorporation of a clinically used antigen into such a pulsatile-release formulation might result in a prolonged immunological response after only a single administration, thereby eliminating the need for booster injections. Although such pulsatile-release formulations that mimic the prime-boost immunization schedule are known to be safe and effective [4,7,8], alternative antigen release kinetics, such as sustained release, have proven to induce strong immune responses as well [9–11]. Moreover, sustained-release formulations are often easier to develop and manufacture and cause fewer side effects than pulsatile-release formulations [12]. As only low levels of antigen are generated upon release from the formulation, there is a limited amount of antigen systemically available during the entire period of release. It is, therefore, worthwhile to investigate the immunological response to such a formulation. In addition, sustained release more closely resembles a natural infection, because the immune system is continuously exposed to an increasing level of antigens during the course of the infection, which is usually several days or weeks [13]. The majority of the single injection vaccine formulations described in the literature are based on the biocompatible and biodegradable polymer poly(DL-lactide-co-glycolide) (PLGA) [4,9]. This polymer has the advantage of being the most extensively investigated polymer in the field of controlled release and has tunable release kinetics [14]. Hydrolytic degradation of PLGA, however, might lead to accumulation of the acidic degradation products lactic acid and glycolic acid, resulting in a pH drop within the microspheres. This might affect the structural integrity and lead to the incomplete release of the incorporated (proteinaceous) antigen [15–17]. Hence, alternative polymers enabling release that is mainly diffusion-controlled are highly desired, as the development of an acidic microclimate is prevented.

In this study, injectable sustained-release microspheres were developed that could serve as a single-injection vaccine formulation. These monolithic microspheres consisted of biodegradable multi-block copolymers in which BSA was incorporated. These phase-separated multi-block copolymers were composed of amorphous, hydrophilic poly(ε-caprolactone)-poly(ethylene glycol)-poly(ε-caprolactone) (PCL-PEG-PCL) blocks and semi-crystalline poly(dioxanone) (PDO) blocks. Such PEG-based polymers swell when brought into an aqueous environment, thereby allowing the gradual release of the model antigen by diffusion and avoiding the accumulation of acidic degradation products [18–20]. An acidic microclimate is, therefore, not formed, in contrast to PLGA-based systems. This, altogether, could allow for sustained release of structurally intact BSA over several weeks. The two multi-block copolymers used in this study differed in the weight ratio of the amorphous and semi-crystalline block, the PEG molecular weight, and the total weight fraction of PEG. We hypothesized that the release duration could be tailored by varying the blend ratio of the polymers. The BSA-loaded microspheres that most closely resembled the target in vitro release profile, that is, a linear or near-linear release over four to six weeks, were subcutaneously (s.c.) administered in mice as an in vivo proof-of-concept study. The induced BSA-specific IgG antibody responses for up to eight weeks and the BSA plasma concentration for up to four weeks were measured to determine whether the microspheres could serve as an alternative to the conventional prime-boost immunization schedule.

2. Materials and Methods

2.1. Materials

p-Dioxanone was obtained from HBCChem, Inc. (San Carlos, CA, USA). Anhydrous 1,4-butanediol (BDO), ε-caprolactone, and PEG with a molecular weight of 1000 g/mol (PEG_{1000}) and 3000 g/mol (PEG_{3000}) were purchased from Thermo Fisher Scientific (Waltham,

MA, USA). Stannous octoate was purchased from Sigma-Aldrich (Zwijndrecht, The Netherlands). 1,4-Butanediisocyanate (BDI) and acetonitrile were obtained from Actu-All Chemicals B.V. (Oss, The Netherlands). Polyvinyl alcohol (PVA; 5-88 EMPROVE®, 85–89% hydrolyzed), hydrogen peroxide, and sulfuric acid were purchased from Merck (Darmstadt, Germany). Sodium azide, Tween 20, dichloromethane (DCM), dimethyl sulfoxide (DMSO), and octane were purchased from Thermo Fisher Scientific (Waltham, MA, USA). BSA, sodium chloride (NaCl), sodium dodecyl sulfate (SDS), and o-phenylenediamine dihydrochloride (OPD) tablets were obtained from Sigma-Aldrich (St. Louis, MO, USA). Sodium hydroxide was obtained from VWR International Ltd. (Leicestershire, UK). Sodium carboxymethyl cellulose (CMC; Blanose™ 7HF PH) was purchased from Ashland (Covington, KY, USA). BSA sample diluent was from Cygnus Technologies (Southport, NC, USA), and horseradish peroxidase (HRP)-linked goat anti-mouse IgG antibody (1 mg/mL) was from Southern Biotech (Birmingham, AL, USA). For the phosphate-perchlorate buffer and the in vitro release medium, sodium dihydrogen phosphate dihydrate ($NaH_2PO_4 \cdot 2H_2O$) and disodium hydrogen phosphate (Na_2HPO_4) were purchased from Thermo Fisher Scientific (Waltham, MA, USA) and sodium perchlorate monohydrate ($NaClO_4 \cdot H_2O$) from VWR International Ltd. (EMSURE®, Leicestershire, UK). For the carbonate-bicarbonate buffer, sodium carbonate (Na_2CO_3) and sodium bicarbonate ($NaHCO_3$) were obtained from Merck (Darmstadt, Germany). For the BSA-specific IgG antibody ELISA, NaCl, potassium dihydrogen phosphate (KH_2PO_4), and Na_2HPO_4 were purchased from Merck (Darmstadt, Germany), sodium dihydrogen phosphate (NaH_2PO_4) from VWR International Ltd. (EMSURE®, Leicestershire, UK), and Tween 20 from Sigma-Aldrich (St. Louis, MO, USA). Gibco™ sterile-filtered 1× phosphate-buffered saline (PBS; 155 mM NaCl, 1.06 mM KH_2PO_4, 2.97 mM $Na_2HPO_4 \cdot 7H_2O$, pH 7.4) was purchased from Thermo Fisher Scientific (Waltham, MA, USA). This PBS was used for all experiments, unless otherwise stated. Sterile 10× PBS (1.5 M NaCl, 20 mM KH_2PO_4, 80 mM NaH_2PO_4, 30 mM KCl, pH 7.4) was obtained from VWR International Ltd. (Leicestershire, UK). Ultrapure water with a resistivity of 18.2 MΩ was obtained from a Millipore Milli-Q Integral 3 (A10) purification system and used for all experiments.

2.2. Polymer Synthesis and Characterization

Poly(ether ester urethane) multi-block copolymers composed of hydrophilic PCL-PEG-PCL and semi-crystalline PDO prepolymer blocks were synthesized and characterized using similar procedures as previously described [18,20].

PDO prepolymer with a target molecular weight of approximately 2800 g/mol was prepared of 356.5 or 228.3 g p-dioxanone in the bulk at 80 °C using 11.5 or 6.7 g anhydrous BDO to initiate the ring-opening polymerization for polymer A and B, respectively. Stannous octoate was used as a catalyst at a monomer/catalyst molar ratio of approximately 25.

[PCL-PEG$_{3000}$-PCL] prepolymer with a target molecular weight of 4000 g/mol and [PCL-PEG$_{1000}$-PCL] prepolymer with a target molecular weight of 2000 g/mol were synthesized similarly using 61.2 g ε-caprolactone, 183.5 g PEG$_{3000}$, and 31.3 mg stannous octoate for [PCL-PEG$_{3000}$-PCL], and 495.9 g ε-caprolactone, 500.9 g PEG$_{1000}$, and 140.1 mg stannous octoate for [PCL-PEG$_{1000}$-PCL]. The mixture was magnetically stirred at 160 °C for 69 h ([PCL-PEG$_{3000}$-PCL]) or 73 h ([PCL-PEG$_{1000}$-PCL]) and then cooled to room temperature.

Thereafter, PDO prepolymer was chain-extended with [PCL-PEG$_{3000}$-PCL] or [PCL-PEG$_{1000}$-PCL] prepolymer using BDI to obtain 20[PCL-PEG$_{3000}$-PCL]-b-80[PDO] or 50[PCL-PEG$_{1000}$-PCL]-b-50[PDO] multi-block copolymer. To this end, approximately 300 g of [PDO] and 75 g of [PCL-PEG$_{3000}$-PCL] were dissolved in dry 1,4-dioxane (80 °C, 30 wt-% solution), after which 20 g of BDI was added to the solution. For 50[PCL-PEG$_{1000}$-PCL]-b-50[PDO], 189.3 g of [PDO] and 189.2 g of [PCL-PEG$_{1000}$-PCL] were dissolved in dry 1,4-dioxane (80 °C, 30 wt-% solution), after which 21.10 g of BDI was added to the solution. Then, the reaction mixture was mechanically stirred for 20 h. Finally, 1,4-dioxane was removed from the reaction mixture by precipitation and vacuum drying. A schematic representation of the composition of the multi-block copolymers is displayed in Figure 1.

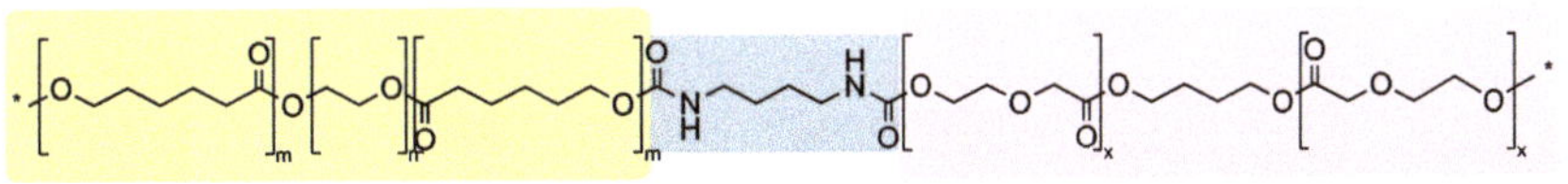

Figure 1. Schematic representation of the general chemical composition of the multi-block copolymers used in this study. In yellow shading: hydrophilic poly(ε-caprolactone)-poly(ethylene glycol)-poly(ε-caprolactone) (PCL-PEG-PCL) block (m: PCL, n: PEG). In blue shading: 1,4-butanediisocyanate (BDI)-based urethane linker. In purple shading: semi-crystalline 1,4-butanediol (BDO)-initiated poly(dioxanone) (PDO) block (x: PDO). The amorphous and semi-crystalline blocks are randomly distributed. The asterisks (*) indicate the possibility of having repeating subunits within the chemical structure. The two polymers used in this study, polymer A and B, differ in the weight ratio of the blocks within the copolymer (PCL-PEG-PCL block vs. PDO block), the molecular weight of PEG, and the total PEG weight fraction.

The synthesized multi-block copolymers 20[PCL-PEG$_{3000}$-PCL]-80[PDO] (polymer A) and 50[PCL-PEG$_{1000}$-PCL]-50[PDO] (polymer B) were analyzed for chemical composition, molecular weight, intrinsic viscosity, residual 1,4-dioxane content, and thermal properties (Table 1). Of polymer A, two different batches were prepared (hereafter referred to as polymer A$_1$ and A$_2$) that differed slightly in their physicochemical characteristics. The caprolactate/PEG and dioxanonate/PEG molar ratios and the weight ratio of the PCL-PEG-PCL/PDO block were determined using ^{1}H NMR analysis. This demonstrated that the actual composition of the multi-block copolymers was in agreement with the targeted composition. The number average molecular weight (M$_n$) and the weight average molecular weight (M$_w$) were determined using gel permeation chromatography, which yielded an M$_n$ of 2.8×10^4 g/mol and M$_w$ of 4.3×10^4 g/mol for polymer A$_1$ and an M$_n$ of 1.5×10^4 g/mol and M$_w$ of 4.5×10^4 g/mol for polymer A$_2$. The M$_n$ and M$_w$ of polymer B were 3.6×10^4 g/mol and 6.7×10^4 g/mol, respectively. The intrinsic viscosity was approximately 0.7 dL/g for polymer A and 0.73 dL/g for polymer B, as determined with an Ubbelohde viscometer. The residual 1,4-dioxane contents as determined by gas chromatography were <18 ppm, indicating successful removal of the solvent. Modulated differential scanning calorimetry (MDSC) was used to determine the thermal behavior of the multi-block copolymers. In brief, 4–8 mg of sample was heated from −85 to 120 °C at a rate of 2 °C/min and a modulation amplitude of 0.42 °C/80 s. The glass transition temperature (T$_g$, midpoint) and melting temperature (T$_m$, maximum of endothermic peak) were determined using the reversed heat flow curve. Polymer A exhibited a T$_g$ at approximately −15 °C, which is attributed to the amorphous PCL-PEG-PCL segments. Polymer B exhibited two T$_g$ values at −57 and −23 °C, which can be ascribed to the amorphous PCL-PEG-PCL segments and the amorphous domains of the PDO block, respectively. Both multi-block copolymers exhibited a T$_m$ at approximately 88 °C due to melting of the crystalline PDO segments. Polymer A exhibited another T$_m$ at 34 °C, which is attributed to melting of PEG crystals.

Table 1. Characterization of the multi-block copolymers used in this study.

	Polymer A$_1$	Polymer A$_2$	Polymer B
	20[PCL-PEG$_{3000}$-PCL]-80[PDO]		50[PCL-PEG$_{1000}$-PCL]-20[PDO]
Molar caprolactate/PEG ratio (^{1}H NMR)	6.8 (6.4 in-weight)	6.4 (6.4 in-weight)	8.3 (8.6 in-weight)
Molar dioxanonate/PEG ratio (^{1}H NMR)	141.6 (147.6 in-weight)	155.2 (147.5 in-weight)	18.5 (18.9 in-weight)

Table 1. Cont.

	Polymer A$_1$	Polymer A$_2$	Polymer B
	20[PCL-PEG$_{3000}$-PCL]-80[PDO]		50[PCL-PEG$_{1000}$-PCL]-20[PDO]
Weight ratio PCL-PEG-PCL/PDO block (^{1}H NMR)	21.2/78.8	19.6/80.4	49.9/50.1
M$_n$ ($\times 10^4$ g/mol)	2.8	1.5	3.6
M$_w$ ($\times 10^4$ g/mol)	4.3	4.5	6.7
Intrinsic viscosity (dL/g)	0.70	0.69	0.73
1,4-dioxane content (ppm)	<18	<18	<18
T$_g$ (°C)	−15	−14	−57 and −23
T$_m$ (°C)	34 and 88	34 and 89	88

2.3. Microsphere Production

BSA-loaded and placebo microspheres with a target diameter of 40 µm were produced by a membrane-assisted water-in-oil-in-water emulsion solvent extraction/evaporation method, similar to a previously described method [21]. In brief, the polymer solution was prepared by dissolving polymer A and B in the desired weight ratio in DCM to obtain a 15 wt-% solution, and filtering the solution over a 0.2 µm polytetrafluoroethylene filter. The BSA solution was prepared by dissolving BSA in PBS at a concentration of 200 mg/mL and filtering the solution over a 0.22 µm polyethersulfone filter. Subsequently, the polymer solution was homogenized with the 200 mg/mL solution of BSA in PBS (for BSA-loaded microspheres) or PBS only (for placebo microspheres) using an Ultra-Turrax®. The volume of BSA solution to be added was calculated to obtain a 5 wt-% target BSA loading, which resulted in a polymer solution to BSA solution ratio of 21 v/v. For the placebo microspheres, the volume of PBS to be added was calculated based on this volume ratio. The resulting primary emulsion, i.e., the dispersed phase, was injected into a continuous phase consisting of 0.4 wt-% PVA and 5 wt-% NaCl in water, by pumping the emulsion through a stainless steel membrane with 20 µm pores (20 µm × 200 µm, hydrophilic ringed stainless steel membrane; Micropore Technologies, Redcar, UK). The primary emulsion was injected at a speed of 1.3 mL/min using a Nexus 3000 syringe pump (Chemyx Inc., Stafford, TX, USA). For all formulations, a dispersed phase to continuous phase ratio of 150 v/v was used. The secondary emulsion was stirred at room temperature with a magnetic stirrer to extract and evaporate DCM. Next, the solidified microspheres were washed five times with 250 mL water and collected on a 5 µm hydrophilic polyvinylidene fluoride filter. Microspheres were freeze-dried using a Christ Alpha 2–4 LSC plus freeze-dryer (Martin Christ Gefriertrocknungsanlagen GmbH, Osterode am Harz, Germany) according to a program previously described and then stored at −20 °C [6]. The formulation and process parameters that were not mentioned above can be found in Table 2. The theoretical PEG, PCL, PDO, BDO, and BDI content of the microspheres prepared from different blend ratios of polymer A and B as determined from the in-weights is shown in Table 3.

2.4. Microsphere Size Analysis

For all microsphere formulations, the particle size expressed as the volume median diameter (d50) and the particle size distribution expressed as the coefficient of variation (CV) were determined with a laser diffraction particle size analyzer (Horiba LA-960, HORIBA Ltd., Kyoto, Japan). Before measurement, microspheres were dispersed in demineralized water and the obtained suspension was added to a fraction cell equipped with a magnetic stirrer to prevent sedimentation of the particles. All samples were measured immediately after addition to the cell, after which a volume-weighted size distribution plot was established according to the Fraunhofer diffraction theory. The d10 and d90 of the particle size distribution were reported as well, indicating the particle diameter at which 10% and 90%

of the distribution, respectively, falls below. The CV was calculated from the d50 and the standard deviation (SD) of the distribution according to Equation (1).

$$CV = \frac{SD}{d50} \times 100\% \tag{1}$$

Table 2. Experimental parameters and settings of different bovine serum albumin (BSA)-loaded and placebo microsphere formulations.

Formulation Parameters		Formulation					
		A	B	C	D	E	F
Weight ratio polymer A:polymer B [1]		100:0	92.5:7.5	85:15	75:25	50:50	92.5:7.5
Target BSA loading (wt-%)		5	5	5	5	5	n.a. [2]
Batch size (g)		1.5	3.5	3.5	3.5	1.5	3.5
Ultra-Turrax®	Speed (rpm)	21,000	25,000	25,000	25,000	21,000	25,000
	Time (s)	40	60	60	60	40	60
	Vessel size (L)	2	5	5	5	2	5
Extraction	Stirrer type	Anchor-type stirring shaft	Stirring bar (10.8 × 2.6 cm)	Stirring bar (10.8 × 2.6 cm)	Stirring bar (10.8 × 2.6 cm)	Anchor-type stirring shaft	Stirring bar (10.8 × 2.6 cm)
	Stirrer speed (rpm)	200	75	75	75	200	75
	Airflow (L/min)	5	10	10	10	5	10
	Time (h)	3	4	4	4	3	4

[1] Polymer A_1 was used for the preparation of formulation A and E; polymer A_2 was used for formulation B, C, D, and F. [2] Formulation F consisted of placebo microspheres that did not contain any BSA.

Table 3. Theoretical PEG, PCL, PDO, BDO, and BDI content of microspheres prepared from different weight ratios of polymer A and B.

Ratio Polymer A: Polymer B	Total PEG (wt-%)	PEG_{3000} (wt-%)	PEG_{1000} (wt-%)	PCL (wt-%)	PDO (wt-%)	BDO (wt-%)	BDI (wt-%)
100:0	15	15	0	4	73	3	5
92.5:7.5	15.675	13.875	1.8	5.425	70.975	2.925	5
85:15	16.35	12.75	3.6	6.85	68.95	2.85	5
75:25	17.25	11.25	6	8.75	66.25	2.75	5
50:50	19.5	7.5	12	13.5	59.5	2.5	5

2.5. Morphology of Microspheres

The surface morphology of the dried microspheres was examined using a NeoScope JCM-5000 scanning electron microscope (SEM; JEOL Ltd., Tokyo, Japan) under high vacuum and a secondary electron detector. SEM images were taken at different magnifications ranging from 50× to 1500×. The acceleration voltage was set at 10 kV, the probe current to standard, and the filament setting to long life. Prior to imaging, the microspheres were fixed onto metal sample stubs using double-sided adhesive carbon tape and sputter-coated with gold. The internal morphology was examined by mixing the microspheres with an organic solvent-free adhesive (UHU® Twist & Glue Renature, Bühl, Germany). After air-drying for 2 days and cooling for 30 min at −70 °C, the samples were cut with a razor blade into five equal pieces. The obtained cross sections were imaged with SEM as described above.

2.6. Protein Content of Microspheres

The actual BSA loading of the microspheres was determined with the bicinchoninic acid (BCA) assay. To this end, 10 mg of microspheres was accurately weighed in triplicate in a glass tube with screw cap. Next, 1 mL of DMSO was added, and the tubes were placed in a heating block at 80 °C and vortexed to completely dissolve the polymer. After dissolution, 5 mL of 0.5 wt-% SDS in 0.05 M sodium hydroxide was added, and the tubes were placed on a roller mixer (60 rpm) overnight at room temperature to solubilize and degrade the protein. Subsequently, 100 µL of the resulting solution was pipetted into another glass tube for further analysis. BCA working reagent was prepared by mixing an alkaline BCA solution with a 4 wt-% aqueous copper(II) sulfate solution (Pierce™ BCA assay kit, Thermo Scientific, Rockford, IL, USA) in a ratio of 50 v/v, and 2 mL of the obtained working reagent was added to the tubes containing the supernatant. The tubes were vortexed and placed in a heating block at 60 °C for 30 min, after which they were cooled to room temperature and again vortexed. Samples were transferred to a plastic cuvette, and the absorbance was immediately measured at 562 nm. An eight-point calibration curve was constructed by spiking known amounts of BSA to a glass tube, and thereafter following the same procedure as described above. The calibration curve was plotted using a quadratic fit and a 1/X weighting factor to determine the actual BSA loading. The actual BSA loading was used to calculate the encapsulation efficiency (EE) according to Equation (2).

$$EE = \frac{\text{Actual loading}}{\text{Target loading}} \times 100\% \qquad (2)$$

2.7. In Vitro Release of Microspheres

The in vitro release of BSA from the microsphere formulations was measured by accurately weighing 20 mg of microspheres in a 2 mL vial and suspending them in 1.8 mL of release medium (100 mM $NaH_2PO_4 \cdot 2H_2O$, 0.2 wt-% NaCl, 0.025 v/v% Tween 20, 0.02 wt-% sodium azide, pH 7.4, 290 mOsm/kg). In order to maintain the release medium at 37 °C, the vials were placed on a roller mixer (40 rpm) in an oven. At predetermined time intervals, the vials were placed in a centrifuge for 5 min at $4000 \times g$. Next, 1.6 mL of the supernatant was collected and replaced by fresh release medium. BSA concentration in the collected release medium was determined by size-exclusion ultra-performance liquid chromatography (SE-UPLC) with fluorescence detection (λ_{ex} = 230 nm and λ_{em} = 330 nm). In brief, an ACQUITY UPLC Protein BEH SEC column (200 Å, 1.7 µm particle size, 4.6 × 150 mm, Waters, Milford, MA, USA) and a mixture of 50 mM phosphate, 0.4 M perchlorate buffer (pH 6.3) and acetonitrile (90:10, v/v) as mobile phase were used for the quantification of BSA. The liquid flow rate of this mobile phase was 0.3 mL/min. The injection volume was 5 µL and the total run time was 8.5 min. The peak areas of the main BSA peak, fragments of BSA, and aggregates of BSA were integrated at a retention time of 4.40 min, 4.67 min, and 2.00 min, respectively. An eight-point calibration curve was plotted using a quadratic fit and a $1/(X \times X)$ weighting factor to determine the BSA concentration in the samples. For quantification of the total BSA concentration, that is, the concentration of all BSA-related compounds together, the areas of all peaks at a retention time of 2.00 to 6.00 min were integrated. As a semi-quantitative measure for the integrity of the released BSA, the BSA concentration calculated from the main BSA peak was divided by the total BSA concentration. All in vitro release curves represent the release of all BSA-related compounds together, unless otherwise stated.

2.8. Residual DCM Content of Microspheres

The residual DCM content in the microspheres was determined with an Agilent 6850 gas chromatograph (GC; Agilent Technologies, Santa Clara, CA, USA) equipped with a flame ionization detector, a CombiPal CTC headspace sampler, and a DB-624 column (30 m × 0.53 mm, 3 µm). As carrier gas, helium with a flow of 7 mL/min was used. The split injection mode was used with a split ratio of 1:15. The initial column temperature was 40 °C maintained for 5 min and then raised (10 °C/min) to 100 °C with a hold time of 1 min. Finally, the temperature was raised to 250 °C with 50 °C/min for 4 min. The syringe and incubation temperatures were 140 °C and 120 °C, respectively. For each formulation, 100 mg of microspheres was accurately weighed in duplicate and dissolved in 5 mL DMSO with 9.4 µg/mL octane as internal standard. Then, 2 mL of the headspace layer was injected into the GC for analysis. An eight-point calibration curve was plotted using a linear fit and a 1/X weighting factor to determine the DCM concentration from the peak area.

2.9. Endotoxin Level in Microspheres

The endotoxin levels in the microsphere formulations that were intended for the in vivo proof-of-concept study were determined with the Limulus amoebocyte lysate (LAL) test using a chromogenic kinetic method at a sensitivity of 0.005 EU/mL. To this end, 1 mL of DMSO was added to 50 mg of accurately weighed microspheres in duplicate, heated to 70 °C in a water bath for 1 min, and vortexed for 20 s to completely dissolve the sample. After dissolution, LAL reagent water was added to the sample (1:50 dilution), and the diluted sample and LAL/substrate reagent were added to each well of a microtiter plate. Then, the absorbance of each well was read at 405 nm and 37 °C, and this initial reading was used as the blank for the corresponding well. Subsequently, the absorbance of each well was read continuously throughout the assay. The time elapsed until the appearance of a yellow color, i.e., an increase of 0.2 absorbance units from the initial reading, was determined for each well, and this reaction time was inversely proportional to the endotoxin level in the sample. A standard curve of reaction time vs. endotoxin concentration was used to calculate the endotoxin concentration in the unknown samples. LAL reagent water was included as a negative control, and a positive product control (PPC) was prepared at a final concentration of 0.5 EU/mL. All standards and controls were assayed in duplicate as well.

2.10. Animal Experiments

Female CB6F1 (C57Bl/6 × BALB/c F1) mice were obtained from Charles River Laboratories (Sulzfeld, Germany). At the start of the study, the mice were eight to nine weeks old and weighed approximately 20 g. The animals were co-housed with a total number of three to six mice in individually ventilated cages and received a 12 h light/dark cycle. All animals received the rodent diet SAFE® A40 (SAFE Diets, Augy, France) and tap water ad libitum. At least five days before the start of the experiment, the mice were imported to the laboratory to assure proper acclimatization. All in vivo experiments were conducted in accordance with Timeline Bioresearch AB ethical permit number 5.8.18-20232/2020.

For the in vivo proof-of-concept study, 48 mice were divided into nine groups. The treatment groups (groups A, B, and C) and positive control (plus treatment or placebo) groups (groups D to G) all contained 6 mice. The negative control groups (groups H and I) contained 3 mice. An overview of the experimental groups and the corresponding formulations used for the immunization study is given in Table 4. All formulations were administered as a 100 or 200 µL s.c. injection in the scruff of the neck under isoflurane anesthesia, and were given at day 0, unless otherwise stated. For the microspheres, 0.6 wt-% CMC solution in 10× PBS was used as the injection vehicle, whereas PBS was used for the administration of BSA solution. All treatment groups (groups A to D) were immunized with microspheres of formulation B, and the placebo group (group E) received an injection of microspheres of formulation F. The amount of microspheres to be administered was calculated from the desired dose of BSA (250, 500, or 1000 µg BSA) and the actual BSA loading of the microspheres, corrected for the percentage released in vitro after five weeks of incubation. The microspheres of groups A, B and D, and C are hereafter referred to as 250, 500, and 1000 µg BSA-microspheres, respectively. Mice of groups F and G received an injection of BSA in PBS at weeks 0 and 3, where the timing of the booster immunization was based on the experimental setup of previous immunization studies [7,22,23].

Table 4. Overview of the groups and the corresponding formulations used for the in vivo immunization study in mice.

Group	Type of Group	Formulation Composition	Administration	Total Dose	Average Daily Dose	Week of Administration	Number of Animals
A	Treatment	BSA-MSP in CMC solution [1]	7.28 mg MSP-F in 193 µL CMC solution [1]	250 µg	7.1 µg [2]	0	6
B	Treatment	BSA-MSP in CMC solution	14.6 mg MSP-F in 187 µL CMC solution	500 µg	14.3 µg [2]	0	6
C	Treatment	BSA-MSP in CMC solution	29.2 mg MSP-F in 174 µL CMC solution	1000 µg	28.6 µg [2]	0	6
D	Positive control/treatment	BSA in PBS + BSA-MSP in CMC solution	500 µg BSA in 100 µL PBS + 14.6 mg MSP-B in 87 µL CMC solution [1]	1000 µg (500 µg + 500 µg)	514.3 µg on day 1, 14.3 µg for remaining days [2]	0	6
E	Positive control/placebo	BSA in PBS + placebo MSP in CMC solution	500 µg BSA in 100 µL PBS + 14.6 mg MSP-F in 87 µL CMC solution	500 µg	500 µg on day 1	0	6
F	Positive control (prime-boost)	BSA in PBS	500 µg BSA in 200 µL PBS (at 0 and 3 weeks)	1000 µg (500 µg + 500 µg)	500 µg on day 1, 500 µg on day 22	0 and 3	6
G	Positive control (prime-boost)	BSA in PBS	28.6 µg BSA in 200 µL PBS (at 0 and 3 weeks)	57.1 µg (28.6 µg + 28.6 µg)	28.6 µg on day 1, 28.6 µg on day 22	0 and 3	6
H	Negative control	PBS	200 µL PBS (at 0 and 3 weeks)	-	-	0 and 3	3
I	Negative control	CMC solution	200 µL CMC solution	-	-	0	3

[1] MSP = microspheres, MSP-B = microspheres of formulation B, MSP-F = microspheres of formulation F.
[2] Assuming an in vivo release duration of five weeks.

Blood samples were taken prior to administration and 1, 2, 3, 4, 6, and 8 weeks after the first administration. In total, seven blood samples were obtained from each mouse. At all time points up to six weeks, 100 µL of blood was collected in K3-EDTA tubes by sublingual bleeding and immediately placed on melting ice. During blood sampling, mice were fully conscious as no anesthesia was used, so they were gently restrained by the scruff of the neck. For the last sampling point, mice were euthanized by cervical dislocation, and all blood was collected and processed for further analysis. Then, 40 µL of plasma was prepared by centrifuging the blood samples at $1800 \times g$ and 4 °C for 10 min and collecting the supernatant. The obtained aliquots were placed on dry ice and eventually stored at −80 °C prior to analysis. All plasma samples were analyzed by ELISA to investigate the BSA-specific IgG antibody response of the mice. Plasma samples from weeks 1 to 4 were also tested by ELISA to determine the BSA levels.

2.11. ELISA for BSA-Specific IgG Antibody Titers

BSA-specific IgG antibody titers in plasma were determined by indirect ELISA. Flat-bottom high binding 96-well microplates (Greiner Bio-One, Kremsmünster, Austria) were coated overnight at 37 °C with 0.3 µg BSA (100 µL 3 µg/mL BSA solution in 0.05 M carbonate-bicarbonate buffer, pH 9.6–9.8) per well. PBS composed of 154 mM NaCl, 0.882 mM KH_2PO_4, and 11.4 mM Na_2HPO_4 and the same PBS supplemented with 0.05 $v/v\%$ Tween 20 (PBS-T) were prepared as wash solution. PBS-T was also used to remove detection antibodies. The plates were washed once with the 0.05 M carbonate–bicarbonate buffer and twice with PBS-T. Then, 1:100 dilutions of plasma samples in PBS-T were prepared and added in twofold serial dilutions to the plates, with each well containing 100 µL of a dilution. Untreated wells, i.e., wells that did not contain any plasma sample, were used to determine the plate background. After incubating the plates for 1.5 h at 37 °C, the plates were washed three times with PBS-T. Next, the plates were incubated for 1 h at 37 °C with

100 µL of a 1:5000 v/v dilution of HRP-linked goat anti-mouse IgG antibody in PBS-T to detect bound IgG antibodies. Plates were again washed three times with PBS-T and once with PBS. Then, 100 µL staining solution (20 mg OPD, 20 µL hydrogen peroxide in 100 mL 0.1 M phosphate buffer, pH 5.6) was added to each well and incubated for 30 min at room temperature shielded from light. The colorimetric reaction was stopped by adding 50 µL 2 M sulfuric acid to the wells. Absorbance was measured at 492 nm and OD values were corrected for the mean plate background. IgG antibody titers were expressed as $\log_2$ values of the reciprocal of the plasma sample dilution that corresponded to a corrected OD value of 0.2 at a wavelength of 492 nm, which was determined as the cut-off value. Samples with readings for the least diluted plasma lower than the cut-off value were assigned an IgG antibody titer of 5.64 $\log_2$, corresponding to a dilution of 1:50, which would be one dilution below the starting dilution of 1:100.

2.12. ELISA for BSA Quantification

Plasma BSA levels were determined with a commercial BSA ELISA kit (F030; Cygnus Technologies, Southport, NC, USA) according to the manufacturer's instructions. Due to limited sample volume, plasma samples were diluted at least 1:2 with BSA sample diluent and analyzed only once (n = 1). Absorbance was measured at 450 nm using a microplate reader, and BSA concentrations were determined from a five-point calibration curve (calibration range 0.5–32 ng/mL). Some plasma samples were applied in higher dilutions of up to 1:50 to fall within the working range of the assay.

2.13. Statistical Analysis

All microsphere formulations (A to F, Table 2) were produced once (n = 1). All measurements were performed in triplicate (n = 3), and data were presented as mean ± SD, unless otherwise stated. The IgG titer-time data were analyzed using GraphPad Prism version 9.1.2 (La Jolla, CA, USA). The area under the IgG titer–time curve (AUC) values were obtained, and data were checked for normality using the Shapiro–Wilk test. Differences between all groups were assessed using the ordinary one-way analysis of variance (ANOVA), followed by Tukey's multiple comparisons test for both AUC values and week 8 IgG titers. Differences between the analyzed groups were considered significant if $p < 0.05$ (* $p < 0.05$, ** $p < 0.01$).

3. Results and Discussion

3.1. Properties of Microspheres of Different Polymer Blend Ratios

Blends of polymer A and B with different weight ratios were used to prepare BSA-loaded microspheres with a 5 wt-% target loading and placebo microspheres. The polymer blend ratio and the incorporation of BSA did not seem to affect the microsphere size and size distribution, as can be seen in Table 5. All formulations had an average particle size of approximately 40 µm. This size enables parenteral administration of the microspheres through a small-gauge hypodermic needle while preventing premature uptake by cells engaging in phagocytosis [24,25]. Moreover, all microsphere formulations had a narrow particle size distribution as reflected by the relatively low CV values. This was the result of a well-defined localized shear and geometry-controlled generation of droplets in the membrane-assisted emulsification process [26]. The morphology of the microspheres was examined using SEM. Representative images of BSA-loaded microspheres composed of a 92.5:7.5 polymer blend (formulation B) are depicted in Figure 2, with Figure 2a,b revealing the surface morphology and Figure 2c,d the internal morphology. Figure 2a,b show that the microspheres had a spherical shape and a smooth and non-porous surface. As expected, images of the internal morphology (Figure 2c,d) display a monolithic matrix with numerous small pores, resulting from the fine primary emulsion used in the preparation of the microspheres. The porosity was homogeneous throughout the cross section of the particles, which implies that BSA was homogeneously distributed throughout the microspheres. A non-porous surface, small internal pores, and a homogeneous drug distribution are critical to obtaining a high EE and low initial burst release [27]. Indeed, the EE of BSA was high for all formulations (>85%, Table 5). The high EE can be attributed to the relatively high molecular weight of the polymers (M_w 4.3–6.7 × 10^4 g/mol) and concentration of the polymer solution (15 wt-%), resulting in a relatively high viscosity of the polymer solution [28,29]. The high polymer solution to BSA solution ratio (21 v/v) [30] and the addition of NaCl to the continuous phase probably contributed to these high EE values as well [31].

Table 5. Characteristics of BSA-loaded and placebo microsphere formulations prepared with different polymer blend ratios [1].

Formulation	Ratio Polymer A: Polymer B	d10 (μm)	d50 (μm)	d90 (μm)	CV (%)	Actual Loading (wt-%)	EE (%)
A	100:0	30.4	38.7	50.5	21.0	4.4 ± 0.1	87.4 ± 1.0
B	92.5:7.5	30.8	39.9	52.4	21.8	4.5 ± 0.5	89.9 ± 10.0
C	85:15	30.6	39.5	51.5	21.7	4.9 ± 0.3	97.3 ± 5.5
D	75:25	30.5	39.2	51.4	21.9	4.9 ± 0.2	96.9 ± 4.5
E	50:50	29.9	39.0	51.6	24.5	5.1 ± 1.3	101.7 ± 26.4
F	92.5:7.5	31.2	42.7	58.2	27.4	n.a. [2]	n.a. [2]

[1] Blend ratio 92.5:7.5 (in grey) was selected for the in vivo proof-of-concept study in mice. [2] Formulation F consisted of placebo microspheres that did not contain any BSA.

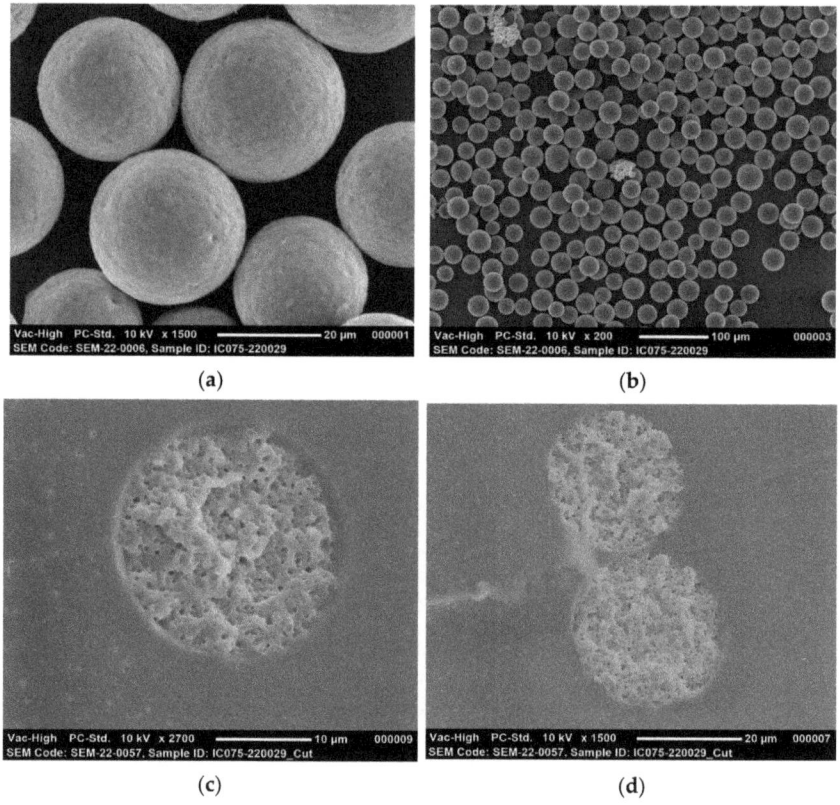

Figure 2. Representative scanning electron microscopy (SEM) images of microspheres loaded with 4.5 wt-% BSA (formulation B): (**a**) 1500× magnification; (**b**) 200× magnification; (**c**) Cross-sectioned microsphere at 2700× magnification; (**d**) Cross-sectioned microspheres at 1500× magnification.

3.2. In Vitro Release of BSA from Microspheres of Different Polymer Blend Ratios

We investigated the suitability of a blend of multi-block copolymers A and B in obtaining microspheres with a low initial burst and linear or near-linear in vitro release of the complete BSA payload within four to six weeks. The effect of the polymer blend ratio on the in vitro release of BSA from the microspheres is presented in Figure 3. For all formulations, the initial burst release, defined as the percentage of BSA released after one day, was minimal (1 to 6%). Moreover, all release profiles showed a similar trend with an initial slow release followed by a faster release after which the release again slowed down. In particular, the microspheres composed of a relatively high percentage of polymer B exhibited such a sigmoidal release profile. The in vitro release rate was clearly influenced by the polymer blend ratio, as the release rate decreased with an increasing weight fraction of polymer B. Formulation A, which was composed of 100% of polymer A, demonstrated the highest release rate, with a cumulative release of approximately 80% after four weeks. The lowest release rate was obtained with formulation E, composed of a 50:50 polymer blend that exhibited a cumulative BSA release of only 20% after four weeks.

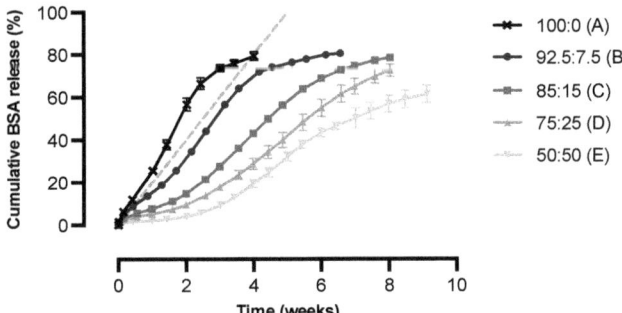

Figure 3. Cumulative in vitro release of BSA from microspheres composed of polymer A and polymer B in different blend ratios (n = 3). The cumulative release is expressed as the percentage of the total amount of BSA incorporated into the microspheres. The dashed line represents the target release profile of the microspheres with a linear release of BSA over a period of five weeks.

For bulk degrading polymers such as the polymers used in this study, drug release from the polymeric matrix is determined by the drug solubility, drug diffusion, drug load, polymer swelling, polymer degradation, or a combination of these factors [19,32]. For a hydrophilic protein with a high molecular weight, such as BSA (6.6 × 10^4 g/mol), diffusion through the hydrated polymer matrix is dependent on the degree of swelling and degradation of the polymer matrix, as these determine the mesh size of the matrix [19]. If a mesh size larger than the protein size is reached through swelling and/or degradation, the protein will be released from the polymer matrix [19,33]. To obtain a better understanding of the in vitro release profile, it is important to determine whether the prepared microspheres exhibit diffusion- or degradation-controlled release.

In previous studies, controlled-release microspheres [20,21,34] and implants [19] were prepared from semi-crystalline, phase-separated multi-block copolymers similar to the polymers used in this study. These polymers also consisted of amorphous PCL-PEG-PCL blocks, but the semi-crystalline blocks were composed of poly(L-lactide) (PLLA) [20,21,34] or PCL [19] instead of PDO. In two of these studies, in vitro release and polymer degradation were assessed to gain insight into the release mechanisms in play. Results suggested that in vitro release was primarily driven by diffusion [19,21]. In vitro release data of several proteins were fitted into different kinetic models and in most cases, diffusion-controlled release was indicated. For the in vitro degradation studies, polymer-only microspheres [21] and implants [19] were incubated in a release medium at 37 °C, and the mass loss was determined over time. Although mass loss only gives an indication of the formation of water-soluble degradation products and degradation products that are not (yet) soluble in water will have formed as well, it does give information on the contribution of polymer degradation to the release kinetics. Only a slight mass loss was observed during the first week after incubation, which was ascribed to the preferential hydrolysis of the PEG-PCL bonds, and the subsequent dissolution and diffusion of PEG. During the remainder of the study (i.e., three [21] and nineteen [19] weeks), the sample mass hardly changed, and the molecular weight of the polymers decreased only slowly. This indicated that hydrolysis of ester bonds in the PLLA and PCL blocks was limited and that no substantial degradation had occurred within the timeframe of the degradation studies, due to slow in vitro degradation of PLLA and PCL and its copolymers. Based on the extrapolation of previously obtained data, the anticipated in vitro degradation time of PLLA-based multi-block copolymers is three to four years [35]. For the PCL-based multi-block copolymers, this is expected to be the same [36]. Therefore, the release from such multi-block copolymers was assumed to be mainly driven by other mechanisms than degradation.

In order to obtain faster degrading microspheres with a more acceptable balance between BSA release and polymer erosion, the faster degrading polymer PDO was used as the semi-crystalline block. The homopolymer has a degradation time of six months [36–38], and in vitro degradation of PDO-based multi-block copolymers is anticipated to be 9 to 24 months [35]. Although PDO-based multi-block copolymers degrade significantly faster than PLLA- and PCL-based multi-block copolymers, it is not expected that degradation of the semi-crystalline PDO block played a significant role in the in vitro release of BSA, as substantial degradation is unlikely to have occurred within the timeframe of the in vitro release studies (i.e., four to nine weeks) [36–38]. Therefore, as in previous studies, the release of BSA from the microspheres was mainly controlled by the amorphous PCL-PEG-PCL block. It is assumed that the release was partially driven by diffusion, as the high swelling degree and water solubility of the PEG blocks within the multi-block copolymer allowed the initial, diffusion-controlled release of BSA [18]. This occurred via dissolution and subsequent diffusion of the antigen through the swollen polymer matrix [19,21]. Release, however, was probably not solely diffusion-controlled but involved some degradation of the PCL-PEG-PCL block as well, which is also reflected in the sigmoidal release profile that was observed for the different microsphere formulations (Figure 3). It is assumed that ongoing degradation of the PCL-PEG-PCL blocks further increased the mesh size of the polymer matrix, which eventually accelerated the release. Especially for the formulations composed of a relatively high amount of polymer B, swelling of the polymer matrix was insufficient to cause an initial fast release of the high molecular weight BSA due to the presence of small-sized PEG blocks (Table 3). This resulted in a sort of lag phase directly after the start of the in vitro release study, after which the release rate increased. Apparently, some degradation and/or increased swelling of the polymer matrix over time was required for BSA to be released from the microspheres.

As expected, the BSA release rate from microspheres composed of polymer A and B was dependent on the polymer blend ratio, as the release rate decreased with an increasing weight fraction of polymer B (Figure 3). The slower release induced by polymer B can be explained by the fact that this polymer is less swellable and degrades slower than polymer A. As the release of BSA from the microspheres is assumed to be both diffusion- and degradation-controlled, the release rate is determined by an interplay between the PEG molecular weight, the total PEG content, the PCL content, and the PDO content of the polymer blends. The interplay between the PEG molecular weight and the total PEG content was previously described for the PLLA-based multi-block copolymers [20,21]. A comparison of polymer B with polymer A demonstrates a lower PEG molecular weight (1000 vs. 3000 g/mol), which explains the decreased release rate with an increasing weight fraction of polymer B, as PEG blocks swell due to the uptake of water. Due to the lower molecular weight of PEG in the PCL-PEG-PCL blocks, polymer B absorbs less water causing slower hydrolytic cleavage of the polymer backbone and a lower swelling degree. This eventually results in a slower release. The difference between the two polymers was also reflected in the mass loss. After incubation of polymer-only microspheres prepared from polymer A, a minor mass loss of <10% was observed after 30 days and <20% after 50 days [35]. For PDO-based multi-block copolymers comparable to polymer B, this was even less [35]. Polymer B does contain a higher total PEG content (24 vs. 15 wt-%), but this did not compensate for the PEG molecular weight. In this case, a high molecular weight of PEG is apparently more important to create a polymeric network that swells enough to allow the diffusion of the high molecular weight BSA, than a high total PEG content is for the formation of such a hydrated network. Moreover, the PCL content was higher for polymer B than for polymer A (25 vs. 5 wt-%), while the PDO content was lower (50 vs. 80 wt-%), as shown in Table 3. As PCL degrades slower than PDO, polymer B is expected to degrade slower than polymer A, resulting in a lower release rate. A higher PCL content also results in a lower swelling degree due to its hydrophobicity, thereby causing a decreased release rate [39].

We aimed to develop a formulation that exhibited a continuous release of BSA for approximately four to six weeks. Microspheres prepared from a 92.5:7.5 blend of polymer A and B (formulation B) exhibited near-linear release kinetics for up to four weeks, after which the release of BSA continued in a slower fashion for another two weeks. In addition, a high cumulative release of 80% was obtained during the course of the in vitro release study. Since these microspheres best met our target in vitro release profile, this formulation was selected for the in vivo proof-of-concept study. Figure 4a presents the results of the in vitro release study with this formulation, showing both the total and the intact BSA release from the microspheres. Protein denaturation and aggregation are common problems for protein-loaded microspheres, as they are subjected to many stress factors upon incubation, such as hydration and elevated temperatures [4,25]. Although the integrity of the released BSA was not tested directly, we did measure the percentage of BSA that was released as fragments or aggregates, which indicated how well the structural integrity was maintained during incubation. During the first four weeks, the integrity of the released BSA was high (>90%, Figure 4b). Only at the end of the in vitro release study did the integrity decrease drastically, as the release mainly consisted of aggregates of BSA. These aggregates are larger than BSA itself and are, therefore, probably released more slowly. During the major part of the in vitro release study, however, aggregates and fragments of BSA were absent and the cumulative intact release was even >70%.

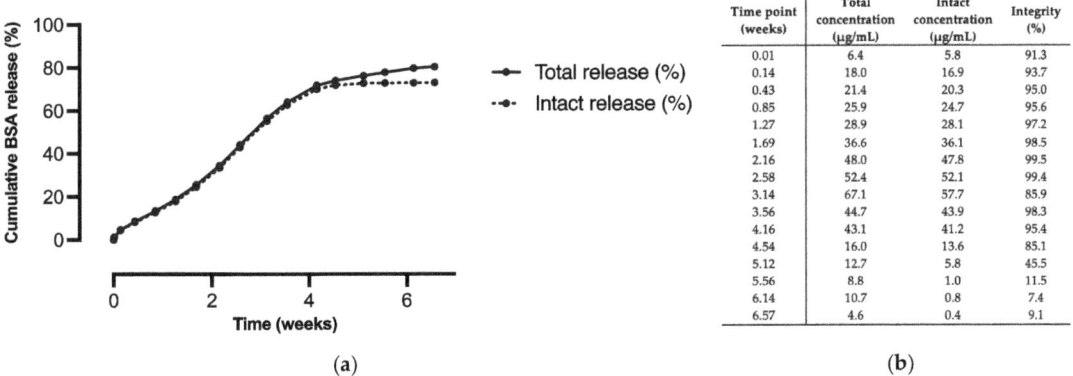

Figure 4. In vitro release of BSA from microspheres composed of polymer A and polymer B in the blend ratio 92.5:7.5 (formulation B, $n = 3$): (**a**) Cumulative total and intact release vs. time. (**b**) Total and intact BSA concentration and corresponding integrity of samples at each individual time point.

Furthermore, the average daily in vitro release from formulation B for different doses of BSA was plotted in Figure 5. A relatively high daily release is visible during the first day of incubation and especially during the first two hours due to a small initial burst release. Apart from day one, the average daily release was rather constant during the first four weeks of the release study. A slight increase in the daily release was observed up to approximately three weeks, followed by a decrease during the remaining weeks of the release study, which is typical for a sigmoidal release profile.

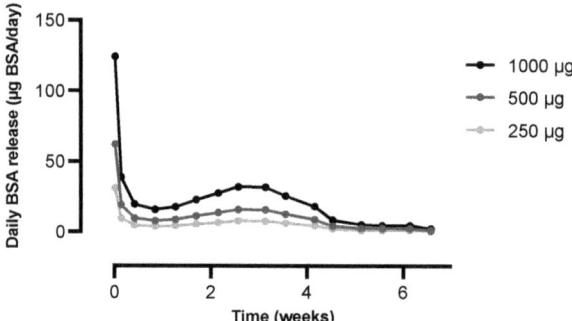

Figure 5. Average daily in vitro release of BSA from microspheres composed of polymer A and polymer B in the blend ratio 92.5:7.5 (formulation B, n = 3). The average daily in vitro release was calculated by dividing the absolute amount of BSA (in µg) that was released between two sampling points by the time between those sampling points. The different curves represent different amounts of microspheres corresponding to a total BSA content of 250, 500, or 1000 µg.

3.3. Residual DCM Content and Endotoxin Analysis of Microspheres Intended for the In Vivo Study

The residual DCM content in the microspheres of formulation B and the corresponding placebo microspheres (formulation F) was measured to determine whether the removal of the toxic organic solvent was effective. The DCM content of formulation B and F was 295 and 294 ppm, respectively, which is well below the ICH concentration limit of 600 ppm [40]. The permissible daily exposure for humans is 6 mg/day [40]. When this value is corrected for the body weight of a mouse (20 g) and for the factor that accounts for the extrapolation between both species (12), a permissible daily exposure of 28.8 µg/day is found for mice. As the highest amount of microspheres to be administered is 29.2 mg, the maximum DCM exposure will be only 8.6 µg, which is below the permissible daily exposure as well. Although there are only limited data available on DCM toxicity after parenteral administration, no increased risk of tumor development was observed in mice after oral administration of DCM doses up to 5 mg/day [41]. Therefore, no carcinogenic effects are expected from the prepared microspheres. In addition, the endotoxin level in both formulations was quantified as it is an important factor for microspheres intended for immunological studies. The LAL test confirmed that both formulations did not contain detectable levels of endotoxin (<5 EU/g microspheres). Therefore, it is not expected that any undefined immune responses will be induced by endotoxins from the microspheres. Overall, both formulations complied with all requirements for use in the in vivo proof-of-concept study.

3.4. IgG Antibody Response and Kinetics of Microspheres In Vivo

Based on the in vitro release results, the BSA-loaded microspheres prepared from a 92.5:7.5 blend of polymer A and B (formulation B) and the corresponding placebo microspheres (formulation F) were chosen for the in vivo proof-of-concept study in mice. The microspheres containing the model antigen BSA were s.c. injected to investigate whether the formulation could elicit a BSA-specific IgG antibody response. Different amounts of the microspheres were injected into the subcutaneous tissue to test the effect of the dose of BSA on the humoral immune response. A positive control/treatment group was included to determine whether priming with BSA in PBS could enhance the antibody response induced by the microspheres. A positive control/placebo group was included to investigate the potential adjuvant effect of the polymers. In addition, two positive controls consisting of a high- and low-dose prime-boost injection of BSA in PBS were included to compare the antibody titers induced by a prime-boost immunization schedule with the titers induced by the microspheres. Two negative controls consisting of PBS and CMC solution were included to confirm that the vehicles did not induce BSA-specific IgG antibodies. For all groups, the BSA-specific IgG antibody titers in the mouse plasma were determined over time, up to eight weeks after administration.

As expected, no IgG antibody response was induced after administration of the injection vehicles to the negative control groups. For the other groups, the systemic BSA-specific IgG antibody titers over time after administration of different BSA and placebo formulations are shown in Figure 6 (see Figure S1 in the Supplementary Materials for the IgG antibody titers of the individual mice). In addition, the final IgG antibody titers as measured at week 8 are shown in Figure 7. The AUC values of the antibody titer vs. time graphs from Figure S1 were calculated for each individual mouse of groups A to G as shown in Figure S2. All mice that received BSA-loaded microspheres had elevated antibody titers from week 1 onwards, which indicates that the microspheres were effective in inducing an immune response. To assess the performance of the sustained-release microspheres in relation to the conventional prime-boost immunization schedule, a high-dose prime and booster injection of BSA in PBS (500 + 500 μg BSA) were administered to mice in group F at weeks 0 and 3, respectively. As expected, antibody titers increased up to week 2, remained steady up to week 3, and again increased and stabilized at week 4 (Figure 6). In other words, the antibody titers spiked following the prime and the booster injection, which demonstrates that the conventional prime-boost immunization schedule was effective as well. Comparison of group C (1000 μg BSA-microspheres) and F (prime-boost 500 + 500 μg BSA) demonstrates that the (week 8) antibody titers as well as the AUC values of both groups were not significantly different. This shows that sustained release of BSA from the microspheres did not result in immunological tolerance toward the model antigen within the tested time frame. The induction of tolerance toward the antigen, causing the vaccine to be ineffective, has previously been related to the sustained release of the antigen from the formulation [42–44]. Clear evidence is, however, lacking [45], and apparently was not found in our study either. When the same total dose of BSA was given, microspheres and a prime-boost injection of BSA in PBS induced a similar IgG antibody response, so the sustained-release microspheres could be a viable alternative to the conventional prime-boost immunization schedule.

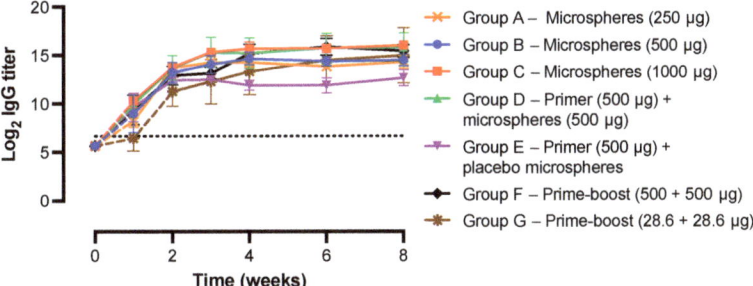

Figure 6. BSA-specific IgG antibody titers in mouse plasma over time after immunization with different BSA formulations (group A to G). The averages of the antibody levels measured in all mice were calculated for each group (n = 6 per group) and presented for all groups together. The dotted line represents the cut-off value for the IgG antibody titer, i.e., a titer of 6.64 $\log_2$, corresponding to the starting dilution of the plasma samples of 1:100. Values below this titer could not be measured.

Samples with a reading for the least diluted plasma (i.e., 100× diluted) lower than the cut-off value were assigned an IgG antibody titer of 5.64 $\log_2$, corresponding to a dilution of 1:50, which would be one dilution below the starting dilution. Dashed lines were used to connect the data points with a titer of 5.64 $\log_2$ to the next data point. The negative control groups receiving PBS (group H) and CMC solution (group I) are not presented in this figure.

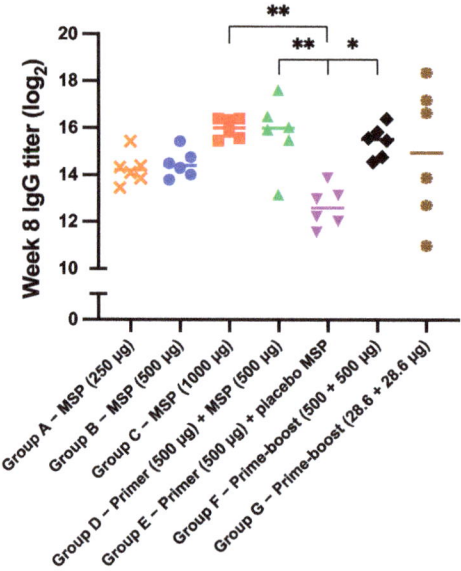

Figure 7. Week 8 IgG titer for each individual mouse of group A to G. Statistical comparisons between the mice of the different groups were performed using the ordinary ANOVA, followed by Tukey's multiple comparisons test (* $p < 0.05$, ** $p < 0.01$). For clarity reasons, statistical comparison is only indicated where $p < 0.05$ (*) or $p < 0.01$ (**), and differences for all other comparisons were non-significant. The negative control groups receiving PBS (group H) and CMC solution (group I) are not presented in this figure. MSP = microspheres.

Interestingly, mice of group E that received a prime injection of 500 μg BSA in PBS and a mock immunization of placebo microspheres demonstrated a rather different immune response. Here, the antibody titers peaked already after two weeks, after which no further increase in titer was observed (Figure 6). For this group, the final IgG antibody titer at week 8 was significantly lower than that of groups C and F ($p < 0.01$ for 1000 μg BSA-microspheres and $p < 0.05$ for prime-boost 500 + 500 μg BSA). The AUC value was also significantly lower than that of group C. Even though the total administered dose of BSA was lower than for groups C and F, these results suggest that a priming dose alone is not sufficient to elicit a strong immune response over time, and that a booster injection or a continuous release of antigen is required. Although the difference was not statistically significant, the fact that the AUC value and week 8 antibody titer of group E were also lower than those of group B (500 μg BSA-microspheres), which did receive the same total dose of BSA, supports this conclusion. A single-injection vaccine formulation such as the microspheres would then have the preference over the conventional prime-boost vaccine. Apart from one outlier, mice that received both a prime injection of 500 μg BSA in PBS and 500 μg BSA-microspheres (group D, Figure 6) showed an antibody response that strongly resembled the response in group C (1000 μg BSA-microspheres), as the total administered dose of BSA was the same. Apparently, priming with BSA in PBS in addition to the sustained-release microspheres does not enhance the antibody response and, therefore, does not have a preference over the administration of microspheres only.

Furthermore, the fact that (week 8) antibody titers and AUC values were similar for groups C and F suggests that the microspheres did not possess any adjuvant activity for the encapsulated model antigen, as was observed previously for PLGA-based single-administration vaccine formulations [7,46,47]. Comparison of group E (500 μg BSA in PBS + placebo microspheres) and F (prime-boost 500 + 500 μg BSA) confirmed this suspicion, as the IgG antibody titer at week 3 was similar for both groups (12.5 ± 0.1 and 13.1 ± 0.6 $\log_2$, respectively).

Mice in the treatment groups (groups A to C) received different amounts of microspheres that were expected to deliver an amount of 250, 500, and 1000 μg BSA, respectively, into the subcutaneous tissue. The antibody responses measured in these groups all followed a similar trend, with an increasing titer up to four weeks, after which it leveled off (Figure 6). A clear difference between the groups is, however, visible at week 1, which demonstrates that the development of high antibody titers takes more time at lower doses. Moreover, the week 8 antibody titer in group C was 3.1- and 2.8-fold higher than in group A and B, respectively (Figure 7), although the differences were not significant ($p > 0.05$). The AUC values raised by immunization with different doses of BSA-loaded microspheres were not significantly different either (Figure S2). Possibly, the difference between the administered doses was not large enough and the doses were all relatively high, which caused only a small difference in immune response. In another study with BSA-loaded microspheres, the influence of the dose on the magnitude of the induced antibody response was more clearly visible [8]. Here, a high dose of BSA (431 μg) elicited 13- and 8-fold higher antibody titers than a low dose of BSA (i.e., 64 μg) at the first and last time point of the in vivo study, respectively. It should, however, be noted that the microspheres in this specific study displayed a pulsatile release of BSA instead of sustained release, which impedes direct comparison.

Finally, mice receiving a high- and a low-dose prime-boost injection of BSA in PBS were compared in terms of IgG antibody response. The dose of the high-dose prime-boost injection (500 + 500 μg BSA, group F) was based on the total dose of the sustained-release microspheres from group C, and the dose of the low-dose prime-boost injection (28.6 + 28.6 μg BSA, group G) was based on the average daily dose of the microspheres. All mice in the high-dose prime-boost group developed high titers of BSA-specific IgG antibodies. However, high variability in antibody titers was observed in the low-dose prime-boost group. These results are in line with a study by Guarecuco et al., where a greater variability in antibody response was observed for a low-dose than for a high-dose BSA formulation [8]. This probably indicates that in some mice of group G, the amount of antigen reaching the draining lymph nodes was sufficient for B cell activation, while in other mice this was not the case [48].

For most of the mice from the treatment groups (groups A to C), IgG antibody titers continued to increase up to four weeks after administration of the formulations, which can be considered an indirect indication of sustained release of BSA from the microspheres. After these four weeks, antibody titers hardly increased, which suggests that the release of BSA from the microspheres had ceased. These results are in line with the in vitro release data (Figure 4a), where the vast majority of the encapsulated BSA was released in a near-linear fashion over a period of four weeks. The development of antigen-specific antibodies, however, takes approximately one week [7,49]. An increase in IgG antibody titers up to four weeks, therefore, suggests an in vivo release duration of only three weeks. This indicates that the release of BSA was faster in vivo than in vitro, probably due to accelerated microsphere degradation in vivo, for instance, caused by increased liquid uptake into the polymer and foreign body responses [8,50,51]. Lipids and other biological molecules can act as plasticizers or affect the surface tension, which enhances water uptake. Moreover, free radicals, acidic products, or enzymes produced by macrophages that form around the microspheres can accelerate polymer degradation. To gain more insight into the in vivo pharmacokinetics of BSA, plasma samples from weeks 1 to 4 of groups A to G were analyzed for BSA levels as well (Figure 8). Sustained release of BSA from the microspheres into the systemic circulation was demonstrated, with plasma BSA concentrations being dependent on the administered dose, as expected. Peak plasma concentrations were 1429 ± 397, 2214 ± 99, and 2762 ± 127 ng BSA/mL for 250, 500, and 1000 µg BSA, respectively. For most of the mice receiving BSA-loaded microspheres, the highest plasma BSA concentration was measured one week after administration, followed by a strong decline in the concentration (Figure 8a–d). After four weeks, only low levels of BSA were still measured. In contrast, the highest release rate in vitro was reached after three weeks of incubation (Figure 5), which indicates that the release of BSA from the microspheres was indeed faster in vivo than in vitro. It is, however, also possible that the decline in BSA plasma concentration after one week was due to antibody formation, as was previously observed by van Dijk et al. after injection of sustained-release microspheres containing a human serum albumin construct [34]. Likewise, in our study, the induced antibodies might have formed a complex with BSA, which prevented the model antigen from binding to the capture antibodies of the ELISA and, thus, from being detected with the assay. Furthermore, the theoretical plasma BSA concentrations of weeks 2 to 4 can be calculated based on the actual plasma BSA concentrations of the previous week, assuming a BSA half-life of 1 day [52,53]. For almost all mice of groups B to D, the actual plasma BSA concentrations of weeks 2 to 4 were higher than the theoretical concentrations. This suggests that at least some release of BSA from the microspheres was still ongoing during these weeks.

Altogether, these findings demonstrate that single-injection microspheres providing a sustained release of BSA can induce strong humoral immune responses in mice, with antibody titers similar to the immune response induced by a prime-boost injection of BSA in PBS. Sustained-release microspheres, therefore, might be a viable alternative to the conventional prime-boost immunization schedule. Further research is, however, needed to determine whether the developed microspheres are also suitable for the delivery of a clinically relevant vaccine and which dose of antigen is optimal for strong antibody induction. In this study, relatively high doses of BSA were administered, while lower doses might have been sufficient as well. Once a clinically relevant antigen has been incorporated, IgG subclasses (e.g., IgG1 and IgG2a) and cellular immune responses could be determined in addition to total IgG. This will provide insight into qualitative aspects of the immune response induced by sustained-release microspheres. Moreover, tailoring the release duration to the specific needs of a vaccine is essential for the use of the sustained-release microspheres for a broad variety of vaccines. According to the in vitro release results, the release duration could be varied by varying the blend ratio of the polymers used but changing the composition of the polymers is an option as well. However, establishing an in vitro-in vivo correlation remains difficult, as there are many factors in play that affect the pharmacokinetics of an antigen. Examples are plasma clearance and antibody formation, but also lymphatic uptake and metabolism, interference of components of the s.c. extracellular matrix, and protein degradation at the injection site [34]. Determining the in vivo release or the plasma concentration as a surrogate indicator of release is, therefore, recommended.

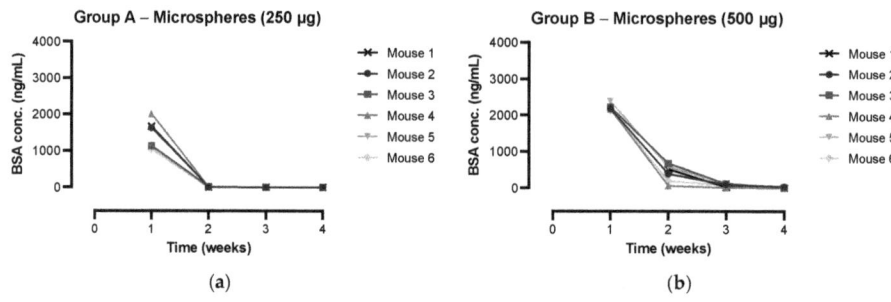

Figure 8. Cont.

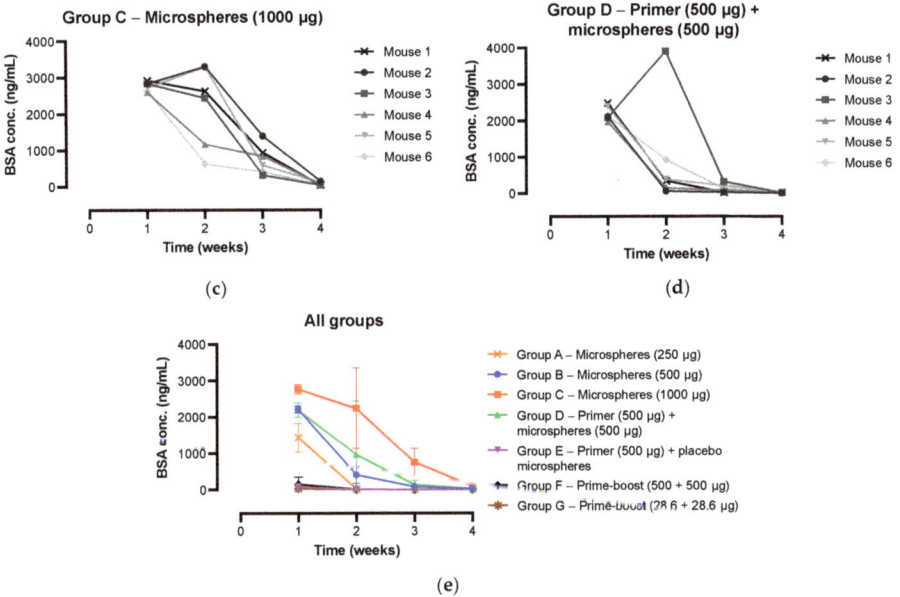

Figure 8. BSA levels in mouse plasma over time after immunization with different BSA formulations (group A to D). Mice (n = 6 per group) were immunized with: (**a**) 250 µg BSA-microspheres in CMC solution; (**b**) 500 µg BSA-microspheres in CMC solution; (**c**) 1000 µg BSA-microspheres in CMC solution; and (**d**) 500 µg BSA in PBS together with 500 µg BSA-microspheres in CMC solution. (**e**) The averages of the BSA levels measured in all mice were calculated for each group (group A to G) and presented for all groups together.

4. Conclusions

Novel multi-block copolymers composed of amorphous, hydrophilic PCL-PEG-PCL blocks and semi-crystalline PDO blocks were used to produce sustained-release microspheres containing the model antigen BSA. The membrane emulsification method enabled the production of uniformly sized particles with the desired size and morphology and high EE. In vitro release studies showed that the release rate could be modulated by adjusting the blend ratio of the two multi-block copolymers. All formulations exhibited sustained release of BSA with low initial burst. Microspheres consisting of a 92.5:7.5 polymer blend released BSA in vitro in a near-linear fashion over a period of approximately four weeks, after which BSA continued to slowly diffuse out for another two weeks. We demonstrated that these microspheres were able to induce a strong BSA-specific IgG antibody response in vivo after s.c. administration in mice. The immune response was equal to that elicited by a prime-boost injection of BSA in PBS administered at 0 and 3 weeks, and the IgG titers followed the same pattern as the in vitro BSA release. Pharmacokinetic analysis of the microspheres demonstrated that in vivo release of BSA was probably ongoing up to at least four weeks as well, although peak plasma concentrations were already reached one week after administration and after four weeks only low levels of BSA were still detected. This suggests that the release of BSA was faster in vivo than in vitro, although the early decline in plasma BSA concentration might also have been caused by the formation and subsequent elimination of antigen–antibody complexes. Converting in vitro release and plasma concentration profiles into in vivo release profiles, thus, remains a challenge. This research shows the potential of sustained-release microspheres as an alternative to the conventional prime-boost immunization schedule. Ultimately, this technology could contribute to the development of single-injection vaccines and improvements in global vaccination coverage.

Further studies with a clinically relevant antigen are, however, necessary to evaluate the clinical potential of the microspheres.

Supplementary Materials: The following supporting information can be downloaded at: https://www.mdpi.com/article/10.3390/pharmaceutics15020676/s1. Figure S1: BSA-specific IgG antibody titers in mouse plasma over time after immunization with different BSA formulations (group A to G). Mice (n = 6 per group) were immunized with (a) 250 µg BSA-microspheres in carboxymethyl cellulose (CMC) solution; (b) 500 µg BSA-microspheres in CMC solution; (c) 1000 µg BSA-microspheres in CMC solution; (d) 500 µg BSA in phosphate-buffered saline (PBS) together with 500 µg BSA-microspheres in CMC solution; (e) 500 µg BSA in PBS together with placebo microspheres in CMC solution; (f) 500 + 500 µg BSA in PBS, prime injection (week 0) and booster injection (week 3); and (g) 28.6 + 28.6 µg BSA in PBS, prime injection (week 0) and booster injection (week 3). The dotted lines represent the cut-off value for the IgG antibody titer, i.e., a titer of 6.64 $\log_2$, corresponding to the starting dilution of the plasma samples of 1:100. Values below this titer could not be measured. Samples with a reading for the least diluted plasma (i.e., 100× diluted) lower than the cut-off value were assigned an IgG antibody titer of 5.64 $\log_2$, corresponding to a dilution of 1:50, which would be one dilution below the starting dilution. For these samples, dashed lines were used to connect the data point below the cut-off value with the next time point. The negative control groups receiving PBS (group H) and CMC solution (group I) are not presented in this figure. Figure S2: Area under the IgG titer–time curve (AUC) values of the BSA-specific IgG antibody titer vs. time graph (Figure S1). Statistical comparisons between the mice of the different groups were performed using the ordinary ANOVA, followed by Tukey's multiple comparisons test (* p < 0.05, ** p < 0.01). For clarity reasons, statistical comparison is only indicated where p < 0.05 (*) or p < 0.01 (**), and differences for all other comparisons were non-significant. The negative control groups receiving PBS (group H) and CMC solution (group I) are not presented in this figure. MSP = microspheres.

Author Contributions: Conceptualization, R.S.v.d.K., J.Z., R.S., H.W.F. and W.L.J.H.; methodology, R.S.v.d.K., M.B., A.L.W.H., J.Z., R.S., H.W.F. and W.L.J.H.; validation, R.S.v.d.K.; formal analysis, R.S.v.d.K. and M.B.; investigation, R.S.v.d.K. and M.B.; resources, R.S. and H.W.F.; data curation, R.S.v.d.K.; writing—original draft preparation, R.S.v.d.K.; writing—review and editing, R.S.v.d.K., M.B., A.L.W.H., J.Z., R.S., H.W.F. and W.L.J.H.; visualization, R.S.v.d.K.; supervision, A.L.W.H., J.Z., R.S., H.W.F. and W.L.J.H.; project administration, R.S.v.d.K. All authors have read and agreed to the published version of the manuscript.

Funding: This research is funded by the European Regional Development Fund (ERDF) through the Northern Netherlands Alliance (SNN) under grant agreement number OPSNN0325. The funders had no role in the design and execution of the research, decision to publish or preparation of the manuscript.

Institutional Review Board Statement: The animal study protocol was approved by the Ethics Committee of Timeline Bioresearch AB under the ethical permit number 5.8.18-20232/2020.

Informed Consent Statement: Not applicable.

Data Availability Statement: Not applicable.

Acknowledgments: The authors thank Jeroen Blokzijl for performing the SE-UPLC analysis and Kim Staal for performing the GC analysis. Furthermore, they thank Kimberly Banus and Daan Wimmers for their technical assistance during the production of the microspheres.

Conflicts of Interest: The authors declare no conflict of interest.

References

1. WHO. Immunization Coverage. 2022. Available online: https://www.who.int/news-room/fact-sheets/detail/immunization-coverage (accessed on 14 December 2022).
2. Ali, H.A.; Hartner, A.M.; Echeverria-Londono, S.; Roth, J.; Li, X.; Abbas, K.; Portnoy, A.; Vynnycky, E.; Woodruff, K.; Ferguson, N.M.; et al. Vaccine equity in low and middle income countries: A systematic review and meta-analysis. *Int. J. Equity Health* **2022**, *21*, 82. [CrossRef] [PubMed]
3. WHO. Immunization Agenda 2030. 2021. Available online: https://www.who.int/docs/default-source/immunization/strategy/ia2030/ia2030-document-en.pdf (accessed on 25 October 2022).

4. McHugh, K.J.; Guarecuco, R.; Langer, R.; Jaklenec, A. Single-injection vaccines: Progress, challenges, and opportunities. *J. Control. Release* 2015, *219*, 596–609. [CrossRef] [PubMed]
5. Cleland, J.L.; Lim, A.; Barrón, L.; Duenas, E.T.; Powell, M.F. Development of a single-shot subunit vaccine for HIV-I: Part 4. Optimizing microencapsulation and pulsatile release of MN rgp120 from biodegradable microspheres. *J. Control. Release* 1997, *47*, 135–150. [CrossRef]
6. van der Kooij, R.S.; Steendam, R.; Zuidema, J.; Frijlink, H.; Hinrichs, W.L.J. Microfluidic production of polymeric core-shell microspheres for the delayed pulsatile release of bovine serum albumin as a model antigen. *Pharmaceutics* 2021, *13*, 1854. [CrossRef] [PubMed]
7. Amssoms, K.; Born, P.A.; Beugeling, M.; De Clerck, B.; Van Gulck, E.; Hinrichs, W.L.J.; Frijlink, H.W.; Grasmeijer, N.; Kraus, G.; Sutmuller, R.; et al. Ovalbumin-containing core-shell implants suitable to obtain a delayed IgG1 antibody response in support of a biphasic pulsatile release profile in mice. *PLoS One* 2018, *13*, e0202961. [CrossRef] [PubMed]
8. Guarecuco, R.; Lu, J.; McHugh, K.J.; Norman, J.J.; Thapa, L.S.; Lydon, E.; Langer, R.; Jaklenec, A. Immunogenicity of pulsatile-release PLGA microspheres for single-injection vaccination. *Vaccine* 2018, *36*, 3161–3168. [CrossRef] [PubMed]
9. Cleland, J.L. Single-administration vaccines: Controlled-release technology to mimic repeated immunizations. *Trends Biotechnol.* 1999, *17*, 25–29. [CrossRef] [PubMed]
10. Feng, L.; Qi, X.R.; Zhou, X.J.; Maitani, Y.; Wang, S.C.; Jiang, Y.; Nagai, T. Pharmaceutical and immunological evaluation of a single-dose hepatitis B vaccine using PLGA microspheres. *J. Control. Release* 2006, *112*, 35–42. [CrossRef]
11. Singh, M.; Singh, A.; Talwar, G.P. Controlled delivery of diphtheria toxoid using biodegradable poly(d,l-lactide) microcapsules. *Pharm. Res.* 1991, *8*, 958–961. [CrossRef]
12. Du, G.; Sun, X. Current advances in sustained release microneedles. *Pharm. Front.* 2020, *2*, e11–e22. [CrossRef]
13. Li, W.; Meng, J.; Ma, X.; Lin, J.; Lu, X. Advanced materials for the delivery of vaccines for infectious diseases. *Biosaf. Health* 2022, *4*, 95–104. [CrossRef]
14. Makadia, H.K.; Siegel, S.J. Poly lactic-co-glycolic acid (PLGA) as biodegradable controlled drug delivery carrier. *Polymers* 2011, *3*, 1377–1397. [CrossRef] [PubMed]
15. Duque, L.; Körber, M.; Bodmeier, R. Improving release completeness from PLGA-based implants for the acid-labile model protein ovalbumin. *Int. J. Pharm.* 2018, *538*, 139–146. [CrossRef] [PubMed]
16. Giteau, A.; Venier-Julienne, M.C.; Aubert-Pouëssel, A.; Benoit, J.P. How to achieve sustained and complete protein release from PLGA-based microparticles? *Int. J. Pharm.* 2008, *350*, 14–26. [CrossRef]
17. Houchin, M.L.; Topp, E.M. Chemical degradation of peptides and proteins in PLGA: A review of reactions and mechanisms. *J. Pharm. Sci.* 2008, *97*, 2395–2404. [CrossRef] [PubMed]
18. Stanković, M.; de Waard, H.; Steendam, R.; Hiemstra, C.; Zuidema, J.; Frijlink, H.W.; Hinrichs, W.L.J. Low temperature extruded implants based on novel hydrophilic multiblock copolymer for long-term protein delivery. *Eur. J. Pharm. Sci.* 2013, *49*, 578–587. [CrossRef]
19. Stanković, M.; Tomar, J.; Hiemstra, C.; Steendam, R.; Frijlink, H.W.; Hinrichs, W.L.J. Tailored protein release from biodegradable poly(ε-caprolactone-PEG)-b-poly(ε-caprolactone) multiblock-copolymer implants. *Eur. J. Pharm. Biopharm.* 2014, *87*, 329–337. [CrossRef]
20. Teekamp, N.; Van Dijk, F.; Broesder, A.; Evers, M.; Zuidema, J.; Steendam, R.; Post, E.; Hillebrands, J.L.; Frijlink, H.W.; Poelstra, K.; et al. Polymeric microspheres for the sustained release of a protein-based drug carrier targeting the PDGFβ-receptor in the fibrotic kidney. *Int. J. Pharm.* 2017, *534*, 229–236. [CrossRef]
21. Scheiner, K.C.; Maas-Bakker, R.F.; Nguyen, T.T.; Duarte, A.M.; Hendriks, G.; Sequeira, L.; Duffy, G.P.; Steendam, R.; Hennink, W.E.; Kok, R.J. Sustained release of vascular endothelial growth factor from poly(ε-caprolactone-PEG-ε-caprolactone)-b-poly(l-lactide) multiblock copolymer microspheres. *ACS Omega* 2019, *4*, 11481–11492. [CrossRef]
22. Igartua, M.; Hernández, R.M.; Esquisabel, A.; Gascón, A.R.; Calvo, M.B.; Pedraz, J.L. Enhanced immune response after subcutaneous and oral immunization with biodegradable PLGA microspheres. *J. Control. Release* 1998, *56*, 63–73. [CrossRef]
23. Conway, B.R.; Eyles, J.; Alpar, H.O. A comparative study on the immune responses to antigens in PLA and PHB microspheres. *J. Control. Release* 1997, *49*, 1–9. [CrossRef]
24. Lemperle, G. Biocompatibility of injectable microspheres. *Biomed. J. Sci. Tech. Res.* 2018, *2*, 2296–2306. [CrossRef]
25. Ye, M.; Kim, S.; Park, K. Issues in long-term protein delivery using biodegradable microparticles. *J. Control. Release* 2010, *146*, 241–260. [CrossRef]
26. Vladisavljević, G.T. Structured microparticles with tailored properties produced by membrane emulsification. *Adv. Colloid Interface Sci.* 2015, *225* (Suppl. C), 53–87. [CrossRef] [PubMed]
27. Qi, F.; Wu, J.; Fan, Q.; He, F.; Tian, G.; Yang, T.; Ma, G.; Su, Z. Preparation of uniform-sized exenatide-loaded PLGA microspheres as long-effective release system with high encapsulation efficiency and bio-stability. *Colloids Surfaces B Biointerfaces* 2013, *112*, 492–498. [CrossRef]
28. Bodmeier, R.; McGinity, J.W. Solvent selection in the preparation of poly(dl-lactide) microspheres prepared by the solvent evaporation method. *Int. J. Pharm.* 1988, *43*, 179–186. [CrossRef]
29. Rafati, H.; Coombes, A.G.A.; Adler, J.; Holland, J.; Davis, S.S. Protein-loaded poly(dl-lactide-co-glycolide) microparticles for oral administration: Formulation, structural and release characteristics. *J. Control. Release* 1997, *43*, 89–102. [CrossRef]

30. Mao, S.; Xu, J.; Cai, C.; Germershaus, O.; Schaper, A.; Kissel, T. Effect of WOW process parameters on morphology and burst release of FITC-dextran loaded PLGA microspheres. *Int. J. Pharm.* **2007**, *334*, 137–148. [CrossRef]
31. Arakawa, T.; Timasheff, S.N. Preferential interactions of proteins with salts in concentrated solutions. *Biochemistry* **1982**, *21*, 6545–6552. [CrossRef]
32. Fu, Y.; Kao, W.J. Drug release kinetics and transport mechanisms of non-degradable and degradable polymeric delivery systems. *Expert Opin. Drug Deliv.* **2010**, *7*, 429–444. [CrossRef]
33. van Dijkhuizen-Radersma, R.; Métairie, S.; Roosma, J.R.; de Groot, K.; Bezemer, J.M. Controlled release of proteins from degradable poly(ether-ester) multiblock copolymers. *J. Control. Release* **2005**, *101*, 175–186. [CrossRef]
34. Van Dijk, F.; Teekamp, N.; Beljaars, L.; Post, E.; Zuidema, J.; Steendam, R.; Kim, Y.O.; Frijlink, H.W.; Schuppan, D.; Poelstra, K.; et al. Pharmacokinetics of a sustained release formulation of PDGFβ-receptor directed carrier proteins to target the fibrotic liver. *J. Control. Release* **2018**, *269*, 258–265. [CrossRef]
35. Haitjema, H.; Steendam, R.; Hiemstra, C.; Zuidema, J.; Doornbos, A.; Nguyen, T. Biodegradable, Phase Separated, Thermoplastic Multi-Block Copolymer. PCT Patent No. WO 2021/066650 A1, 8 April 2021.
36. Middleton, J.C.; Tipton, A.J. Synthetic biodegradable polymers as orthopedic devices. *Biomaterials* **2000**, *21*, 2335–2346. [CrossRef] [PubMed]
37. Heene, S.; Thoms, S.; Kalies, S.; Wegner, N.; Peppermüller, P.; Born, N.; Walther, F.; Scheper, T.; Blume, C.A. Vascular network formation on macroporous polydioxanone scaffolds. *Tissue Eng. Part A* **2021**, *27*, 1239–1249. [CrossRef] [PubMed]
38. Zilberman, M.; Nelson, K.D.; Eberhart, R.C. Mechanical properties and in vitro degradation of bioresorbable fibers and expandable fiber-based stents. *J. Biomed. Mater. Res. Part B Appl. Biomater.* **2005**, *74B*, 792–799. [CrossRef] [PubMed]
39. Kotcharat, P.; Chuysinuan, P.; Thanyacharoen, T.; Techasakul, S.; Ummartyotin, S. Development of bacterial cellulose and polycaprolactone (PCL) based composite for medical material. *Sustain. Chem. Pharm.* **2021**, *20*, 100404. [CrossRef]
40. European Medicines Agency ICH Guideline Q3C (R8) on Impurities: Guideline for Residual Solvents. 2021. Available online: https://www.ema.europa.eu/en/documents/regulatory-procedural-guideline/ich-guideline-q3c-r8-impurities-guideline-residual-solvents-step-5_en.pdf (accessed on 25 October 2022).
41. Serota, D.G.; Thakur, A.; Ulland, B.; Kirschman, J.; Brown, N.; Coots, R.H. A two-year drinking-water study of dichloromethane in rodents. II. Mice. *Food Chem. Toxicol.* **1986**, *24*, 959–963. [CrossRef]
42. Dresser, D.W.; Gowland, G. Immunological paralysis induced in adult rabbits by small amounts of a protein antigen. *Nature* **1964**, *203*, 733–736. [CrossRef]
43. Dixon, F.J.; Maurer, P.H. Immunologic unresponsiveness induced by protein antigens. *J. Exp. Med.* **1955**, *101*, 245–257. [CrossRef]
44. Mitchison, N.A. Induction of immunological paralysis in two zones of dosage. *Proc. R. Soc. Lond. B* **1964**, *161*, 275–292.
45. Lofthouse, S. Immunological aspects of controlled antigen delivery. *Adv. Drug Deliv. Rev.* **2002**, *54*, 863–870. [CrossRef] [PubMed]
46. Lavelle, E.C.; Yeh, M.K.; Coombes, A.G.A.; Davis, S.S. The stability and immunogenicity of a protein antigen encapsulated in biodegradable microparticles based on blends of lactide polymers and polyethylene glycol. *Vaccine* **1999**, *17*, 512–529. [CrossRef] [PubMed]
47. O'Hagan, D.T.; Rahman, D.; McGee, J.P.; Jeffery, H.; Davies, M.C.; Williams, P.; Davis, S.S.; Challacombe, S.J. Biodegradable microparticles as controlled release antigen delivery systems. *Immunology* **1991**, *73*, 239–242. [PubMed]
48. Heesters, B.A.; van der Poel, C.E.; Das, A.; Carroll, M.C. Antigen presentation to B cells. *Trends Immunol.* **2016**, *37*, 844–854. [CrossRef]
49. Leo, O.; Cunningham, A.; Stern, P.L. Vaccine immunology. *Perspect. Vaccinol.* **2011**, *1*, 25–59. [CrossRef]
50. Sandor, M.; Harris, J.; Mathiowitz, E. A novel polyethylene depot device for the study of PLGA and P(FASA) microspheres in vitro and in vivo. *Biomaterials* **2002**, *23*, 4413–4423. [CrossRef]
51. Tracy, M.A.; Ward, K.L.; Firouzabadian, L.; Wang, Y.; Dong, N.; Qian, R.; Zhang, Y. Factors affecting the degradation rate of poly(lactide-co-glycolide) microspheres in vivo and in vitro. *Biomaterials* **1999**, *20*, 1057–1062. [CrossRef]
52. Nguyen, A.; Reyes, A.E.; Zhang, M.; McDonald, P.; Wong, W.L.T.; Damico, L.A.; Dennis, M.S. The pharmacokinetics of an albumin-binding Fab (AB.Fab) can be modulated as a function of affinity for albumin. *Protein Eng. Des. Sel.* **2006**, *19*, 291–297. [CrossRef]
53. Stevens, D.; Eyre, R.; Bull, R. Adduction of hemoglobin and albumin in vivo by metabolites of trichloroethylene, trichloroacetate, and dichloroacetate in rats and mice. *Fundam. Appl. Toxicol.* **1992**, *19*, 336–342. [CrossRef]

Disclaimer/Publisher's Note: The statements, opinions and data contained in all publications are solely those of the individual author(s) and contributor(s) and not of MDPI and/or the editor(s). MDPI and/or the editor(s) disclaim responsibility for any injury to people or property resulting from any ideas, methods, instructions or products referred to in the content.

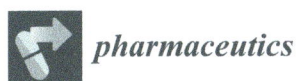

Article

Deferasirox Nanosuspension Loaded Dissolving Microneedles for Intradermal Delivery

Hafsa Shahid Faizi [1], Lalitkumar K. Vora [1], Muhammad Iqbal Nasiri [1,2], Yu Wu [1], Deepakkumar Mishra [1], Qonita Kurnia Anjani [1], Alejandro J. Paredes [1], Raghu Raj Singh Thakur [1], Muhammad Usman Minhas [3,*] and Ryan F. Donnelly [1,*]

[1] School of Pharmacy, Queen's University Belfast, Medical Biology Centre, 97 Lisburn Road, Belfast BT9 7BL, UK
[2] Department of Pharmaceutics, Hamdard Institute of Pharmaceutical Sciences, Hamdard University, Islamabad 45550, Pakistan
[3] College of Pharmacy, University of Sargodha, Sargodha 40100, Pakistan
* Correspondence: usman.minhas@uos.edu.pk (M.U.M.); r.donnelly@qub.ac.uk (R.F.D.)

Abstract: Microneedles are minimally invasive systems that can deliver drugs intradermally without pain and bleeding and can advantageously replace the hypodermal needles and oral routes of delivery. Deferasirox (DFS) is an iron chelator employed in several ailments where iron overload plays an important role in disease manifestation. In this study, DFS was formulated into a nanosuspension (NSs) through wet media milling employing PVA as a stabilizer and successfully loaded in polymeric dissolving microneedles (DMNs). The release studies for DFS-NS clearly showed a threefold increased dissolution rate compared to pure DFS. The mechanical characterization of DFS-NS-DMNs revealed that the system was sufficiently strong for efficacious skin penetration. Optical coherence tomography images confirmed an insertion of up to 378 μm into full-thickness porcine skin layers. The skin deposition studies showed 60% drug deposition from NS-DMN, which was much higher than from the DFS-NS transdermal patch (DFS-NS-TP) (without needles) or pure DFS-DMNs. Moreover, DFS-NS without DMNs did not deposit well inside the skin, indicating that DMNs played an important role in effectively delivering drugs inside the skin. Therefore, it is evident from the findings that loading DFS-NS into novel DMN devices can effectively deliver DFS transdermally.

Keywords: nanocrystals; nanosuspension; dissolving microneedles; deferasirox; intradermal delivery

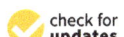

Citation: Faizi, H.S.; Vora, L.K.; Nasiri, M.I.; Wu, Y.; Mishra, D.; Anjani, Q.K.; Paredes, A.J.; Thakur, R.R.S.; Minhas, M.U.; Donnelly, R.F. Deferasirox Nanosuspension Loaded Dissolving Microneedles for Intradermal Delivery. *Pharmaceutics* 2022, 14, 2817. https://doi.org/10.3390/pharmaceutics14122817

Academic Editor: Heather Benson

Received: 19 September 2022
Accepted: 8 December 2022
Published: 15 December 2022

Publisher's Note: MDPI stays neutral with regard to jurisdictional claims in published maps and institutional affiliations.

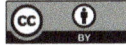

Copyright: © 2022 by the authors. Licensee MDPI, Basel, Switzerland. This article is an open access article distributed under the terms and conditions of the Creative Commons Attribution (CC BY) license (https://creativecommons.org/licenses/by/4.0/).

1. Introduction

In recent times, the inadequacy of drugs' cross through the skin barrier, the stratum corneum (SC), remains a major limitation of transdermal delivery [1,2]. This problem has been addressed by introducing micron-scale needles that can enhance skin permeability, thus increasing effective transdermal delivery [3,4]. Microneedles (MNs) that employ a combination of hypodermic needles and transdermal patches are painless and negligibly invasive devices that can bypass the SC [5,6]. As the *SC* contains no nociceptors and MNs do not invade deeper where nerve endings are present, they are capable of carrying drugs to the permeable regions of skin without provoking nerves responsible for pain [7,8]. MNs can also obviate the first pass effect, which is a classic drawback of oral drug delivery, by effectively delivering drugs via the intradermal route [9,10].

DFS is an iron chelator employed in iron toxicity for various diseases [11]. It is highly effective in treating iron overload in thalassemic patients caused by blood transfusions [12,13]. DFS has also been investigated for reducing oxidative stress and inflammation in patients where iron is responsible for the development of inflammation and tissue damage through the production [14] of reactive oxygen species (ROS). It forms a stable complex with Fe(III) ions with 2:1 binding to eliminate iron. DFS, due to its iron-chelating properties, is proven to be safe and effective in the treatment of a skin condition called porphyria cutanea tarda [15].

Other studies found that DFS presented antitumor activity for treating solid tumors [16,17]. DFS is a Class II compound, according to the biopharmaceutics classification system (BCS), exhibiting low solubility and high permeability [12,18]. Current oral drug delivery can result in the short duration of action, resulting in a higher dosing frequency with lower patient compliance. In addition to the fact that first pass effect decreases the bioavailability of drug, it can also be unsuitable for patients who are unconscious and/or vomiting. Therefore, an alternative drug delivery route is highly desirable. To avoid the stated drawbacks for oral route, intradermal delivery improved therapy due to the maintenance of plasma levels up to the end of the dosing interval compared to a decline in plasma levels with oral delivery, making it a major advantage of the former. However, impermeable skin barrier could not allow the delivery of the hydrophobic drug as its absorption in the viable layers of the skin is negligible. One drug delivery strategy that could be considered to improve the delivery of this hydrophobic DFS into the skin are MNs, which circumvent the protective barrier of the SC by physically piercing this outermost layer of the skin [19–21].

However, unlike hydrophilic drugs, the formation of nanosuspensions (NSs) of hydrophobic drugs is necessary for inclusion into polymeric MNs for uniform distribution inside MNs [19,22–24]. NSs refer to a nanosized (1–1000 nm) liquid dispersion of drug particles coated by a stabilizer layer, for example, a surfactant or polymer [25–27]. Additionally, the advantages of increased surface area, greater dissolution rates, better absorption and, hence, higher bioavailability, make nanosuspension a desirable and widely employed technique for hydrophobic drugs [28–30]. Moreover, NS can yield high drug loading because of the smaller amount of surfactants needed to stabilize nanosized drug molecules, unlike polymeric nanoparticles, where the use of larger amounts of polymeric excipients is essential to encapsulate the drug molecules [31,32].

In this study, two concepts of drug nanosizing and microneedle-based intradermal drug delivery were combined to enhance the efficient delivery of the poorly water-soluble drug DFS. The goal of this work was the incorporation of DFS NSs into polymeric MNs for effective intradermal delivery as opposed to oral delivery, as it presents numerous drawbacks. First, DFS NSs were prepared using wet media milling. Afterward, the DFS-NS were subsequently loaded into the DMNs. The newly formed MNs, after effective loading of drug NSs, were assessed for particle size, polydispersity index (PDI), mechanical strength, skin insertion, drug content, and ex vivo skin deposition of the drug.

2. Materials and Methods

2.1. Materials

Deferasirox (DFS) was purchased from Cangzhou Enke Pharma-tech Co., Ltd., Guangzhou, China. Poly(vinyl alcohol) (PVA) (9000–10,000 mol wt) was purchased from Sigma Aldrich (Poole, Dorset, UK). Poly(vinyl pyrrolidone) (PVP) with a molecular weight of 58,000 Da (K-29/32) and a PVP molecular weight of 111. A total of 143 Da (K-90) were purchased from Ashland Industries (Wilmington, DE, USA). The purified water utilized in all experiments was obtained from ELGA® DV 25, Purelab Option, water purification System (ELGA-Q, USA). All other chemicals used were of analytical reagent grade.

2.2. Preparation of Drug-Loaded Nanosuspension

DFS NSs were prepared with the wet media milling method, as presented in Figure 1, using beads (ceramic beads, 0.2 mm diameter) with slight modifications, as reported previously [33]. This preparation method was chosen because of its easy and solvent-free operation and high drug loading [1]. PVA was selected as a stabilizer for the NS. One hundred milligrams of DFS was accurately weighed in a 7 mL volume glass vial, followed by the addition of 6 mL of 1% w/w PVA solution. Approximately 2 mL of beads was added to this mixture, and two magnetic stirring bars of dimensions (25 mm × 8 mm) were placed in the vial. The vial containing drug, stabilizer, ceramic beads (particle size of 0.1 mm) and magnetic stirrers was placed on a magnetic stirring plate running at a speed of 1000 rpm and 1500 rpm for 6–12 h. The resulting NS were retrieved after 24 h of milling, kept at −80 °C for 6–8 h and freeze-dried at −40 °C for 26 h to remove all water content. The effect of an increase in milling speed and milling time on particle size was also recorded.

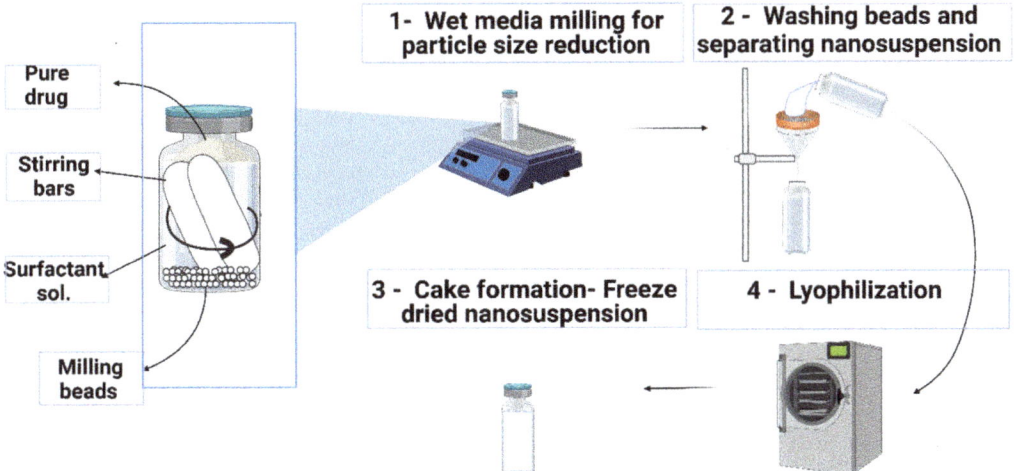

Figure 1. Schematic representation of the fabrication of the DFS-NS.

2.3. Particle Size and Surface Charge Analysis

The hydrodynamic size, zeta potential, and polydispersity index (PDI) of freshly prepared and lyophilized DFS-NS were determined using a NanoBrook Omni (Brookhaven Instrument, Holtsville, NY, USA). PDI shows uniformity in the size distribution of particles within a sample, and zeta potential gives us information on the stability of the given formulation. Freshly prepared DFS-NS samples were taken at 6, 12, 24 and 48 h to monitor particle size reduction as a function of milling time. Briefly, samples were diluted suitably in water prior to measurement. An electric field was applied across the DFS-NS solutions using the technique of phase analysis light scattering (PALS) procedure for measuring zeta potential. Particle size and PDI were analyzed by employing the dynamic light scattering (DLS) method. Folded capillary cells were used for holding samples, and the temperature was maintained at 25 ± 2 °C for each measurement. All experimental runs were performed in triplicate to obtain mean data.

2.4. Particle Size Analysis for Pure Drug

For determination of DFS particle size, a Mastersizer® 3000 equipped with a Hydro® cell (Malvern Panalytical Ltd., Worcestershire, UK) was used employing laser diffraction phenomenon, as previously described [34]. A total of 20 mg of coarse drug was accurately weighed and mixed with 10 mL of 2% w/v poloxamer 188 by employing vortex mixing for adequate disaggregation of particles, followed by dispersion in 500 mL of water. The agitation of the Hydro® cell was set at 2000 rpm for 3 min, after which the sample was further sonicated for 30 s. The samples were measured six times, and the results were expressed in terms of the De Brouckere and Sauter mean diameters ([D4,3] and [D3,2], respectively) and D10, D50 and D90.

2.5. Differential Scanning Calorimetry Analysis

Differential scanning calorimetry (DSC) studies of pure DFS, pure PVA (stabilizer), a physical mixture of DFS and PVA, and DFS-NS were carried out using a DSC Q100 (TA Instruments, Surrey, UK). Weighed samples of 3.0–5.0 mg were sealed in aluminum pans (nonhermetic). A flow rate of 50 mL per minute was set, and the heating rate was kept at

10.0 °C/min in nitrogen. To calibrate the DSC, the melting temperature of indium was set at 156.6 °C.

2.6. X-ray Diffraction Measurements

The study was carried out using a benchtop X-ray diffractometer (Miniflex™, Rigaku Corporation, Kent, UK). Radiation was from Ni-filtered Cu Kβ, with a wavelength of 1.39 Å at a voltage of 30 kV, a current of 15 mA, and at room temperature. DFS, PVA, a physical mixture of DFS and PVA and DFS-NS were packed into the rotating sample holder. The obtained data were typically collected by scanning a range of 0–60° with a scanning rate of 2°/min.

2.7. FTIR Measurements

Fourier transform infrared (FTIR) spectral analysis of DFS, PVA (10 kDa) and DFS-NS was conducted to study the drug–excipient interaction. The absorption spectra were recorded from 4000 to 400 cm^{-1} using an FTIR spectrometer (Accutrac FT/IR-4100™ Series, Jasco, Essex, UK).

2.8. Drug Content Analysis for DFS-NS

The drug content analysis for DFS-NS was performed in triplicate by dissolving accurately weighed (10 mg) freeze-dried NS into 1 mL of dimethyl sulfoxide (DMSO) and sonicating for 15 min. Then, 100 µL of the resulting solution was added to 900 µL of acetonitrile and centrifuged (12,000× g) for 10 min. Then, 100 µL supernatant was carefully collected and further diluted with 900 µL of phosphate buffer (PBS) containing 0.5% Tween 80 solution, followed by HPLC analysis. The % recovery of the drug was calculated using the following formula.

$$\% \text{ Recovery of drug} = \frac{\text{known amount loaded}}{\text{amount detected via analysis}} \times 100 \quad (1)$$

2.9. In Vitro Release Studies for DFS NS

Release studies were performed using high retention cellulose dialysis tubing (2.3 mm, 0.9 inches). A total of 20 milligrams of accurately weighed drug and MNs were dispersed separately in 1 mL of PBS solution (in triplicate) and filled inside the dialysis membrane, secured with clips on both ends to contain the samples. These filled dialysis bags were then placed in 100 mL of PBS solution and incubated at 37 °C with mild shaking (40 rpm). A 500 µL sample of released media was taken at different time intervals of 2, 4, 6, 12, 24, 48, and 72 h, and 500 µL of the same media was replaced to maintain the volume. The samples were diluted by adding 500 µL of acetonitrile and centrifuged (2000× g) for 10 min to remove the polymer. Moreover, 100 µL of the supernatant was diluted with 900 µL of 0.5% of Tween 80 in PBS solution and injected into the HPLC for analysis.

2.10. Preparation of DFS-NS Loaded Dissolving Microneedles (DFS-NS DMN)

MN arrays were prepared using a silicone mold design, as presented in Figure 2, with microneedle heights of 700 µm, base widths of 300 µm and interspacing of 15 µm (a total of 600 arrays). These silicone molds were generously provided by LTS Lohmann (Germany). The polymers used for the preparation of the casting gel were PVA (9000–1000 MW) and PVP (K32/29). First, freeze-dried NS containing 300 mg of DFS was mixed with 1 ml of deionized water using a SpeedMixer™ (DAC 150.1 FVZ-K, Synergy Devices Ltd., UK) to form a homogeneous blend. This blend was then poured into 0.75 g of 40% PVP solution (K32/29). This mixture was homogenized again using SpeedMixer™ at 3500 rpm for 5 min to obtain a homogenous casting gel for MN fabrication. Here, 180 mg PVA is already present in the DFS-NS added. The DFS-NS casting gel was then poured onto the top surface of the MN molds and was subjected to a high-pressure tank at 60 psi for 3 min. The excess gel was removed by scraping lightly with a spatula, and the molds were again placed for 30 min in the pressure tank at the same pressure. After that, the molds were kept at room temperature for 24 h, and then 30% PVP (K90) solution was applied as a second layer (baseplate casting), followed by centrifugation (3500 rpm) for 8 min to remove any air bubbles. The MNs were removed from the molds after an additional 48 h of drying at room temperature and subjected to further studies.

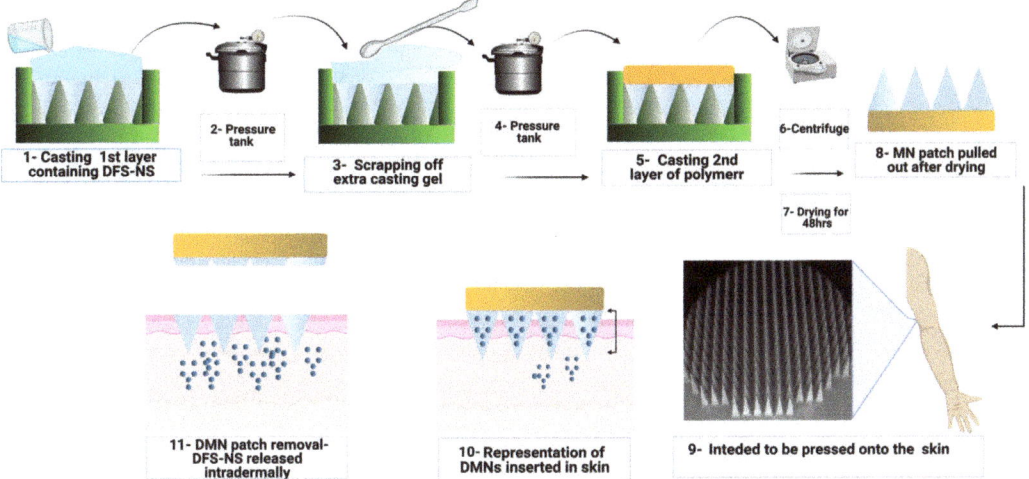

Figure 2. Schematic representation of the fabrication of DFS-NS DMNs and their application.

2.11. Determination of Insertion Properties and Mechanical Strength of DFS-NS DMN Arrays

Parafilm M®, an elastic thermoplastic film made with a material resembling olefin (Bemis Company Inc., Soignies, Belgium), was used as a skin mimetic for the insertion of DFS-NS-DMNs. Initially, the height of the DMN arrays was recorded by stereomicroscopy prior to the application of compression force. For insertion studies, eight layers of Parafilm M® sheet were placed onto the horizontal aluminum block under the movable probe and followed the same procedure as explained above. After the application of 32 N force, the DMNs were removed, and each layer of Parafilm M® was observed under a microscope to count the number of holes created in each layer. The heights of DMNs after penetration into Parafilm M® were noted using a Leica EZ4 D digital microscope to evaluate the reduction in height. The percentage insertion was calculated by the following formula:

$$\text{Percentage insertion} = \frac{\text{Number of holes created}}{\text{Number of microneedles in a patch}} \times 100 \quad (2)$$

The mechanical properties of DFS-NS-DMNs and DFS-DMNs were studied using Texture Analyser (TA. XT-Plus, Stable Microsystem, Haslemere, UK) used in compression mode, as reported in earlier research [35,36]. The pre- and post-test speeds were 1 mm/s, while the trigger force was set at 0.049 N. A Leica EZ4 D digital microscope (Leica Microsystems, Wetzlar, Germany) was employed to study the morphological appearance of DFS-NS-DMNs before compression. Later, the DMN patches were fixed on the bottom of a movable probe using double-sided tape with needles facing down. The probe was run/declined against a horizontal, leveled block of aluminum at a rate of 0.5 mm s^{-1}, and 32 N force was applied to the DMN patch for 30 s. After application of the desired force, DFS-NS-DMNs were examined for any size reduction using a Leica EZ4 D digital microscope, and the percentage reduction in height was calculated as follows:

$$\% \text{ height reduction} = \frac{\text{mean height before compression} - \text{mean height after compression}}{\text{mean height before compression}} \times 100 \qquad (3)$$

2.12. High-Performance Liquid Chromatography (HPLC) Analysis

Reversed phase HPLC (Agilent, 1260 Infinity II VWD, Germany) was used for analytical quantification of DFS using a C18 column (5 μm pore size, 4.6 × 100 mm) (Phenomenex, Macclesfield, UK). The flow rate was set at 1. ml/min, the oven temperature was set at 35 °C and analysis was performed with UV detection at 245 nm The mobile phase was composed of acetonitrile:phosphate buffer (pH 3.0), 50%:50%, and the injection volume was 10 μL. The standard calibration curve was plotted by making appropriate dilutions in the range of 0.096 to 100 μg/mL, and an R^2 of 0.999 exhibited good linearity [37].

2.13. Drug Content Analysis for DFS-NS-DMNs

Drug content was analyzed by dissolving accurately weighed DFS-NS-DMN arrays as well as DFS-DMNs in 3 mL of water and sonicating for 15 min. Then, 2 mL DMSO was added, and the mixture was sonicated for 30 min for efficient extraction of the drug. Furthermore, 200 μL of this solution was mixed with 0.9 mL acetonitrile to allow precipitation of PVP polymer while the drug remained dissolved. This dispersion was centrifuged at 12,000× g for 10 min, and 100 μL of the supernatant was collected to further be diluted with 1.9 mL of mobile phase, which was then injected for HPLC analysis. Studies were performed in triplicate.

2.14. Digital Microscopy and SEM Imaging of DFS-NS-DMNs

The surface morphology and shape of DFS-NS-DMNs were examined using a Keyence VHX-700F Digital Microscope (Keyence, Osaka, Japan) and a TM3030 benchtop scanning electron microscope (SEM) (Hitachi, Krefeld, Germany). The latter was used in low vacuum mode at a voltage of 15 kV.

2.15. Insertion Studies in Excised Porcine Skin by Optical Coherence Tomography

It has been established earlier that the skin of neonatal pigs acts similarly to human skin [38]; hence, it was used to study the insertion of DFS-NS-DMNs. The skin was obtained from stillborn piglets and excised within 24 h of birth using a scalpel. The skin was then refrigerated at −20 °C for storage after being enclosed in aluminum foil until use. Prior to use, skin was defrosted and then thawed in phosphate-buffered saline (PBS) of pH 7.4, after which fine hair was removed carefully using a razor and washed thoroughly with PBS solution again. Absorbent tissue paper was used to dry the skin, and the skin was laid down flat on a weighing boat. Using the Texture Analyzer, DMN arrays were then pressed onto the porcine skin (force 32 N for 30 s). Optical coherence tomography (OCT) images were captured immediately upon insertion using an OCT Microscope (EX1301, Michelson Diagnostics Ltd., Kent, UK) to evaluate the successful insertion of MN arrays into the skin.

2.16. Dissolution Studies of DFS-NS-DMNs in Excised Porcine Skin

Dissolution of DMNs was determined by taking images by a Leica EZ4 D digital microscope at 10, 15, 30 and 60 min after insertion of the DMN patch into excised porcine skin following incubation at 37 °C. These images showed how much time DFS-NS-DMNs took to completely dissolve inside porcine skin. They also show the morphology of DMNs after each time point, depicting the gradual process of microneedle dissolution over time.

2.17. Ex Vivo Porcine Skin Deposition Study of DFS-NS-DMNs

Drug deposition for DFS-NS-DMNs was investigated using full thickness neonatal porcine skin, as described previously [34,39]. After thawing in phosphate-buffered saline (PBS) (pH 7.4), the skin was carefully shaved using a razor and washed with PBS before use. The skin surface was dried using tissue paper and placed dermis side down on paper sheets to provide support, and the underside of the skin was bathed in PBS (pH 7.4) at 37 °C for 30 min to equilibrate. After insertion of the MN patch, a cylindrical 12.0 g stainless steel weight was placed onto the top of the MN array patch to prevent MN expulsion and placed inside the oven at 37 ± 2 °C for 24 h. These pieces of skin along with the applied MNs were placed at 37 °C for 24 h. To prevent skin drying, another weighing boat was placed on the top, and 10 mL PBS (pH 7.4) solution was added to maintain skin hydration. Following applications, MNs remaining on the skin surface were carefully removed, and then the skin surface was thoroughly cleaned by applying 3 × 1 mL of PBS (pH 7.4) solution and gently wiped with wet paper tissue. The skin at the MN application site was then visualized using a Leica EZ4 W stereo microscope, and the MN-applied skin part was harvested using a scalpel. These harvested skins were cut into small pieces and placed into 2 mL Eppendorf tubes containing 0.5 mL water. The samples were bead milled using TissueLyser LT (QIAGEN®, Manchester, UK) for 15 min to solubilize the remaining MN shafts deposited in the skin. Subsequently, 1 mL of acetonitrile was added to each sample, and the mixture was homogenized for another 15 min again to solubilize the drug. The resulting mixture was then sonicated for 30 min and centrifuged at 48,000 rpm for 10 min to settle down the skin pieces. One hundred microliters of the supernatant was pipetted out into another 2 mL Eppendorf tube, and 900 µL of acetonitrile was added to it to precipitate out any polymers. After vortexing, the mixture was centrifuged again at 16,000 rpm for 10 min to settle down the precipitated polymer, and the supernatant was injected into the HPLC for analysis. Skin deposition studies were performed with DFS-NS-DMNs as well as pure drug-loaded DMN arrays. In addition, DFS-NS Transdermal patch (TP) and plain DFS-NS were investigated for drug deposition for comparison by following the same procedure as above.

3. Results and Discussion

DMN patches were fabricated with hydrophobic drug-loaded nanosystems to deliver the drug intradermally. DMN acts as a drug reservoir and is self-implanted subcutaneously to release drugs regionally and sustainably without producing systemic side effects. The DMN is applied on the skin surface and painlessly pierces the epidermis, creating microscopic aqueous pores through which drugs diffuse to the dermal microcirculation.

3.1. Characterization of DFS-NS

DFS-NS were prepared using the wet bead milling technique, and the pure drug was suspended in the medium with the help of a stabilizer. This method converted the pure drug into a nanosized range with a particle size in the 200 nm range. The particle size reduction increases the surface area and dissolution rate and, hence, enhances penetration of the drug through the skin [40]. A suitable stabilizer is necessary for producing a stable nanosuspension, as nanoparticles can be unstable due to higher Gibb's energy, which interns because of their larger surface area [41].

PVA (9000–10,000 mol wt.) was selected as a stabilizer for the nanosuspension, as it is more compatible with polymeric microneedle arrays. Initially, 3% w/w PVA solutions (DFS-NS-1) were used as stabilizers, which were later reduced to 1% (DFS-NS-2) as the particle size and PDI were almost the same for both nanosuspensions. This can be attributed to the fact that a small change in the amount of surfactant seldom influences the particle size of the nanosuspension rather than the type of stabilizer, which is more important [42].

The bead size affected NSs formation to a great extent, as a rule of thumb exists that states that a 1000-fold particle size reduction is obtained in relation to the bead size. This seems to be true as a particle size in the range of 200 nm was obtained in the existing study with the 0.2 mm beads used. This indicates that bead size is directly proportional to particle size obtained after milling. This can be attributed to the fact that the ability of smaller beads to gnaw drug crystals is greater as they are more fast-moving. Nevertheless, extremely small beads are difficult to separate after milling and may also pose a risk of aggregation due to excess unutilized energy (not employed in size reduction) [43].

Moreover, DFS-NS-2 was taken for DMN array fabrication, as higher drug loading is possible due to the lower concentration of PVA compared to the drug in the NS. With milling speeds of 1000 rpm and 1500 rpm, the mean particle sizes after 24 h of milling were 280.92 ± 18.72 nm and 230.92 ± 1.73 nm, respectively, as shown in Figure 3A. This clearly indicates that the milling speed has a huge impact on the particle size. The PDI was also improved from 0.20 ± 0.02 mV to 0.16 ± 0.02 mV after an increase in milling speed, indicating a more uniform size reduction at higher speeds.

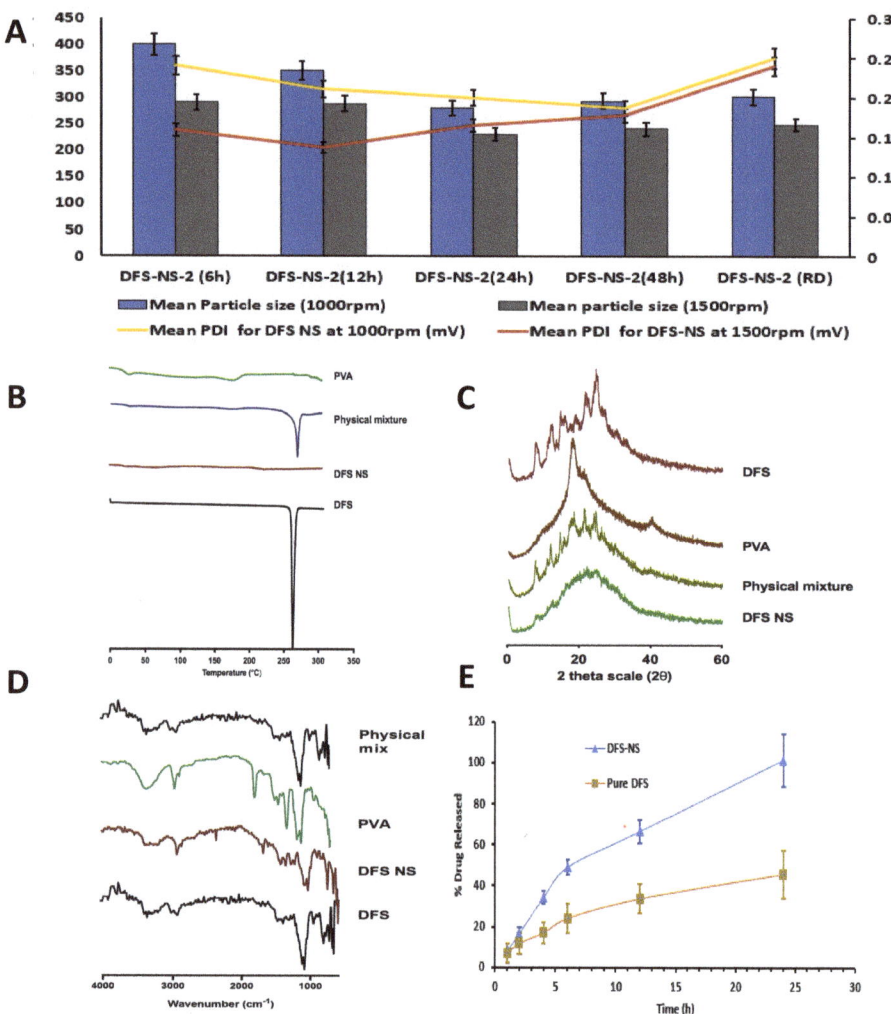

Figure 3. Particle size and PDI at 6, 12, 24, 48 h of milling and RD after freeze-drying at (**A**) 1000 rpm and 1500 rpm milling speed expressed as means + SDs, $n = 3$. (**B**) Differential scanning calorimetry thermogram of PVA, physical mixture of DFS and PVA, DFS-NS and DFS, (**C**) Powder X-ray diffraction of plain DFS, PVA, physical mixture of DFS and PVA and DF-NS, (**D**) Fourier transform infrared analysis of DFS, PVA, and DFS-NS. (**E**) In vitro release profile of DFS-NS and pure DFS by employing dialysis membrane and PBS as release media, expressed as the means ± SDs, $n = 3$.

The effect of milling time was also quite clear, as samples taken after 6 h of milling (at 1500 rpm speed) exhibited a particle size of 291.32 ± 4.54 nm with a PDI of 0.159 ± 0.020 mV, while at 24 h, it was further reduced to 230.92 ± 1.02 nm with a PDI of 0.125 ± 0.023 mV. Therefore, particle size was reduced as a function of milling time, as samples taken at 6 h, 12 h, and 24 h showed a consistent reduction in particle size, as shown in Figure 3B, with an almost constant PDI below 0.2. However, the particle size did not show any considerable reduction in samples taken at 48 h of milling, which shows that 24 h of milling is more suitable for efficient and maximum particle size reduction. Moreover, the particle size increased in most of the samples to 240.92 ± 4.03 nm after 48 h of milling because further exposure to high energy increases the kinetic energy of the crystalline material, resulting in aggregation rather than a reduction in size.

The zeta potentials for both DFS-NS-1 and DFS-NS-2 were −19.46 mV ± 1.56 and −20.51 mV ± 3.46, respectively, which shows that PVA formed a surface adsorption layer on the particles, preventing aggregation and therefore providing sufficient stabilization. After freeze-drying, the particle size and PDI were checked, and a slight increase in particle size (248.95 nm ± 10.81) was observed. The zeta potential value of redispersed (RD) DFS-NS-2 was −19.46 mV ± 5.61, which shows good stability. The particle size profile of DFS showed a wider particle size range than that of DFS-NS-2, which clearly indicates that the DFS-NS particle size is more uniformly distributed. DFS had a particle size of D [2–36] 2.46 μm, D [9] 6.71 μm, Dv (10) 1.12 μm, Dv (50) 3.90 μm, and Dv (90) 7.98 μm. DFS-NS-2 was selected for further formulation into DMNs, which will be referred to as DFS-NS-DMN in the upcoming text.

3.2. Characterization Using Differential Scanning Calorimetry, X-ray Diffraction and FTIR

The physical state of DFS before and after being manufactured into NS was determined by DSC. As shown in Figure 3B, the DSC thermogram of DFS exhibited a characteristic sharp endothermic peak at 260 °C, which corresponds to the melting point of DFS in the crystalline state. This characteristic peak was observed in the physical mixture but was absent in the lyophilized DF-NS, which shows its amorphous nature.

To verify the obtained DSC results and to reconfirm the crystalline state of the lyophilized DFS-NS, XRD analysis was carried out, and the peaks of DFS, PVA, and the physical mixture of DFS and DFS NS are presented in Figure 3C. The diffractogram of pure DFS displayed several sharp peaks at the diffraction angles (2θ) of 10.47°, 14.61°, 23.97° and 26.67°, indicating that DFS is present in a crystalline form. In contrast, there were no distinguished peaks in the XRD diffractograms of the NS form, indicating that the NS formulations present an amorphous structure. Overall, when taking both the DSC and XRD results into account, it can be concluded that the crystalline structure of DFS was largely amorphized following bead milling.

The FTIR spectra of DFS showed the presence of peaks at ~1750 cm^{-1} indicating the presence of the carboxylic acid group, along with the presence of a peak at ~1100 cm^{-1} confirming the presence of phenyl structure. The peak at ~3350 cm^{-1} prominently indicated a phenol hydroxyl group. Similar peaks were observed in DFS NS samples confirming the presence of DFS. However, DFS NS also showed the characteristic peaks of PVA ~2900 cm^{-1} and ~2850 cm^{-1} indicating the asymmetric and symmetric C-H stretching vibrations which could also be observed in the PVA sample. The FTIR spectra of DFS NS presented the prominent peaks of Both DFS and PVA; however, no peak shifting and generation of the new peak was observed, suggesting limited chemical and physical interaction between both chemicals. The FTIR spectra of the physical mix showed the presence of characteristic peaks of DFS and PVA; however, no major change in the peak was observed to indicate any chemical interaction between DFS and PVA.

SEM images were obtained for DFS, DFS-NS and DFS NS-loaded MN tips by SEM with a Quanta FEG 250 (FEI, Hillsboro, OR, USA). SEM images showed that DFS-NS-DM arrays were formed well structurally. The resulting needles measured 700 μm in height and displayed sharp tips.

3.3. Drug Content and In Vitro Release Study

The percentage recovery of the drug in DFS-NS was found to be 85% ± 6.5%, which suggested that some drug was lost while separating the nanosuspension from the milling beads. A dialysis membrane is widely used for the release study of various drugs, and a skin condition is critical for the true assessment of drug release, independent of saturation effects and dissolution media volume. The skin condition was maintained at three times the volume of dissolution media (PBS) compared to the solubility of DFS in PBS. The drug release kinetics of DFS-NS were conducted to assess whether nanosizing led to an increase in the dissolution rate. The dissolution profile of the pure drug dispersed in PVA (prepared using the same method as adopted for DFS-NS) exhibited a lower dissolution rate, as only 40.6% of the drug was solubilized/released into the media after 24 h, whereas the DFS-NS showed 99.89% release until 24 h, as shown in Figure 3E. This can be attributed to the reduction in particle size, which increases the specific surface, which, according to the Noyes–Whitney equation, leads to an increase in the dissolution rate [25]. Many other reports in the literature have shown similar results for poorly soluble drugs [44]. Moreover, the wettability and saturation solubility of the drug in the nanosuspension form are also increased [20,45,46].

3.4. Characterization of DFS-NS-DMN Arrays

An aqueous hydrogel of PVA and PVP was used in combination to prepare the DMN casting gel. PVA and PVP have been extensively employed for DMNs owing to their hydrophilicity, biocompatibility, and strength for durable fabrication. Additionally, densely packed DMNs are formed due to their adhesive property. PVA alone caused DMNs to bend because they were too soft, while too much PVP triggered the brittleness of needles. The correct combination of the two was found in 30% w/w PVA and 20% w/w PVP.

The aqueous blend was prepared by adding different concentrations of lyophilized DFS-NS to attain the highest achievable drug loading for the system while maintaining the strength of the DMN arrays. For the second layer, only PVP without drug was used, as previous studies have shown that drugs in the baseplate, as well as needles, result in poor mechanical strength. Moreover, it helps in the efficient use of the drug, as drugs in the baseplate seldom deposit inside the skin [47,48].

The formation of homogenous MN arrays with sharp tips was confirmed by viewing them under a microscope with a length of 700 μm. The morphology was further investigated using a digital microscopy and SEM imaging, as shown in Figure 4A–F, displaying uniform needle formation throughout the MN patch. The mean drug loading in the MN array was 1459.20 ± 15.44 μg drug in an entire MN array of 700 needles, which means 2.08 μg in each needle. The particle size and PDI were measured by dispersing in purified water each time before (248.95 nm ± 10.81) and after (291.13 nm ± 12.72) loading the DFS-NS into the DMN arrays.

3.5. Determination of Insertion Properties and Mechanical Strength of DFS-NS DMN

The insertion properties of the DMNs were also adequate, as the needles penetrated three layers of Parafilm M® with 100% penetration in the first layer, 85% in the second and 15% in the third layer, as revealed in Figure 4G. It has already been proven that penetration up to 330 μm is insufficient for effective deposition of drugs across the skin. The thickness of each layer of Parafilm M® was approximately 126 μm. There was no height reduction, and the needle length that was inserted was approximately 378 μm, which is equal to 56% of the total height of the MNs. Meanwhile, DFS-DMN penetrated up to two layers.

The reduction in size of the DFS-NS-DMNs was calculated to be 11.5%, as shown in Figures 4H and 5A,B. This value depicts excellent strength, as the needles were able to bear the 32 N force without exhibiting a loss in height of more than 11.5%. It has been established previously that 32 N equates to the mean force applied by human subjects to insert microneedles into their skin. The DFS-DMNs exhibited an 18% (Figures 4I and 5C,D) reduction in the height of needles after compression, which shows inadequate strength to be inserted into human skin. Therefore, DFS-DMNs will likely fail to deliver drugs intradermally because of the lack of sufficient mechanical strength required for penetration into the skin.

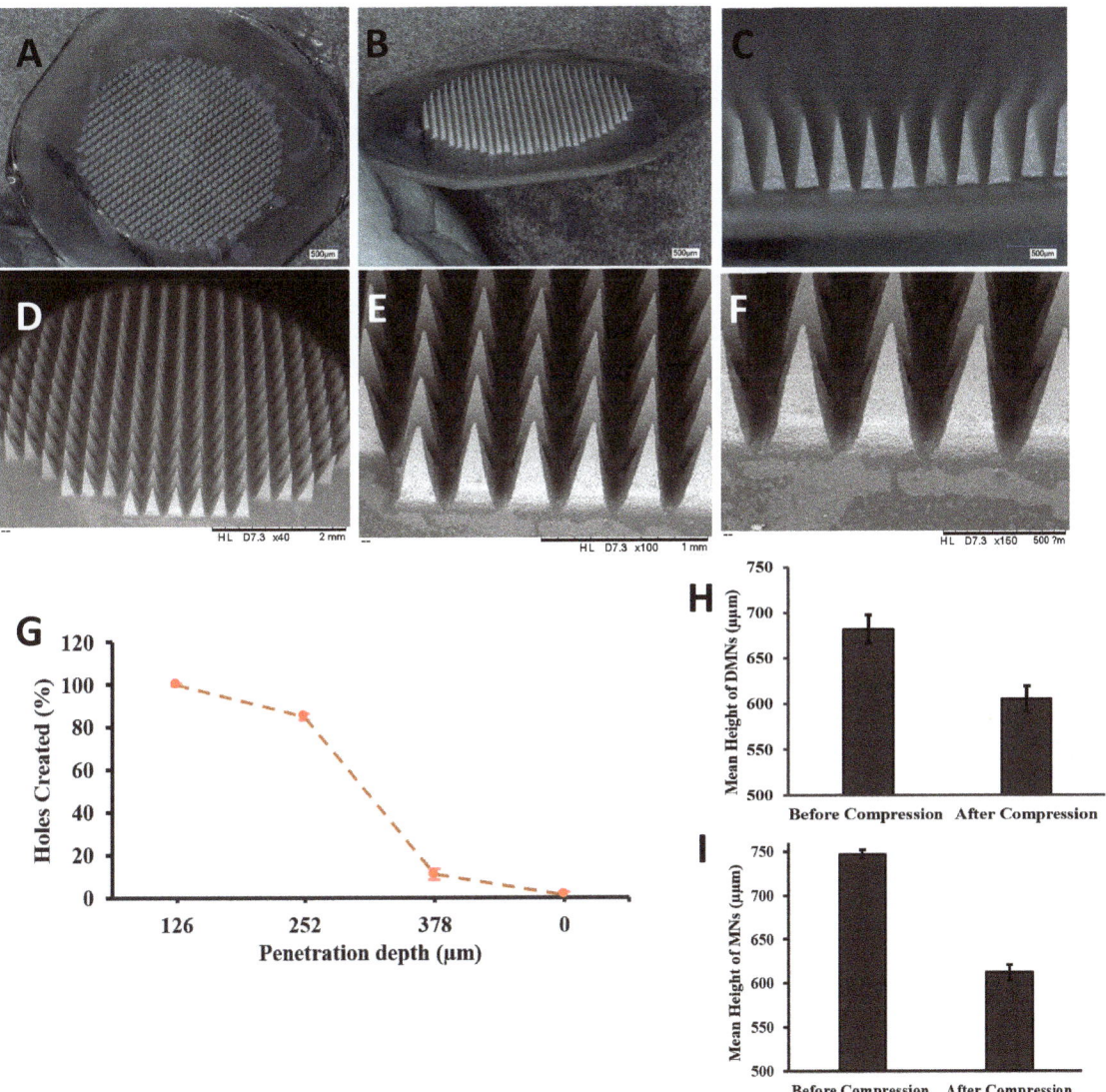

Figure 4. (A–C) Digital images of DFS-NS-DMNs at different magnifications. (D–F) SEM images of DFS-NS-DMNs. (G) The percentage of holes created in Parafilm M® layers and the corresponding approximate insertion depth. Mechanical strength determination of DMNs by a texture analyzer by applying a force of 32 N for 30 s (mean ± SD, n = 6). (H) Mean height reduction of DFS-NS-DMNs, (I) Mean height reduction of DFS-DMNs.

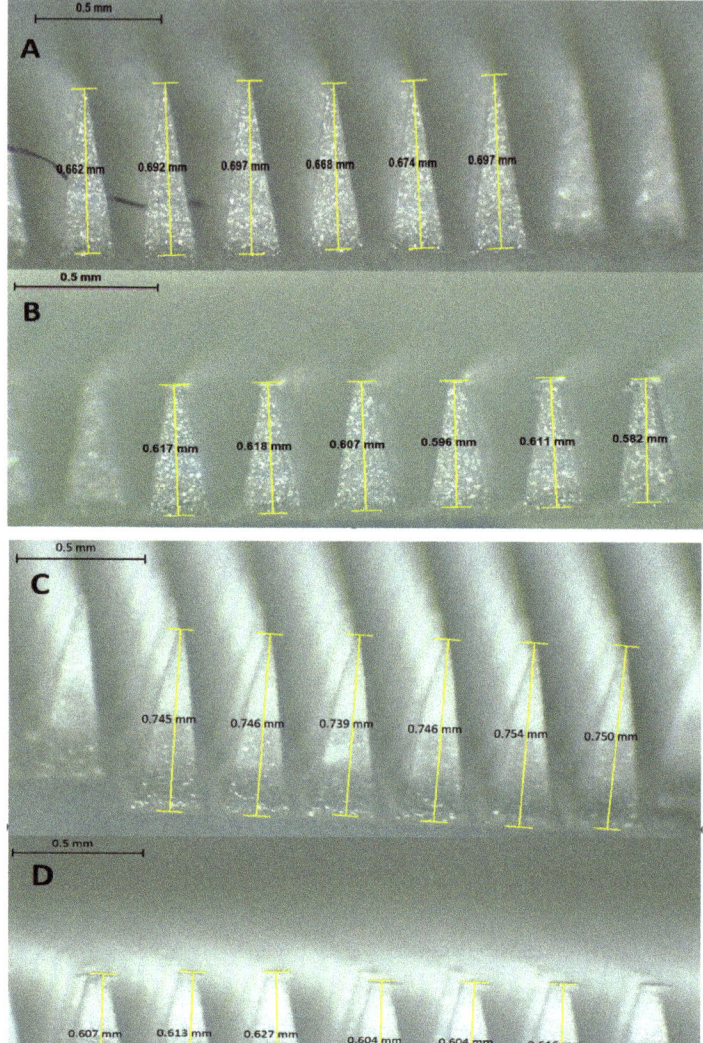

Figure 5. Mechanical strength determination of DMNs by a texture analyzer by applying a force of 32 N for 30 s (mean ± SD, $n = 6$). (**A**) Heights of DFS-NS-DMNs before compression; (**B**) Heights of DFS-NS-DMNs after compression; (**C**) Heights of DFS-DMNs before compression; (**D**) Heights of DFS-DMNs after compression.

3.6. Scanning Electron Microscopy

SEM images showed the acicular crystalline structure of pure DFS (Figure 6A) with quite large particle size (20 μm to 50 μm), while freeze-dried DFS-NS in Figure 6B depicted the spherical particle size with sizes ranging from approximately 200 nm. SEM image (Figure 6C) of broken single MN tip with exposed outer surface (upper half image) as well as internal cross-section (lower half image) showed a smooth surface and uniform distribution of DFS-NS in the PVA/PVP DMN matrix, respectively, without any evident particle aggregation.

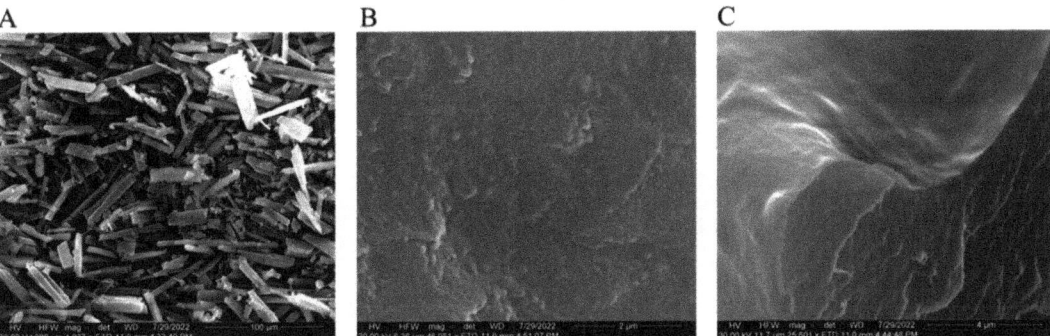

Figure 6. Scanning electron micrographs of (**A**) DFS crystals, (**B**) freeze-dried DFS-NS before DMN loading, and (**C**) magnified image of DFS-NS embedded into the DMN tips.

3.7. Dissolution of DFS-NS-DMN Arrays

Dissolution studies of the DFS-NS-DMN array were performed using porcine skin. The DMNs were applied for 60 min, and the dissolution time of DMNs was observed at different time intervals of 10, 15, 30 and 60 min. DMNs were completely dissolved within 30 min, as shown in Figure 7A–D, revealing that DMNs were fabricated properly. The rapid dissolution profile of these MAP formulations in intradermal fluid may be attributed to the hydrophilic nature of the needles with the easily dispersible nanosuspension form of DFS.

3.8. Determination of Skin Penetration

OCT images revealed how DFS-NS-MNs were inserted into the parafilm layers as well as excised porcine skin [49,50]. These arrays were capable of penetrating to a great extent through the layers of parafilm (Figure 7E,F) and porcine skin (Figure 7G,H). A significant length of microneedles can be seen inside the parafilm layers, and needles were inserted up to the 4th layer (378 μm), which reiterates what was observed previously in penetration studies. The holes created on porcine skin can be seen in Figure 7G. The skin is flexible in nature, so the pores seem to close up after a while, leaving a print of the inserted DMNs behind.

3.9. Deposition Study on Excised Porcine Skin

The deposition study indicates the amount of drug that is deposited inside the skin from the DFS-NS-DMNs. The mean drug content deposited inside the skin was 632.47 ± 16.5 μg, comparing approximately 60% of the total drug loaded in DMNs. Drug deposition from DFS-DMNs into skin was calculated as 345 ± 12.5 μg. This clearly indicates that a greater amount of drug was deposited into porcine skin from DFS-NS-DMNs. This can be due to a greater dissolution rate of DFS-NS into the interstitial fluid of porcine skin compared with pure DFS, as demonstrated earlier in release studies. This might also be due to higher drug loading into DMNs, since nanosuspensions of hydrophobic drug allow a more homogeneous loading along the entire length of polymeric microneedles compared to the pure hydrophobic drug [9]. Pure DFS has a particle size of D [9] 2.46 μm, D [9], 6.71 μm Dv (10), 1.12 μm, Dv (50) 3.90 μm and Dv (90) 7.98 μm, as measured by DLS, and the results are expressed in terms of the De Brouckere and Sauter mean diameters, which are much larger than the DFS-NS particle size (248 nm).

The amount of drug deposited from DFS-NS-TP (without needles) was 30.56 ± 3.56 μg, and the amount of drug deposited by the application of DFS-NS alone was only 10 ± 4.32 μg.

These values indicate that DMNs can deliver a significantly larger amount of drug as they can penetrate the stratum corneum, unlike DFS-NS-TP and DFS-NS, as shown in Figure 7I.

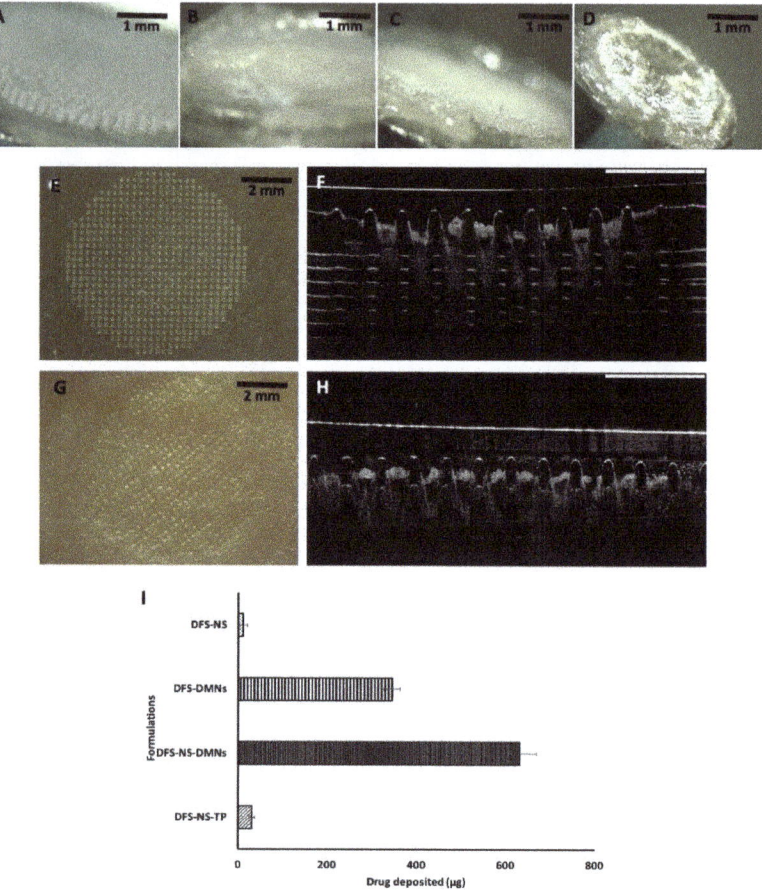

Figure 7. Dissolution study of DFS-NS-DMNs after insertion into excised porcine skin. Images taken after (**A**) 10 min of insertion, (**B**) 15 min of insertion, (**C**) 30 min of insertion, and (**D**) 60 min of insertion. Digital and OCT images of DFS-NS-DMNs; (**E,F**) DFS-NS-DMNS inserted in parafilm layers, (**G,H**) DFS-NS-DMNs inserted into excised porcine skin. (**I**) DFS deposited in excised porcine skin following the insertion of DFS-NS, DFS-DMNs, DFS-NS-DMNs, and DFS-NS-TP (without needles). Data are expressed as the mean ± SD, n = 3.

Therefore, the DMN facilitates higher DFS delivery across the skin. Additionally, the reduced particle size of DFS allows the homogeneous distribution of DFS into the DMN lower end of the tips, which also greatly influences drug deposition in the skin. This NS form of DFS also allows for increased surface area, greater dissolution rates and subsequently better absorption intradermally.

Nevertheless, the drug deposition study conducted in this research from full-thickness porcine skin did not depict the level of drug in each layer of the skin (SC, epidermis and dermis); therefore, it is difficult to predict the DFS gradient and availability of DFS for immediate systemic release or sustained effect of the DFS. However, based on previous work from our research group with similar type of hydrophobic drugs (cabotegravir, rilpivirine), DFS NS deposited intradermally with dissolution as well as skin rate-limiting factor for the sustained release [51–54] could allow the reduction of the frequency of DFS dose administration. However, to prove the sustained delivery effect, further in vivo research is needed.

In the current work, we successfully formulated dissolving MAPs loaded with an optimized NS of DFS. These formulations have been shown to display acceptable mechanical properties enabling effective skin penetration, as evidenced from the Parafilm® M and ex vivo skin insertion study. To develop an MN-based formulation for the management of iron toxicity, we prefer the dissolving MN approach relative to other types of MNs [49,55]. With a dissolving MAP approach, we can easily administer DFS in a single-step application process with a short wear time. This single MN application with delivered dose could be high enough for localized site-specific application. However, single MN would not be adequate for use in humans to deliver the enough systemic dose to get the therapeutic response; therefore, multiple MN within one larger patch need to be formulated and investigated in vivo to prove the usefulness of this delivery route in iron toxicity management [56].

4. Conclusions

An iron chelator DFS was incorporated for the first time in DMNs successfully in the form of a nanosuspension, exhibiting appropriate mechanical strength for effective skin insertion. Deposition studies revealed that DFS can be proficiently deposited into porcine skin for local and possible systemic delivery without the use of hypodermic needles and intervention of healthcare professionals, as well as evading side effects of the oral route. Moreover, DFS-NS showed a greater dissolution rate than pure DFS for probable subsequent uptake by the rich dermal microcirculation. Thus, the results support the claim that DFS-NS-DMNs can prove to be significant alternatives to conventional routes of delivery. This proof-of-concept study provides the basis for further investigation through in vivo studies to explore the therapeutic efficacy and expansion of this work by forming larger DMN patches for loading higher drug doses.

Author Contributions: H.S.F.: Investigation, Methodology, Formal analysis, Writing—original draft, Writing—review and editing; L.K.V.: Supervision, Investigation, Methodology, Formal analysis, Writing—review and editing; M.I.N.: Investigation, Methodology, Formal analysis; Y.W.: Investigation, Methodology, Formal analysis; D.M.: Supervision, Methodology; Q.K.A.: Methodology, analysis, Formal analysis, Writing—review and editing; A.J.P.: Supervision, Methodology; R.R.S.T.: Supervision, Methodology, Resources, Funding acquisition; M.U.M.: Supervision, Methodology; R.F.D.: Supervision, Methodology, Resources, Funding acquisition, Writing—review and editing. All authors have read and agreed to the published version of the manuscript.

Funding: The authors gratefully acknowledge the financial support from the Punjab Higher Education Commission (HEC) of Pakistan.

Institutional Review Board Statement: Not applicable.

Informed Consent Statement: Not applicable.

Data Availability Statement: Not applicable.

Acknowledgments: We are also thankful to the School of Pharmacy, Queen's University Belfast, Northern Ireland, United Kingdom, for their technical support and for providing research facilities. We also acknowledge the College of Pharmacy, University of Sargodha, Sargodha, Pakistan for their kind support and encouragement to complete this research work.

Conflicts of Interest: The authors declare no conflict of interest.

References

1. Luo, Z.; Sun, W.; Fang, J.; Lee, K.; Li, S.; Gu, Z.; Dokmeci, M.R.; Khademhosseini, A. Biodegradable Gelatin Methacryloyl Microneedles for Transdermal Drug Delivery. *Adv. Healthc. Mater.* **2019**, *8*, e1801054. [CrossRef] [PubMed]
2. Yadav, P.R.; Munni, M.N.; Campbell, L.; Mostofa, G.; Dobson, L.; Shittu, M.; Pattanayek, S.K.; Uddin, M.J.; Das, D.B. Translation of Polymeric Microneedles for Treatment of Human Diseases: Recent Trends, Progress, and Challenges. *Pharmaceutics* **2021**, *13*, 1132. [CrossRef] [PubMed]

3. Chen, Y.; Chen, B.Z.; Wang, Q.L.; Jin, X.; Guo, X.D. Fabrication of Coated Polymer Microneedles for Transdermal Drug Delivery. *J. Control. Release* **2017**, *265*, 14–21. [CrossRef] [PubMed]
4. Volpe-Zanutto, F.; Ferreira, L.T.; Permana, A.D.; Kirkby, M.; Paredes, A.J.; Vora, L.K.; Bonfanti, A.P.; Charlie-Silva, I.; Raposo, C.; Figueiredo, M.C.; et al. Artemether and Lumefantrine Dissolving Microneedle Patches with Improved Pharmacokinetic Performance and Antimalarial Efficacy in Mice Infected with Plasmodium Yoelii. *J. Control. Release* **2021**, *333*, 298–315. [CrossRef] [PubMed]
5. Vora, L.K.; Donnelly, R.F.; Larrañeta, E.; González-Vázquez, P.; Thakur, R.R.S.; Vavia, P.R. Novel Bilayer Dissolving Microneedle Arrays with Concentrated PLGA Nano-Microparticles for Targeted Intradermal Delivery: Proof of Concept. *J. Control. Release* **2017**, *265*, 93–101. [CrossRef]
6. Kulkarni, D.; Damiri, F.; Rojekar, S.; Zehravi, M.; Ramproshad, S.; Dhoke, D.; Musale, S.; Mulani, A.A.; Modak, P.; Paradhi, R.; et al. Recent Advancements in Microneedle Technology for Multifaceted Biomedical Applications. *Pharmaceutics* **2022**, *14*, 1097. [CrossRef]
7. Gowda, B.H.J.; Ahmed, M.G.; Sahebkar, A.; Riadi, Y.; Shukla, R.; Kesharwani, P. Stimuli-Responsive Microneedles as a Transdermal Drug Delivery System: A Demand-Supply Strategy. *Biomacromolecules* **2022**, *23*, 1519–1544. [CrossRef]
8. McAlister, E.; Kirkby, M.; Domínguez-Robles, J.; Paredes, A.J.; Anjani, Q.K.; Moffatt, K.; Vora, L.K.; Hutton, A.R.; McKenna, P.E.; Larrañeta, E. The Role of Microneedle Arrays in Drug Delivery and Patient Monitoring to Prevent Diabetes Induced Fibrosis. *Adv. Drug Deliv. Rev.* **2021**, *175*, 113825. [CrossRef]
9. Yadav, P.R.; Dobson, L.J.; Pattanayek, S.K.; Das, D.B. Swellable Microneedles Based Transdermal Drug Delivery: Mathematical Model Development and Numerical Experiments. *Chem. Eng. Sci.* **2022**, *247*, 117005. [CrossRef]
10. Vora, L.K.; Moffatt, K.; Donnelly, R.F. 9—Long-Lasting Drug Delivery Systems Based on Microneedles. In *Long-Acting Drug Delivery Systems*; Larrañeta, E., Raghu Raj Singh, T., Donnelly, R.F., Eds.; Woodhead Publishing: Cambridge, UK, 2022; pp. 249–287, ISBN 978-0-12-821749-8.
11. Galeotti, L.; Ceccherini, F.; Fucile, C.; Marini, V.; Di Paolo, A.; Maximova, N.; Mattioli, F. Evaluation of Pharmacokinetics and Pharmacodynamics of Deferasirox in Pediatric Patients. *Pharmaceutics* **2021**, *13*, 1238. [CrossRef]
12. Akdağ, Y.; Izat, N.; Öner, L.; ŞahiN, S.; Gülsün, T. Effect of Particle Size and Surfactant on the Solubility, Permeability and Dissolution Characteristics of Deferasirox. *JRP* **2019**, *23*, 851–859. [CrossRef]
13. Calabrese, C.; Panuzzo, C.; Stanga, S.; Andreani, G.; Ravera, S.; Maglione, A.; Pironi, L.; Petiti, J.; Shahzad Ali, M.; Scaravaglio, P.; et al. Deferasirox-Dependent Iron Chelation Enhances Mitochondrial Dysfunction and Restores P53 Signaling by Stabilization of P53 Family Members in Leukemic Cells. *Int. J. Mol. Sci.* **2020**, *21*, 7674. [CrossRef]
14. Saigo, K.; Kono, M.; Takagi, Y.; Takenokuchi, M.; Hiramatsu, Y.; Tada, H.; Hishita, T.; Misawa, M.; Imoto, S.; Imashuku, S. Deferasirox Reduces Oxidative Stress in Patients with Transfusion Dependency. *J. Clin. Med. Res.* **2013**, *5*, 57–60. [CrossRef]
15. Pandya, A.G.; Nezafati, K.A.; Ashe-Randolph, M.; Yalamanchili, R. Deferasirox for Porphyria Cutanea Tarda: A Pilot Study. *Arch. Dermatol.* **2012**, *148*, 898–901. [CrossRef]
16. Carter, A.; Racey, S.; Veuger, S. The Role of Iron in DNA and Genomic Instability in Cancer, a Target for Iron Chelators That Can Induce ROS. *Appl. Sci.* **2022**, *12*, 10161. [CrossRef]
17. Chen, C.; Wang, S.; Liu, P. Deferoxamine Enhanced Mitochondrial Iron Accumulation and Promoted Cell Migration in Triple-Negative MDA-MB-231 Breast Cancer Cells Via a ROS-Dependent Mechanism. *Int. J. Mol. Sci.* **2019**, *20*, 4952. [CrossRef]
18. Lui, G.Y.L.; Obeidy, P.; Ford, S.J.; Tselepis, C.; Sharp, D.M.; Jansson, P.J.; Kalinowski, D.S.; Kovacevic, Z.; Lovejoy, D.B.; Richardson, D.R. The Iron Chelator, Deferasirox, as a Novel Strategy for Cancer Treatment: Oral Activity against Human Lung Tumor Xenografts and Molecular Mechanism of Action. *Mol. Pharm.* **2013**, *83*, 179–190. [CrossRef]
19. Abdelghany, S.; Tekko, I.A.; Vora, L.; Larrañeta, E.; Permana, A.D.; Donnelly, R.F. Nanosuspension-Based Dissolving Microneedle Arrays for Intradermal Delivery of Curcumin. *Pharmaceutics* **2019**, *11*, 308. [CrossRef]
20. Vora, L.K.; Moffatt, K.; Tekko, I.A.; Paredes, A.J.; Volpe-Zanutto, F.; Mishra, D.; Peng, K.; Raj Singh Thakur, R.; Donnelly, R.F. Microneedle Array Systems for Long-Acting Drug Delivery. *Eur. J. Pharm. Biopharm.* **2021**, *159*, 44–76. [CrossRef]
21. Rojekar, S.; Vora, L.K.; Tekko, I.A.; Volpe-Zanutto, F.; McCarthy, H.O.; Vavia, P.R.; Donnelly, R.F. Etravirine-Loaded Dissolving Microneedle Arrays for Long-Acting Delivery. *Eur. J. Pharm. Biopharm.* **2021**, *165*, 41–51. [CrossRef]
22. Alkilani, A.Z.; Nasereddin, J.; Hamed, R.; Nimrawi, S.; Hussein, G.; Abo-Zour, H.; Donnelly, R.F. Beneath the Skin: A Review of Current Trends and Future Prospects of Transdermal Drug Delivery Systems. *Pharmaceutics* **2022**, *14*, 1152. [CrossRef] [PubMed]
23. Larrañeta, E.; Vora, L. Delivery of Nanomedicines Using Microneedles. Available online: https://onlinelibrary.wiley.com/doi/abs/10.1002/9781119305101.ch6 (accessed on 19 April 2022).
24. Altuntaş, E.; Tekko, I.A.; Vora, L.K.; Kumar, N.; Brodsky, R.; Chevallier, O.; McAlister, E.; Kurnia Anjani, Q.; McCarthy, H.O.; Donnelly, R.F. Nestorone Nanosuspension-Loaded Dissolving Microneedles Array Patch: A Promising Novel Approach for "on-Demand" Hormonal Female-Controlled Peritcoital Contraception. *Int. J. Pharm.* **2022**, *614*, 121422. [CrossRef] [PubMed]
25. Kalhapure, R.S.; Palekar, S.; Patel, K.; Monpara, J. Nanocrystals for Controlled Delivery: State of the Art and Approved Drug Products. *Expert Opin. Drug Deliv.* **2022**, *19*, 1303–1316. [CrossRef] [PubMed]
26. McGuckin, M.B.; Wang, J.; Ghanma, R.; Qin, N.; Palma, S.D.; Donnelly, R.F.; Paredes, A.J. Nanocrystals as a Master Key to Deliver Hydrophobic Drugs via Multiple Administration Routes. *J. Control. Release* **2022**, *345*, 334–353. [CrossRef] [PubMed]

27. Paredes, A.J.; McKenna, P.E.; Ramöller, I.K.; Naser, Y.A.; Volpe-Zanutto, F.; Li, M.; Abbate, M.T.A.; Zhao, L.; Zhang, C.; Abu-Ershaid, J.M.; et al. Microarray Patches: Poking a Hole in the Challenges Faced When Delivering Poorly Soluble Drugs. *Adv. Funct. Mater.* **2021**, *31*, 2005792. [CrossRef]
28. Wu, X.; Chen, Y.; Gui, S.; Wu, X.; Chen, L.; Cao, Y.; Yin, D.; Ma, P.; Wong, J.; Brugger, A.; et al. Nanosuspensions for the Formulation of Poorly Soluble Drugs. *Int. J. Pharm.* **2004**, *3*, 785–796. [CrossRef]
29. Wu, Y.; Vora, L.K.; Mishra, D.; Adrianto, M.F.; Gade, S.; Paredes, A.J.; Donnelly, R.F.; Singh, T.R.R. Nanosuspension-Loaded Dissolving Bilayer Microneedles for Hydrophobic Drug Delivery to the Posterior Segment of the Eye. *Biomater. Adv.* **2022**, *137*, 212767. [CrossRef]
30. Gigliobianco, M.R.; Casadidio, C.; Censi, R.; Di Martino, P. Nanocrystals of Poorly Soluble Drugs: Drug Bioavailability and Physicochemical Stability. *Pharmaceutics* **2018**, *10*, 134. [CrossRef]
31. Vora, L.K.; Vavia, P.R.; Larrañeta, E.; Bell, S.E.J.; Donnelly, R.F. Novel Nanosuspension-Based Dissolving Microneedle Arrays for Transdermal Delivery of a Hydrophobic Drug. *J. Interdiscip. Nanomed.* **2018**, *3*, 89–101. [CrossRef]
32. Jacob, S.; Nair, A.B.; Shah, J. Emerging Role of Nanosuspensions in Drug Delivery Systems. *Biomater. Res.* **2020**, *24*, 3. [CrossRef]
33. Permana, A.D.; Paredes, A.J.; Zanutto, F.V.; Amir, M.N.; Ismail, I.; Bahar, M.A.; Sumarheni; Palma, S.D.; Donnelly, R.F. Albendazole Nanocrystal-Based Dissolving Microneedles with Improved Pharmacokinetic Performance for Enhanced Treatment of Cystic Echinococcosis. *ACS Appl. Mater. Interfaces* **2021**, *13*, 38745–38760. [CrossRef]
34. Paredes, A.J.; Volpe-Zanutto, F.; Permana, A.D.; Murphy, A.J.; Picco, C.J.; Vora, L.K.; Coulter, J.A.; Donnelly, R.F. Novel Tip-Loaded Dissolving and Implantable Microneedle Array Patches for Sustained Release of Finasteride. *Int. J. Pharm.* **2021**, *606*, 120885. [CrossRef]
35. Tekko, I.A.; Vora, L.K.; Volpe-Zanutto, F.; Moffatt, K.; Jarrahian, C.; McCarthy, H.O.; Donnelly, R.F. Novel Bilayer Microarray Patch-Assisted Long-Acting Micro-Depot Cabotegravir Intradermal Delivery for HIV Pre-Exposure Prophylaxis. *Adv. Funct. Mater.* **2022**, *32*, 2106999. [CrossRef]
36. Cárcamo-Martínez, Á.; Mallon, B.; Anjani, Q.K.; Domínguez-Robles, J.; Utomo, E.; Vora, L.K.; Tekko, I.A.; Larrañeta, E.; Donnelly, R.F. Enhancing Intradermal Delivery of Tofacitinib Citrate: Comparison between Powder-Loaded Hollow Microneedle Arrays and Dissolving Microneedle Arrays. *Int. J. Pharm.* **2021**, *593*, 120152. [CrossRef]
37. Saravanan, S.; Swetha, R. Method Development and Validation for Determination of Impurities in Deferasirox by RP-HPLC Technique. *J. Drug Deliv. Ther.* **2012**, *2*, 148–152. [CrossRef]
38. Cilurzo, F.; Minghetti, P.; Sinico, C. Newborn Pig Skin as Model Membrane in In Vitro Drug Permeation Studies: A Technical Note. *AAPS PharmSciTech* **2007**, *8*, 2–5. [CrossRef]
39. Li, M.; Vora, L.K.; Peng, K.; Donnelly, R.F. Trilayer Microneedle Array Assisted Transdermal and Intradermal Delivery of Dexamethasone. *Int. J. Pharm.* **2022**, *612*, 121295. [CrossRef]
40. Pireddu, R.; Schlich, M.; Marceddu, S.; Valenti, D.; Pini, E.; Fadda, A.M.; Lai, F.; Sinico, C. Nanosuspensions and Microneedles Roller as a Combined Approach to Enhance Diclofenac Topical Bioavailability. *Pharmaceutics* **2020**, *12*, 1140. [CrossRef]
41. Rachmawati, H.; Rahma, A.; Al Shaal, L.; Müller, R.H.; Keck, C.M. Destabilization Mechanism of Ionic Surfactant on Curcumin Nanocrystal against Electrolytes. *Sci. Pharm.* **2016**, *84*, 685–693. [CrossRef]
42. Powar, T.A.; Hajare, A.A. Lyophilized Ethinylestradiol Nanosuspension: Fabrication, Characterization and Evaluation of in Vitro Anticancer and Pharmacokinetic Study. *Indian J. Pharm. Sci.* **2020**, *82*, 54–59. [CrossRef]
43. Kakran, M.; Shegokar, R.; Sahoo, N.G.; Al Shaal, L.; Li, L.; Müller, R.H. Fabrication of Quercetin Nanocrystals: Comparison of Different Methods. *Eur. J. Pharm. Biopharm.* **2012**, *80*, 113–121. [CrossRef] [PubMed]
44. Mokale, V. Glyburide Nanosuspension: Influence of Processing and Formulation Parameter on Solubility and in Vitro Dissolution Behavior. *Asian J. Pharm.* **2013**, *7*, 111–117. [CrossRef]
45. Jarvis, M.; Krishnan, V.; Mitragotri, S. Nanocrystals: A Perspective on Translational Research and Clinical Studies. *Bioeng. Transl. Med.* **2019**, *4*, 5–16. [CrossRef] [PubMed]
46. Agrawal, Y.; Patel, V. Nanosuspension: An Approach to Enhance Solubility of Drugs. *J. Adv. Pharm. Technol. Res.* **2011**, *2*, 81. [CrossRef] [PubMed]
47. Rein-Weston, A.; Tekko, I.; Vora, L.; Jarrahian, C.; Spreen, B.; Scott, T.; Donnelly, R.; Zehrung, D. LB8. Microarray Patch Delivery of Long-Acting HIV PrEP and Contraception. *Open Forum Infect. Dis.* **2019**, *6*, S996. [CrossRef]
48. Demartis, S.; Anjani, Q.K.; Volpe-Zanutto, F.; Paredes, A.J.; Jahan, S.A.; Vora, L.K.; Donnelly, R.F.; Gavini, E. Trilayer Dissolving Polymeric Microneedle Array Loading Rose Bengal Transfersomes as a Novel Adjuvant in Early-Stage Cutaneous Melanoma Management. *Int. J. Pharm.* **2022**, *627*, 122217. [CrossRef]
49. Vora, L.K.; Courtenay, A.J.; Tekko, I.A.; Larrañeta, E.; Donnelly, R.F. Pullulan-Based Dissolving Microneedle Arrays for Enhanced Transdermal Delivery of Small and Large Biomolecules. *Int. J. Biol. Macromol.* **2020**, *146*, 290–298. [CrossRef]
50. Peng, K.; Vora, L.K.; Domínguez-Robles, J.; Naser, Y.A.; Li, M.; Larrañeta, E.; Donnelly, R.F. Hydrogel-Forming Microneedles for Rapid and Efficient Skin Deposition of Controlled Release Tip-Implants. *Mater. Sci. Eng. C* **2021**, *127*, 112226. [CrossRef]
51. Tekko, I.; Vora, L.; McCrudden, M.; Jarrahian, C.; Rein-Weston, A.; Zehrung, D.; Giffen, P.; McCarthy, H.; Donnelly, R. Novel Dissolving Bilayer Microarray Patches as a Minimally Invasive, Efficient Intradermal Delivery System for a Long-Acting Cabotegravir Nanosuspension. In Proceedings of the 2019 Controlled Release Society Annual Meeting & Exposition, Valencia, Spain, 21–24 July 2019.

52. Paredes, A.J.; Permana, A.D.; Volpe-Zanutto, F.; Amir, M.N.; Vora, L.K.; Tekko, I.A.; Akhavein, N.; Weber, A.D.; Larrañeta, E.; Donnelly, R.F. Ring Inserts as a Useful Strategy to Prepare Tip-Loaded Microneedles for Long-Acting Drug Delivery with Application in HIV Pre-Exposure Prophylaxis. *Mater. Des.* **2022**, *224*, 111416. [CrossRef]
53. Volpe-Zanutto, F.; Vora, L.K.; Tekko, I.A.; McKenna, P.E.; Permana, A.D.; Sabri, A.H.; Anjani, Q.K.; McCarthy, H.O.; Paredes, A.J.; Donnelly, R.F. Hydrogel-Forming Microarray Patches with Cyclodextrin Drug Reservoirs for Long-Acting Delivery of Poorly Soluble Cabotegravir Sodium for HIV Pre-Exposure Prophylaxis. *J. Control. Release* **2022**, *348*, 771–785. [CrossRef]
54. Moffatt, K.; Tekko, I.A.; Vora, L.; Volpe-Zanutto, F.; Hutton, A.R.J.; Mistilis, J.; Jarrahian, C.; Akhavein, N.; Weber, A.D.; McCarthy, H.O.; et al. Development and Evaluation of Dissolving Microarray Patches for Co-Administered and Repeated Intradermal Delivery of Long-Acting Rilpivirine and Cabotegravir Nanosuspensions for Paediatric HIV Antiretroviral Therapy. *Pharm. Res.* **2022**. [CrossRef]
55. Ita, K. Dissolving Microneedles for Transdermal Drug Delivery: Advances and Challenges. *Biomed. Pharmacother.* **2017**, *93*, 1116–1127. [CrossRef]
56. Ripolin, A.; Quinn, J.; Larrañeta, E.; Vicente-Perez, E.M.; Barry, J.; Donnelly, R.F. Successful Application of Large Microneedle Patches by Human Volunteers. *Int. J. Pharm.* **2017**, *521*, 92–101. [CrossRef]

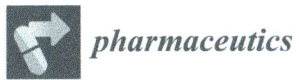

Article

Formulated Phospholipids as Non-Canonical TLR4 Agonists

Hong Liang [1], William R. Lykins [1], Emilie Seydoux [1], Jeffrey A. Guderian [1], Tony Phan [1], Christopher B. Fox [1,2,*] and Mark T. Orr [1,2]

[1] Access to Advanced Health Institute (AAHI), 1616 Eastlake Ave E, Suite 400, Seattle, WA 98102, USA
[2] Department of Global Health, University of Washington, 3980 15th Ave NE, Seattle, WA 98195, USA
* Correspondence: christopher.fox@aahi.org; Tel.: +1-206-858-6027

Abstract: Immunogenic agents known as adjuvants play a critical role in many vaccine formulations. Adjuvants often signal through Toll-like receptor (TLR) pathways, including formulations in licensed vaccines that target TLR4. While TLR4 is predominantly known for responding to lipopolysaccharide (LPS), a component of Gram-negative bacterial membranes, it has been shown to be a receptor for a number of molecular structures, including phospholipids. Therefore, phospholipid-based pharmaceutical formulations might have off-target effects by signaling through TLR4, confounding interpretation of pharmaceutical bioactivity. In this study we examined the individual components of a clinical stage oil-in-water vaccine adjuvant emulsion (referred to as a stable emulsion or SE) and their ability to signal through murine and human TLR4s. We found that the phospholipid 1,2-dimyristoyl-sn-glycero-3-phosphocholine (DMPC) activated TLR4 and elicited many of the same immune phenotypes as canonical TLR4 agonists. This pathway was dependent on the saturation, size, and headgroup of the phospholipid. Interestingly, DMPC effects on human cells were evident but overall appeared less impactful than emulsion oil composition. Considering the prevalence of DMPC and other phospholipids used across the pharmaceutical space, these findings may contextualize off-target innate immune responses that could impact preclinical and clinical development.

Keywords: oil-in-water emulsions; phospholipids; adjuvants; Toll-like receptor agonists

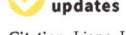

Citation: Liang, H.; Lykins, W.R.; Seydoux, E.; Guderian, J.A.; Phan, T.; Fox, C.B.; Orr, M.T. Formulated Phospholipids as Non-Canonical TLR4 Agonists. *Pharmaceutics* **2022**, *14*, 2557. https://doi.org/10.3390/pharmaceutics14122557

Academic Editors: Vibhuti Agrahari and Prashant Kumar

Received: 28 October 2022
Accepted: 21 November 2022
Published: 22 November 2022

Publisher's Note: MDPI stays neutral with regard to jurisdictional claims in published maps and institutional affiliations.

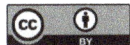

Copyright: © 2022 by the authors. Licensee MDPI, Basel, Switzerland. This article is an open access article distributed under the terms and conditions of the Creative Commons Attribution (CC BY) license (https://creativecommons.org/licenses/by/4.0/).

1. Introduction

Adjuvanted protein vaccines represent a large and growing fraction of the vaccine marketplace, including but not limited to approved products from Dynavax (the Heplisav-B vaccine against hepatitis B) and GSK (the Shingrix vaccine against shingles) and products in clinical development against severe acute respiratory syndrome coronavirus 2 (SARS-CoV-2) from Novavax and Sanofi-GSK among others [1–3]. The immunogenicity of adjuvanted protein vaccines depends on molecular agents known as adjuvants, which stimulate the innate immune system to program a more effective adaptive immune response to the delivered protein antigen [4]. Three broad classes of adjuvants are currently used with licensed human vaccines: aluminum-containing adjuvants (e.g., Alhydrogel and AS04), oil-in-water emulsions (e.g., MF59 and AS03), and Toll-like receptor (TLR) agonists (e.g., AS01b and CpG-1018), often formulated with aluminum or lipid-based particles [5]. Aluminum and emulsion adjuvants primarily augment antibody responses to vaccine antigens by elongating germinal center exposure, whereas the combination adjuvants with TLR agonists also promote CD4[+] T cell responses [5,6]. In the context of SARS-CoV-2, TLR-agonist adjuvanted peptide vaccines that can elicit both CD4[+] and CD8[+] T cell responses were found to be effective against a wide range of emerging variants [7].

TLRs are pattern recognition receptors (PRRs) capable of recognizing specific pathogen-associated molecular patterns (PAMPs) conserved among micro-organisms and stimulate inflammatory signaling cascades. Since the discovery of TLR pathways in the 1990s and the identification of lipopolysaccharide (LPS) as the canonical agonist of the TLR4 pathway, numerous studies have identified alternative agonists and antagonists [8–13]. These alternate signaling molecules can be small molecules, LPS mimics, or a range of other structures. Additionally, compounds have been identified that act on up- or downstream components of the TLR4 signaling pathway, which are often derived from metabolic byproducts but can also be exogenously derived [13]. This has led to a library of hundreds to potentially thousands of molecular agents with known activity in the TLR4 pathway. Substantial progress has been made in the last several years in defining the mechanisms of action for many of these compounds. This knowledge has enabled rational development of next-generation adjuvants and more informative clinical evaluation of new adjuvanted vaccines [14]. Among their potential mechanisms of action, adjuvants can act on antigen-presenting cells (APCs) through inflammasome and/or TLR-mediated pathways. Inflammasome activation via TLR4 requires two signals: First, signal 1 engages TLR4 through the adaptor proteins myeloid differentiation factor 2 (MD-2), LPS-binding protein, and CD14 to activate nuclear factor-κB (NF-κB) to produce nucleotide-binding domain-like receptor protein 3 (NLRP3) and pro-interleukin-1β (pro-IL-1β). Next, signal 2 stimulates NLRP3, pro-caspase-1, and the adaptor protein apoptosis-associated speck-like protein containing a caspase activation and recruitment domain (ASC) assembly, which subsequently cleaves the pro-caspase into its active form caspase-1, which then cleaves pro-IL-1β and pro-IL-18 (constitutively expressed) into active, secretory forms [15,16].

Glucopyranosyl lipid adjuvant (GLA) is a synthetic TLR4 agonist that, when formulated with a phospholipid-stabilized squalene-in-water stable emulsion (SE), forms a safe and effective vaccine adjuvant, which has advanced to Phase 2 clinical testing [17,18]. The combination adjuvant GLA-SE promotes strong TH1 cellular and balanced IgG1/IgG2 antibody responses to a variety of vaccine antigens in animal models and human clinical studies and provides protective immunity against infections such as tuberculosis and leishmaniasis [15,19]. The adjuvanticity of GLA is critically dependent on its formulation in SE [20]. We have found that GLA-SE mediates TH1 induction via myeloid differentiation factor 88 (MyD88) and Toll/IL-1 receptor domain-containing adaptor protein inducing interferon-β (TRIF) signaling and produces IL-18 in draining lymph nodes, suggesting the inflammasome is involved [21,22]. We have further demonstrated that SE induces APC recruitment in the draining lymph nodes, which drives the development of adaptive immunity. The adjuvanticity of SE was substantially impaired in $ASC^{-/-}$ or $NLPR3^{-/-}$ mice, suggesting that SE functions in an inflammasome-dependent manner [15]. These findings further support a two-step mechanism of action for the combination GLA-SE adjuvant to activate the inflammasome in which (1) GLA, signaling via TLR4, increases expression of the inflammasome components NLRP3 and ASC and the inflammasome substrates pro-IL-1β and pro-IL-18, and (2) SE activates the NLRP3-dependent inflammasome to activate caspase-1 to process the proenzymes into their secreted active forms.

Despite progress, the specific mechanisms by which oil-in-water emulsions engage with the innate immune system are still not completely understood. Recently, fatty acids and oxidized phospholipids that result from cellular damage have been shown to engage with TLR4-dependent pathways in animal models in a pro- or anti-inflammatory manner [12,23–25]. These damage-associated molecular patterns (DAMPs) often result from the partial oxidation of unsaturated fatty acids such as 1-palmitoyl-2-arachidonoyl-phosphatidylcholine (PAPC), leading to a heterogeneous pool of products (i.e., oxidized PAPC [oxPAPC]) [26]. oxPAPC in particular has been shown to block LPS activity in murine models of septic shock by competitively inhibiting LPS binding to CD14 and preventing downstream signaling [23,27]. Further, pre-treatment with oxPAPC can even reduce mouse survival against peritoneal *Escherichia coli* challenge [28]. However, oxPAPC can also induce a prolonged hyper-inflammatory state when dosed after LPS [25]. Additionally, several recent reports have suggested that phosphatidylcholine (PC) molecules may interact with TLR4 [23–25].

Other phospholipids, such as those present in adjuvant emulsions like SE, may also engage with the TLR4 pathway. SE consists of a squalene-in-water emulsion stabilized by non-ionic surfactants and emulsifiers, including poloxamer 188 and the phospholipid 1,2-dimyristoyl-sn-glycero-3-phosphocholine (DMPC), and has been evaluated in a number of clinical-stage vaccine models [29–31]. In this report, we show that DMPC present in SE can stimulate the TLR4 pathway. We demonstrate that DMPC is necessary and sufficient to recapitulate the TLR4 pathway-stimulating effect of SE, and can stimulate the production of antigen-specific antibodies in a TLR4-dependent manner. Additionally, we observed that phospholipid-stimulated IL-1β production in murine bone marrow-derived dendritic cells (BMDCs) was sensitive to the chemical composition of both the phospholipid tail and headgroups. The results of our study may be relevant to the development of phospholipid-containing delivery systems and their characterization in preclinical and clinical models.

2. Materials and Methods
2.1. Reagents

SE (5X concentrate consisting of 10% v/v squalene, 1.9% w/v DMPC, 0.09% w/v poloxamer 188, 1.8% v/v glycerol, and 25 mM ammonium phosphate buffer) was made in-house by high-pressure homogenization as previously described [20]. Grapeseed SE (2X concentrate consisting of 4% v/v grapeseed oil, 0.76% w/v DMPC, 0.036% w/v poloxamer 188, 1.8% v/v glycerol, and 25 mM ammonium phosphate buffer) was prepared by the same high-pressure homogenization method as above. MF59-like emulsion (2X concentrate consisting of 4% v/v squalene, 0.4% w/v sorbitan trioleate, 0.4% w/v polysorbate 80, and 10 mM citrate buffer) was manufactured by high-pressure homogenization as described previously for AAHI's MF59-like EM022 composition [32]. Liposomes containing one of the following PCs were formulated at 1.9% (w/v) in deionized water: 1-palmitoyl-2-oleoyl-sn-glycero-3-phosphocholine (POPC); 1,2-dioleoyl-sn-glycero-3-phosphocholine (DOPC); 1,2-distearoyl-sn-glycero-3-phosphocholine (DSPC); 1,2-dipalmitoyl-sn-glycero-3-phosphocholine (DPPC); DMPC; 1,2-dilauroyl-sn-glycero-3-phosphocholine (DLPC); and 1,2-dimyristoyl-sn-glycero-3-phospho-(1′-rac-glycerol) (DMPG) were obtained from Lipoid (Newark, NJ, USA) or Avanti Polar Lipids (Alabaster, AL, USA). 1,2-dimyristoyl-sn-glycero-3-phosphoethanolamine (DMPE) and 1,2-dimyristoyl-sn-glycero-3-phospho-L-serine (DMPS) were obtained from Sigma Aldrich (St. Louis, MO, USA). The liposome mixture was then bath-sonicated at 65 °C for 20–60 min followed by 0.2-µm filtration. Particle size was determined by diluting an aliquot of each formulation 1:100-fold in deionized water and measuring the scattering intensity-based size average (Z-avg) by dynamic light scattering with a Zetasizer APS (Malvern Panalytical, Malvern, UK). Particle size and polydispersity index for materials used in this study can be found in Supplementary Tables S1 and S2. GLA-AF (5X concentrate consisting of 0.25 mg/mL GLA and 0.21 mg/mL DPPC) was manufactured in-house by sonication as previously described [20]. Ultrapure LPS (*E. coli* 0111:B4), FSL-1, and polymyxin B were obtained from InvivoGen (San Diego, CA, USA). Adenosine 5′-triphosphate (ATP) was purchased from Thermo Fisher Scientific (Waltham, MA, USA).

2.2. Animal Ethics

Female C57BL/6 wild-type (WT), TLR2$^{-/-}$, TLR4$^{-/-}$, MyD88$^{-/-}$, and NLRP3$^{-/-}$ mice aged 6–10 weeks were purchased from The Jackson Laboratory (Harbor, ME, USA). All strains were maintained in specific-pathogen-free (SPF) conditions. All animal experiments and protocols used in this study were approved by the Infectious Disease Research Institute, now AAHI, Institutional Animal Care and Use Committee (IACUC) and the Office of Laboratory Animal Welfare Assurance (Assurance ID A4337-01) effective 25 February 2015, to 28 February 2019.

2.3. Bone Marrow-Derived Dendritic Cell Prime and Stimulation In Vitro

BMDCs derived from WT or TLR2$^{-/-}$, TLR4$^{-/-}$, MyD88$^{-/-}$, or NLRP3$^{-/-}$ mice were cultured following the protocol developed by Lutz et al. [33]. Briefly, BMDCs were derived from bone marrow and allowed to differentiate in IMDM (Iscove's Modified

Dulbecco's Medium) containing 10% fetal bovine serum (FBS), 1% L-glutamine, 1% penicillin/streptomycin, and 20 ng/mL granulocyte-macrophage colony-stimulating factor (GM-CSF). Non-adherent cells were collected between Day 8 and Day 10 for stimulation. Collected cells were centrifuged and resuspended in OptiPRO SFM (Thermo Fisher Scientific). 125,000 cells in 125 µL were plated per well in a 48-well plate. Cells were primed by treatment with LPS (10 µg/mL) or media for 2 h then re-centrifuged prior to treatment as indicated below immediately after plating and incubated at 37 °C with 5% CO_2 for 5 h: SE or MF59-like emulsion with squalene or grapeseed oil at 0.5% oil (v/v), phospholipid and liposomes at 0.095% (w/v), LPS (TLR4 agonist) at 10 µg/mL, and FSL-1 (TLR2/6 agonist) at 100 ng/mL. Following treatment, cells were centrifuged and supernatant was collected and stored at −20 °C until analysis. To recover cell lysates, 125 µL of 1X radioimmunoprecipitation assay (RIPA) buffer with protease inhibitors (Roche, Basel, Switzerland) was added per well and allowed to incubate as per the manufacturer's instructions prior to the collection of lysates. Potential LPS contamination was assessed by pre-treating LPS, SE, and DMPC liposomes with 50 µg/mL polymyxin B for 5 h before addition to BMDC cultures as described above.

2.4. Cytokine Enzyme-Linked Immunosorbent Assays (ELISAs)

To enable qualitative comparison between cytoplasmic (pro-IL-1β) and secreted IL-1β, we chose to use ELISA as opposed to a more direct cellular method, such as intracellular cytokine staining. Supernatants and lysates from primary BMDC assays were assessed for production of IL-1β (supernatant), pro-IL-1β (lysate), IL-18 (lysate), tumor necrosis factor alpha (TNFα, lysate), and IL-12p40 (lysate) via ELISA (Thermo Fisher Scientific) according to the manufacturer's instructions. Cytokine quantification was performed via a standard curve using GraphPad Prism v9 software (San Diego, CA, USA).

2.5. Reporter Cell Assays

HEK-Blue mTLR4, hTLR4, and mTLR7 reporter cells were obtained from InvivoGen (San Diego, CA, USA). For these cells, a secreted embryonic alkaline phosphatase (SEAP) reporter gene is placed under the control of an interferon (IFN)-β minimal promoter fused to five NF-κB and AP-1 binding sites. Stimulation with a TLR4 agonist activates NF-κB and AP-1, which induce the production of SEAP. The production of SEAP induced by NF-κB and AP-1 activation, which is triggered by TLR4 or TLR7 stimulation, is measured at an optical density (OD) of 650 after 6 h following the protocol provided by the manufacturer (InvivoGen). Cells were cultured at 25,000 cells/well and treated with either DMPC (150 µg/mL), GLA-AF (50 µg/mL), 3M-052-AF (1 µg/mL), or media, and incubated at 37 °C for 40 h (hTLR4 and mTLR4) or 44 h (mTLR7). Each stimulation condition was performed in triplicate.

2.6. Human Whole Blood Immunogenicity Assay

SE and MF59-like emulsions comprising squalene or grapeseed oil were evaluated for innate immunostimulatory activity on whole blood from 6 healthy human subjects (3 male and 3 female). The emulsions were incubated directly with heparinized whole blood at 0.4% (v/v) oil for 18–24 h at 37 °C, and production of monocyte chemoattractant protein-1 (MCP-1), IL-8, and macrophage inflammatory protein-1β (MIP-1β) cytokines in supernatants was quantified as described previously [34].

2.7. Mice and Immunizations

Female WT and TLR4$^{-/-}$ mice were immunized via an intramuscular injection in the quadriceps muscles of hind limbs (50 µL per leg) with formulations containing 2.5 µg of recombinant ID97 tuberculosis antigen formulated with a squalene-based MF59-like emulsion or SE both at 2% oil by volume [35]. Blood was collected via terminal cardiac bleeding on Day 21, and serum was isolated prior to storage and analysis.

2.8. Serum Endpoint Titer ELISA

Serum titers against ID97 antigen were evaluated by antibody-capture ELISA. Briefly, Corning high-binding 384-well plates (VWR International, Radnor, PA, USA) were coated overnight at 4 °C with 2 µg/mL ID97 in coating buffer (eBioscience, San Diego, CA, USA), then washed in phosphate-buffered saline (PBS)-Tween 20. Serially diluted serum samples were incubated for 1 h followed by either anti-mouse IgG (H + L)-HRP, IgG1-HRP, or IgG2c-HRP (SouthernBiotech, Birmingham, AL, USA); and 3,3′,5,5′-tetramethylbenzidine (TMB) substrate was applied as per the manufacturer's instructions. Plates were analyzed at 450 nm using an ELx808 Absorbance Reader (Bio-Tek Instruments, Winooski, VT, USA), and endpoints were set as the minimum dilution at which values were lesser than or equal to an OD of 0.5.

2.9. Statistical Analysis

Data were analyzed using GraphPad Prism by one-way ANOVA (with corrections for multiple comparisons applied as indicated in figure captions). Values were considered significantly different with $p < 0.05$ (*), $p < 0.01$ (**), $p < 0.001$ (***), and $p < 0.0001$ (****).

3. Results

3.1. SE Does Not Induce Mature IL-1β Secretion through the Inflammasome

To determine whether SE activates the inflammasome, we treated media or LPS-primed murine BMDCs with SE or the known inflammasome activator ATP [36]. LPS prime and ATP treatment resulted in secretion of mature IL-1β into the supernatant, whereas SE treatment did not cause extracellular IL-1β accumulation (Figure 1A). To our surprise, treatment of naïve, i.e., not LPS-primed, BMDCs with SE caused an accumulation of intracellular pro-IL-1β, similar to LPS priming. The accumulation of pro-IL-1β in the lysate was significantly greater in SE-treated cells compared to untreated or ATP-treated cells. This suggests that SE, or one of its components, can activate signal 1, but not signal 2, of the inflammasome pathway, similar to LPS.

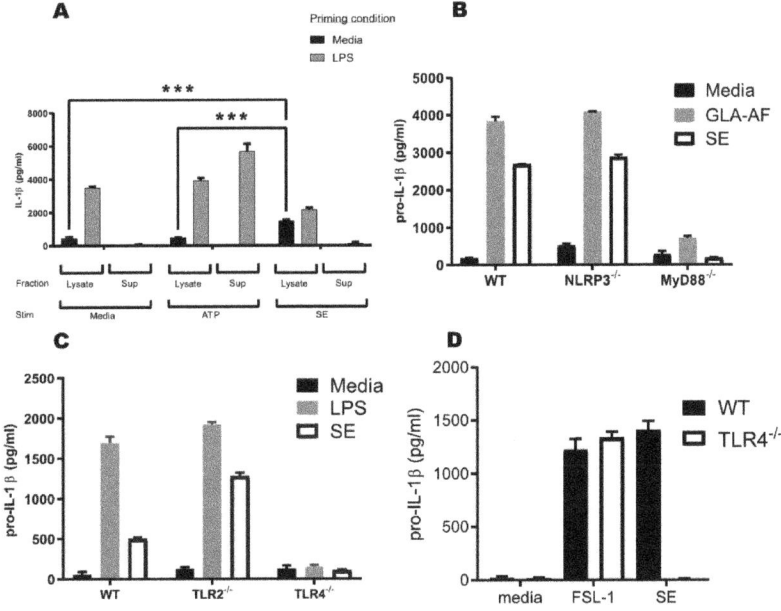

Figure 1. Stable emulsion (SE) elicits pro-IL-1β production in bone marrow-derived dendritic cells (BMDCs) via a TLR4-dependent process. (**A**) SE stimulates signal 1 of the TLR4 inflammasome pathway

in the absence of lipopolysaccharide (LPS). BMDCs from wild-type (WT) mice were primed with media or LPS (10 µg/mL) for 2 h and then stimulated with media, 5 mM ATP, or 0.5% SE. Supernatant (sup) and lysate were collected and assayed for IL-1β or pro-IL-1β, respectively, by enzyme-linked immunosorbent assay (ELISA). (**B**) SE stimulates pro-IL-1β production in a MyD88-dependent process. BMDCs were derived from WT, NLRP3$^{-/-}$, or MyD88$^{-/-}$ mice and stimulated with media, glucopyranosyl lipid adjuvant-aqueous formulation (GLA-AF) (4 µg/mL), or SE for 5 h. Cells were lysed and assayed for pro-IL-1β by ELISA. (**C**) SE stimulates IL-1β production in a TLR4-dependent process. BMDCs were derived from WT, TLR2$^{-/-}$, or TLR4$^{-/-}$ mice and stimulated with media, LPS, or SE for 5 h. Cells were lysed and assayed for pro-IL-1β by ELISA. (**D**) TLR4$^{-/-}$ mice are not generally immune deficient. BMDCs were derived from WT or TLR4$^{-/-}$ mice and stimulated with media, FSL-1 (100 µg/mL), or SE. Cells were lysed and assayed for pro-IL-1β by ELISA. Data are representative of 3–6 experiments with similar results, showing mean ± SEM; statistical significance was determined via one-way ANOVA followed by a Tukey test for multiple comparisons. *** $p < 0.001$.

3.2. TLR4 and MyD88 Are Crucial for the Pro-IL-1β Induction Activity

Most TLRs, except TLR3, depend on the MyD88 adaptor protein to effectively link PAMP recognition to changes in gene expression and to mediate signal 1 of inflammasome activation. Therefore, to understand if SE was specifically interacting with known TLR4 signaling pathways, we employed transgenic MyD88$^{-/-}$ animals and cell lines as negative controls [37]. Consistent with SE being a canonical TLR4 agonist, pro-IL-1β expression was ablated in MyD88$^{-/-}$ BMDCs treated with GLA or SE, whereas the inflammasome molecule NLRP3 was not required for pro-IL-1β expression (Figure 1B). To determine which MyD88-associated receptors recognized SE, we examined responses in TLR4- and TLR2-deficient BMDCs. TLR4$^{-/-}$, but not TLR2$^{-/-}$, BMDCs failed to increase pro-IL-1β expression in response to SE treatment, indicating that SE acts on the TLR4-MyD88 signaling axis (Figure 1C). Importantly, TLR4$^{-/-}$ BMDCs produced normal amounts of pro-IL-1β in response to the TLR2/6 ligand FSL-1, confirming that these cells are not globally defective in pro-IL-1β expression (Figure 1D). This suggests that some component of SE is stimulating pro-IL-1β production specifically via a TLR4 and MyD88-mediated process.

3.3. DMPC, a Component of SE, Is Essential for TLR4 Activity

To determine whether squalene or DMPC is signaling through the TLR4-MyD88 pathway to enhance pro-IL-1β expression, we developed stable oil-in-water emulsions lacking either DMPC or squalene and applied them to murine BDMCs. We have previously found that replacing squalene with other oils, including grapeseed oil, impairs the adjuvant activity of oil-in-water emulsions, allowing us to use grapeseed oil as a non-immunogenic control [38]. Squalene is also a primary component of both the MF59 and AS03 emulsions used in licensed vaccine products. Therefore, an MF59-like emulsion was used as a non-DMPC-containing control for the immunogenicity of squalene. GLA in an aqueous formulation (GLA-AF) was used as a positive control for TLR4 stimulation. The DMPC-containing grapeseed oil SE retained pro-IL-1β activity, whereas the DMPC-free MF59-like emulsion was not active (Figure 2A). Treatment of BMDCs with DMPC formulated as a liposome without squalene was also sufficient to elicit pro-IL-1β production and other pro-inflammatory cytokines including IL-18, TNFα, and IL-6 (Figure 2B). DMPC liposomes and DMPC-containing emulsions were able to elicit inflammatory signals similar to the canonical agonist GLA, suggesting an equivalent immune phenotype.

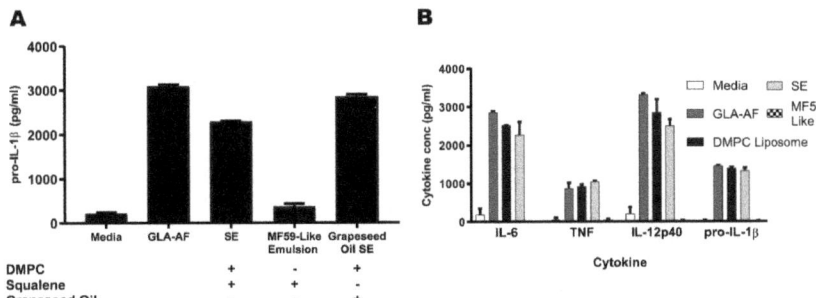

Figure 2. 1,2-dimyristoyl-sn-glycero-3-phosphocholine (DMPC) is necessary and sufficient for pro-IL-1β and cytokine production. WT BMDCs were stimulated with media, GLA-AF, squalene SE, MF59-like emulsion, or grapeseed oil SE for 5 h. (**A**) Pro-IL-1β production is ablated in DMPC-free emulsions. Lysate was collected and assayed for pro-IL-1β by ELISA, using the formulations marked below the axis. (**B**) SE and GLA have similar cytokine profiles. WT BMDCs were stimulated as in (**A**) or with DMPC prepared as a liposome for 5 h. Lysates were assayed for pro-IL-1β, IL-6, TNFα, and IL-12p40 by ELISA. Data are shown as the mean +/− SEM of n = 3–6 replicates. Data are representative of three experiments with similar results.

3.4. DMPC Is an Agonist of the Murine and Human TLR4 Pathways

To further validate the TLR4 activity of DMPC, we employed a TLR4$^{-/-}$ mouse model and a transgenic reporter model for both mouse and human TLR4 activity in a human cell line. As with SE, pro-IL-1β production by DMPC liposome stimulation was ablated in TLR4$^{-/-}$ BMDCs (Figure 3A). These results suggest that DMPC plays an essential role in SE TLR4 activity. However, LPS (endotoxin) is a TLR4 ligand, and its contamination in test reagents could generate false conclusions regarding TLR4 ligands. Polymyxin B is able to selectively bind LPS and neutralize its biological activity [39]. Therefore, to confirm that SE and DMPC are bona fide TLR4 agonists with pro-IL-1β activities and not the result of endotoxin contamination, we treated LPS, SE, and DMPC liposomes with 50 µg/mL polymyxin B before adding them to BMDCs. Addition of polymyxin B was sufficient to abrogate the pro-IL-1β response to LPS but had no impact on the response to DMPC or SE, indicating that their activities are not due to endotoxin contamination (Figure 3B).

Murine and human TLR4s have different specificities for some ligands [40,41]. To determine whether DMPC engages the human TLR4, as well as murine TLR4, we employed HEK-Blue reporter cells transfected with either murine TLR4 (and species-matched adaptor proteins MD-2 and CD14) or human TLR4. Both human and murine TLR4 reporters were strongly responsive to GLA-AF stimulation as a canonical positive control and moderately responsive to DMPC stimulation, whereas a TLR7 reporter system was non-responsive to DMPC but was activated by the known TLR7/8 agonist 3M-052 as a positive control (Figure 3C) [20]. Other studies using HEK-Blue cells overexpressing human or murine TLR4 have shown similar responses to DMPC stimulation [40,42]. These results demonstrate that DMPC is the TLR4 active component of SE, that activity is not due to endotoxin contamination, and that the activity of DMPC is maintained across both murine and human TLR4s.

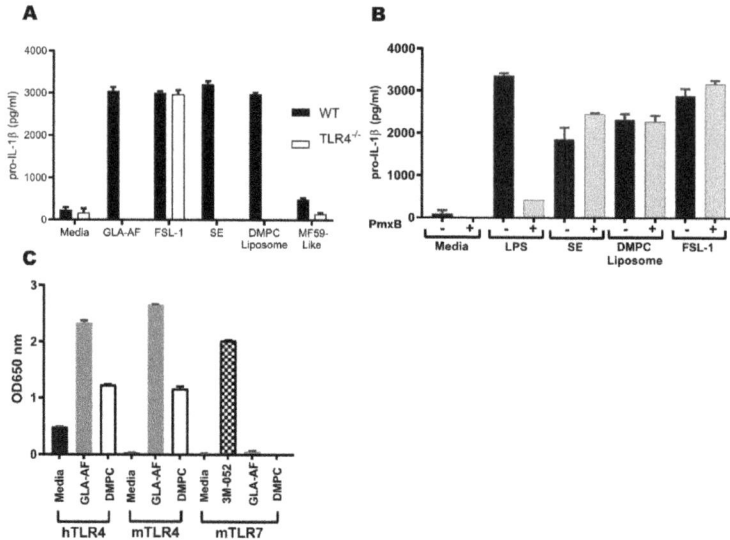

Figure 3. DMPC activates human and murine TLR4 pathway. (**A**) DMPC recapitulates the pro-IL-1β production of SE in a TLR4-dependent manner. WT and TLR4$^{-/-}$ BMDCs were stimulated with media, GLA, SE, DMPC liposomes, or MF59-like emulsion for 5 h. Lysate was collected and assayed for pro-IL-1β by ELISA. (**B**) SE and DMPC stimulation of pro-IL-1β production is not a result of endotoxin contamination. WT BMDCs were stimulated with media, LPS, SE, DMPC liposomes, or MF59-like emulsion pretreated with polymyxin B (PmxB) for 5 h. Lysate was collected and assayed for pro-IL-1β by ELISA. (**C**) DMPC has activity in both human and murine TLR4s. HEK reporter cells transfected with murine (m) or human (h) TLR4 or murine TLR7 were stimulated with media, GLA-AF, DMPC liposomes, or 3M052-AF (TLR7/8 ligand) for 44 h. The production of SEAP induced by NF-κB and AP-1 activation triggered by TLR4 or TLR7 ligand stimulation was measured at OD 650. Data are shown as the mean +/− SEM of a representative with each condition performed in triplicate. Data are representative of three experiments with similar results.

3.5. Emulsion Stimulation of Innate Immune Activity in Human Whole Blood Is Dominated by Oil-Phase Components

Adjuvant immunogenicity varies between species, and the stimulation of chemokine secretion to attract innate immune cell populations is a critical step toward adaptive immunity [8,43–45]. To further understand the activity of DMPC on markers of human innate immunity, we applied SEs and MF59-like emulsions formulated from either squalene or grapeseed oil to human whole blood from 6 donors (3 male and 3 female) for 18–24 h and assayed a panel of secreted cytokines via ELISA. Monocyte chemoattractant protein-1 (MCP-1 or CCL2), IL-8, and macrophage inflammatory protein-1β (MIP-1β or CCL3) were chosen because of their role in early innate immune cell recruitment and because of their previous use in other preclinical vaccine formulation studies [34,46,47]. The squalene-containing formulations (SE and MF59-like emulsion) were more effective at eliciting MCP-1 (Figure 4A) and MIP-1β (Figure 4B) secretion than the grapeseed-containing formulations, regardless of DMPC content. However, the DMPC-containing grapeseed SE stimulated the secretion of more IL-8 than the grapeseed oil MF59-like emulsion (Figure 4C), confirming a TLR4/MyD88/NF-κB-dependent IL-8 secretion previously reported and further validating DMPC as a TLR4 ligand [48,49]. For some markers of human immunogenicity such as production of IL-8, DMPC clearly has some effect when compared to the DMPC-free MF59-like emulsions. However, oil selection (e.g., squalene vs. grapeseed oil) has a more pronounced phenotype.

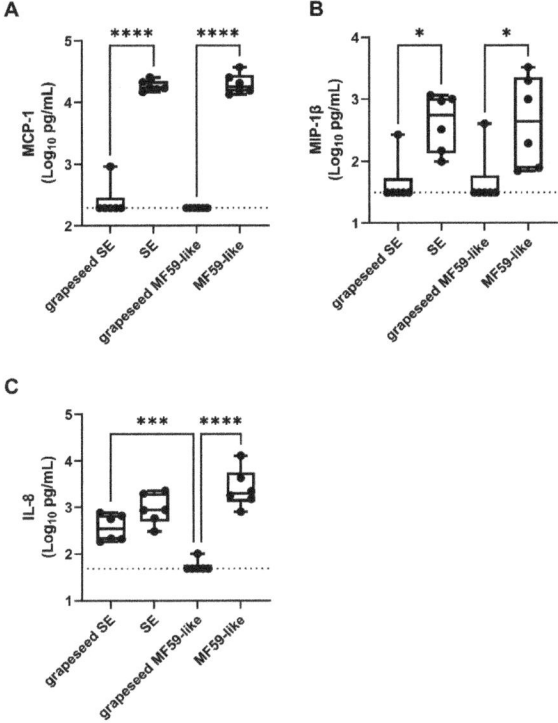

Figure 4. Human whole blood response to emulsion formulations is dominated by oil-phase component. In vitro stimulation of human whole blood with oil-in-water emulsions at 0.4% v/v oil. Squalene-containing formulations led to increased secretion of (**A**) MCP-1, (**B**) MIP-1β, and (**C**) IL-8. Log-transformed cytokine concentrations were measured in supernatants of heparinized blood stimulated by incubation with emulsions. Box and whisker plots indicate 1st–3rd quartiles with whiskers representing the minimum and maximum values from n = 6 donors (3 male and 3 female). Statistical significance was determined by one-way ANOVA followed by Tukey's correction for multiple comparisons. * $p < 0.05$, *** $p < 0.001$, and **** $p < 0.0001$.

3.6. Phospholipid Acyl Chain Length, Saturation State, and Headgroup Structure Are Critical for TLR4 Activity

DMPC contains a PC headgroup and two saturated acyl chains, each containing 14 carbons (14:0). To determine the structural motifs of DMPC that are important for TLR4 engagement, we examined the pro-IL-1β response of BMDCs stimulated with liposomes comprising structural variants of phospholipids with different headgroups or acyl chains (Figure 5A). DLPC, which has the same headgroup as DMPC but shorter acyl chains (C12, 12:0), showed similar pro-IL-1β production activity to DMPC (Figure 5B). Conversely, longer acyl chains with the same phosphocholine headgroup as DMPC, either the fully saturated C16 (16:0) DPPC or C18 (18:0) DSPC, the monounsaturated C18 (18:1) DOPC, or the asymmetrical C16/C18 (16:0/18:1) POPC, all elicited very little pro-IL-1β compared to DMPC (Figure 5B). Among the three saturated C14 phospholipids, DMPC and DMPG induced the production of pro-IL-1β whereas DMPS did not, suggesting that the headgroup structure also impacts TLR4 engagement (Figure 5B). This demonstrates that both acyl chain length and headgroup structure determine the immunogenicity of phospholipids in murine BMDCs.

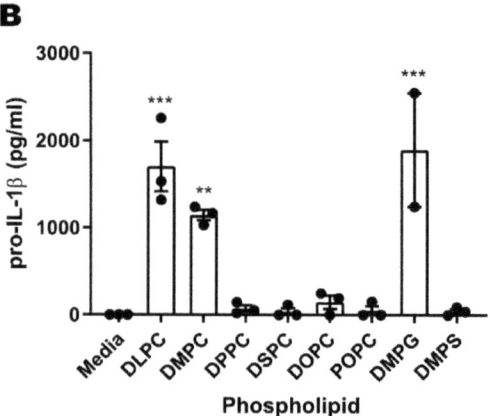

Figure 5. Both the acyl chain length and headgroup structure affect the activity of murine BMDCs. WT BMDCs were stimulated with a panel of phospholipids (**A**) as liposomes. (**B**) Stimulation of pro-IL-1β production is dependent on lipid structure. After 5 h, lysates were collected and assayed for pro-IL-1β by ELISA. Data are shown as the mean +/− SEM of $n = 3$ replicates. Data are representative of three experiments with similar results, showing mean ± SEM. Statistical significance was determined via one-way ANOVA followed by a Dunnett correction for multiple comparisons to the media-only group. ** $p < 0.01$ and *** $p < 0.001$.

3.7. TLR4 Plays a Role in Murine SE-Stimulated Antibody Responses

Finally, to determine if TLR4 engagement by the DMPC-containing SE adjuvant contributes to its ability to augment the adaptive immune response, we immunized WT and TLR4$^{-/-}$ C57BL/6J mice with ID97, a protein tuberculosis antigen, adjuvanted with squalene SE or squalene MF59-like emulsion. Three weeks after immunization, WT mice who received the SE-adjuvanted vaccine showed significantly enhanced serum antigen-specific IgG and IgG1 antibody production compared to TLR4$^{-/-}$ mice who received the same vaccine (Figure 6A,B). In mice that received the SE adjuvant, IgG2c production was not affected by TLR4 knockout (Figure 6C). These differences between WT and TLR4$^{-/-}$ mice were not observed using the MF59-like emulsion, which does not contain DMPC, suggesting that SE acts through TLR4 to promote these antibody responses and that DMPC is the TLR4 active compound (Figure 6A,B). This suggests that the adjuvanting effect of SE is related to the inclusion of DMPC.

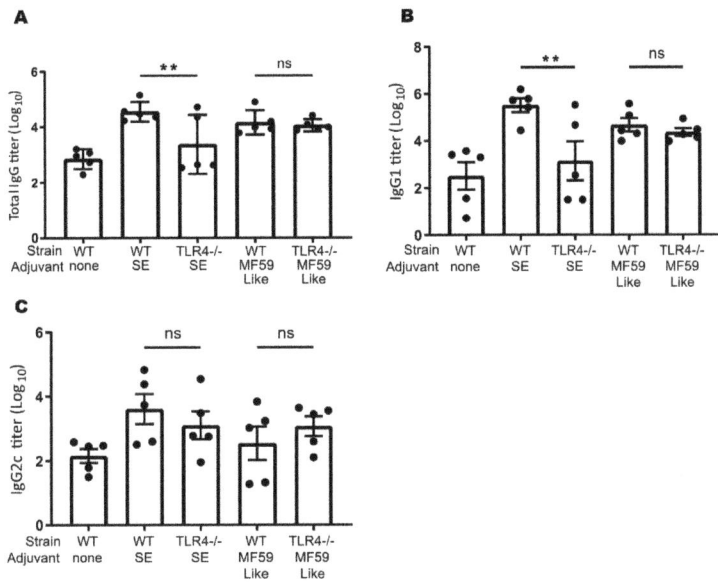

Figure 6. SE acts through TLR4 to augment humoral responses to vaccination. DMPC-containing adjuvants act in a TLR4-dependent process, whereas MF59-like emulsions show TLR4-independent activity. WT and TLR4$^{-/-}$ mice were immunized once with a tuberculosis protein antigen (ID97) either unadjuvanted or adjuvanted with SE or MF59-like emulsion. Three weeks later, peripheral blood was collected. Serum was assayed for antigen-specific (**A**) IgG, (**B**) IgG1, and (**C**) IgG2c by ELISA. Data are shown as the mean +/− SEM of a representative population with each condition performed in triplicate. Data are pooled from two experiments with similar results. ** $p < 0.01$ and ns = not significant.

4. Discussion

In this study, we present evidence that DMPC functions as a TLR4 agonist in the context of the SE adjuvant. We show that DMPC can trigger signal 1 of the TLR4-dependent inflammasome pathway and can induce an immune phenotype similar to canonical TLR4 agonists such as GLA. We additionally show that DMPC can engage with both human and murine TLR4s, although the immunogenicity of DMPC is overshadowed by the impacts of oil selection. Finally, we demonstrate that phospholipid structure impacts its ability to interact with the TLR4 pathway and that DMPC promotes antibody production in adjuvanted protein vaccines in a TLR4-dependent process. Based on our results clarifying the pathway interactions in Figure 1 and our results showing a dependence on chemical structure in Figure 5, we believe that there is a specific molecular interaction between DMPC and TLR4 mediated by MyD88.

Based on previous studies of other lipids associated with TLR4 engagement, DMPC may be stabilized in the MD-2 binding pocket and facilitate the association between MD-2 and TLR4, leading to downstream signaling through MyD88 and/or TRIF [50,51]. This conclusion is supported by the induction of pro-IL-1β production in murine BMDCs after treatment with DMPC-containing SE formulations (regardless of oil composition) (Figure 2A) and by the lack of IL-1β expression after SE or DMPC liposome treatment in TLR4$^{-/-}$ murine BMDCs (Figures 1C,D and 3A). The DMPC-containing grapeseed oil emulsion also stimulates more secretion of IL-8 in human whole blood than the grapeseed oil-based MF59-like emulsion (Figure 4C), demonstrating some impact of DMPC on human immunogenicity. Overall, the results presented in Figures 1–3 suggest that both DMPC-containing emulsions (SE) and DMPC liposomes can signal through TLR4. These results are distinct from previous findings by other groups looking at the TLR4 activity of long-chain saturated fatty acids, such as palmitic acid, due to the inherit spatial structure of an intact phospholipid [52]. Our findings suggest that DMPC engages the TLR4-MyD88 axis but functions in an inflammasome-independent manner as shown by its resilience against NLRP3 knockout (Figure 1B). This supports the conclusion that DMPC is able to trigger TLR4 signal 1, leading to pro-IL-1β production, but is unable to trigger mature IL-1β secretion. Although inflammasome signaling is a canonical pathway by which some adjuvants trigger antibody production, other studies have indicated that TLR4-agonist emulsions lead to strong humoral immune responses through alternative pathways dependent on IL-18 and subcapsular macrophages [22,53]. Because of the limited ability of SE to provide signal 2 of the canonical inflammasome pathway and its independence from NLRP3 (Figure 1B), SE may be functioning via one of these non-canonical processes.

It is important to consider the type of immune response generated by adjuvant systems when evaluating their applied use. This is often accomplished through the use of representative cytokine production panels. We show that DMPC liposomes can elicit similar levels of the pro-inflammatory cytokines TNFα, IL-6, and IL-1β, and the canonical TH1 signal IL-12p40, as SE and GLA (Figure 2B). DMPC can also elicit equivalent cytokine production independent of oil-phase composition (Figure 2A). We have previously shown that oil selection can impact in vivo immunogenicity and that squalene outperforms other common oils in the context of antigen-specific IgG production and long-lived antibody-secreting plasma cell development [38]. The equivalence in pro-IL-1β production we observed between the squalene and grapeseed oil groups (Figure 2A) suggests the lysate pro-IL-1β is primarily due to DMPC signaling through the TLR4 pathway.

Well-known and characterized differences exist between the binding specificity of murine and human TLR4 pathway adaptors, which potentially stifles the translation of results in small animal models to human clinical products [41,54]. While we observed similar IL-1β responses in HEK cells overexpressing murine or human TLR4 after treatment with DMPC (Figure 3C), we only saw effects of DMPC on IL-8 production in human whole blood (Figure 4) and instead found that oil-phase lipid (e.g., squalene or grapeseed oil) dominated the pro-inflammatory cytokine response (MCP-1 and MIP-1β). This suggests that while DMPC may partially engage the human TLR4 pathway, it does not seem to play a substantial role in human immunogenicity. Due in part to the differences in binding pockets between human and murine adaptor proteins (MD-2, TRIF, etc.), agents that are known to be human TLR4 antagonists can be agonists of the murine pathway [40,45]. Therefore, it is unclear at present the manner by which DMPC is interacting with the human TLR4 pathway.

Our results (Figure 5B) further suggest that phospholipid structure may impact the agonist activity of adjuvant systems. Previous studies have shown that saturated lipid chains 10–14 carbons in length are the most effective at activating or suppressing TLR4 signaling and that bioactivity drops off dramatically with longer aliphatic chains and degree of unsaturation [13,33]. We observed that fully saturated 12–14 carbon PC lipids, but not unsaturated or longer chain structures, stimulate pro-IL-1β production in murine BMDCs. In contrast, we have shown that a number of phospholipid-containing emulsions, including both TLR4-active (DMPC) and TLR4-inactive (DOPC, POPC) PCs, have similar adjuvanting properties in mice [55]. This suggests that while DMPC has specific activity in the TLR4 pathway, the downstream biological implications of this are secondary to the adjuvanting effect of intact emulsion formulations [20,56]. Interestingly, DMPS and DMPG liposomes exhibit dramatically different behavior in terms of pro-IL-1β production, despite having identical aliphatic portions and similarly sized headgroups. It is unclear if this is due to DMPS functioning as an antagonist while still engaging with the same binding pocket or if it is entirely precluded from interacting with the TLR4 pathway due to steric hindrance or clashing between charged groups, among other possibilities. It is also unclear if DMPG, which was found to stimulate pro-IL-1β production in murine cells, would have a similar agonistic effect in human models.

Previous studies of the oxidized PC lipid oxPAPC in mice have shown that it interreacts with the TLR4 pathway as an antagonist or agonist depending on the immune context and LPS co-dosing schedule [23–25]. When dosed prior to LPS exposure, oxPAPC can competitively inhibit LPS and sepsis, but when dosed after LPS priming, oxPAPC treatment can lead to prolonged hyperinflammation [23,25,27]. This suggests that immune context has a strong influence on the downstream impact of TLR4-phospholipid interactions. This should be considered when developing lipid-based formulations for biologics or other potentially immunogenic compounds (e.g., polyethylene glycol, polylactic acid, etc.), which might lead to undesirable inflammatory responses or adaptive immunity [57,58].

DMPC-containing SE was found to stimulate the production of antigen-specific antibodies against the tuberculosis antigen ID97 in a mouse model via a TLR4-dependent process (Figure 6) [17]. Further, based on the titer ratio of IgG1 (TH2) and IgG2c (TH1), we observed that both the MF59-like and the SE formulation produced a TH2-biased immune response in mice, whereas GLA-SE is known to induce a more TH1-biased response [59]. Unlike the SE treated mice, the antibody response to MF59-like emulsions was unchanged in the TLR4$^{-/-}$ animals. This is in agreement with previous work showing that MF59 acts in a TLR4-independent, although MyD88-dependent, manner [60]. Interestingly, it has been shown previously that only the complete MF59 adjuvant, and not any individual component, was able to augment antibody responses, suggesting that the particulate formulation presentation in particular is the key to its immunogenicity, emphasizing the need for development of composition and formulation in tandem [56]. Conversely, with SE we observed that the removal of TLR4 specifically impacts antibody production, implying that some TLR4-dependent interaction is promoting adaptive immunity. The TLR4-dependent activity of SE and DMPC has potential implications in the development of drug and vaccine formulations. DMPC is a common component of liposomal and emulsion systems used to deliver small molecules and biologics in preclinical and clinical settings. The potential TLR4 activity of selected phospholipids such as DMPC should be taken into account in preclinical study development and interpretation of the biological activity of drug and vaccine formulations.

5. Conclusions

The contribution of individual formulation components towards innate and adaptive immunity of SE, a squalene-phospholipid emulsion, was evaluated. Compared to an MF59-like emulsion, which does not contain the phospholipid DMPC, SE was found to act in a TLR4-dependent manner, with DMPC being the key pathway agonist. These conclusions were confirmed in in vitro models of murine and human TLR4 and in vivo murine models of TLR4 activity. We also showed that phospholipids similar to DMPC seem to interact with the TLR4 pathway in a chemical structure-dependent manner. These results contribute to the growing body of literature on the mechanisms of action of adjuvant-emulsion and the interactions between formulation components and the innate immune system, and should be considered in the interpretation of preclinical formulation results.

Supplementary Materials: The following supporting information can be downloaded at: https://www.mdpi.com/article/10.3390/pharmaceutics14122557/s1, Table S1: Liposomal particle size and polydispersity index. Table S2: Emulsion and other formulation particle size and polydispersity index.

Author Contributions: Conceptualization, C.B.F., J.A.G., H.L. and M.T.O.; formal analysis, H.L. and W.R.L.; investigation, J.A.G., H.L., M.T.O., T.P. and E.S.; writing—original draft preparation, H.L., W.R.L. and M.T.O.; writing—review and editing, C.B.F. and W.R.L.; visualization, H.L. and W.R.L.; supervision, C.B.F.; funding acquisition, C.B.F. All authors have read and agreed to the published version of the manuscript.

Funding: Research reported in this publication was supported by the National Institute of Allergy and Infectious Diseases of the National Institutes of Health under Contract No. HHSN272201400041C and Grant No. R01AI135673, and by the Bill and Melinda Gates Foundation Grant No. OPP1130379. 30% of the total project costs ($100,000) was financed with federal money, and 70% was financed by nongovernmental sources. The content is solely the responsibility of the authors and does not necessarily represent the official views of the National Institutes of Health.

Institutional Review Board Statement: All animal study protocols were approved by the Infectious Disease Research Institute (IDRI), now AAHI, Institutional Animal Care and Use Committee (IACUC) and were performed according to the IACUC regulations and guidelines.

Informed Consent Statement: Not applicable.

Data Availability Statement: The data presented in this study are available on request from the corresponding author.

Acknowledgments: We thank Amit Khandhar for helpful discussions.

Conflicts of Interest: Christopher B. Fox is an inventor on patents or patent applications describing formulated phospholipids as non-canonical TLR4 agonists. All other authors declare no conflict of interest. The funders had no role in the design of the study, in the collection, analyses, or interpretation of data; in the writing of the manuscript; or in the decision to publish the results.

References

1. Champion, C.R. Heplisav-B: A Hepatitis B Vaccine with a Novel Adjuvant. *Ann. Pharmacother.* **2021**, *55*, 783–791. [CrossRef] [PubMed]
2. Luchner, M.; Reinke, S.; Milicic, A. TLR Agonists as Vaccine Adjuvants Targeting Cancer and Infectious Diseases. *Pharmaceutics* **2021**, *13*, 142. [CrossRef] [PubMed]
3. Keech, C.; Albert, G.; Cho, I.; Robertson, A.; Reed, P.; Neal, S.; Plested, J.S.; Zhu, M.; Cloney-Clark, S.; Zhou, H.; et al. Phase 1–2 Trial of a SARS-CoV-2 Recombinant Spike Protein Nanoparticle Vaccine. *N. Engl. J. Med.* **2020**, *383*, 2320–2332. [CrossRef] [PubMed]
4. O'Hagan, D.T.; Lodaya, R.N.; Lofano, G. The Continued Advance of Vaccine Adjuvants—'We Can Work It Out'. *Semin. Immunol.* **2020**, *50*, 101426. [CrossRef]
5. Shi, S.; Zhu, H.; Xia, X.; Liang, Z.; Ma, X.; Sun, B. Vaccine Adjuvants: Understanding the Structure and Mechanism of Adjuvanticity. *Vaccine* **2019**, *37*, 3167–3178. [CrossRef]
6. Tritto, E.; Mosca, F.; De Gregorio, E. Mechanism of Action of Licensed Vaccine Adjuvants. *Vaccine* **2009**, *27*, 3331–3334. [CrossRef]
7. Heitmann, J.S.; Bilich, T.; Tandler, C.; Nelde, A.; Maringer, Y.; Marconato, M.; Reusch, J.; Jäger, S.; Denk, M.; Richter, M.; et al. A COVID-19 Peptide Vaccine for the Induction of SARS-CoV-2 T Cell Immunity. *Nature* **2022**, *601*, 617–622. [CrossRef]
8. Schroder, K.; Irvine, K.M.; Taylor, M.S.; Bokil, N.J.; Le Cao, K.-A.; Masterman, K.-A.; Labzin, L.I.; Semple, C.A.; Kapetanovic, R.; Fairbairn, L.; et al. Conservation and Divergence in Toll-like Receptor 4-Regulated Gene Expression in Primary Human versus Mouse Macrophages. *Proc. Natl. Acad. Sci. USA* **2012**, *109*, E944–E953. [CrossRef]
9. Qu, G.; Liu, S.; Zhang, S.; Wang, L.; Wang, X.; Sun, B.; Yin, N.; Gao, X.; Xia, T.; Chen, J.J.; et al. Graphene Oxide Induces Toll-like Receptor 4 (TLR4)-Dependent Necrosis in Macrophages. *ACS Nano* **2013**, *7*, 5732–5745. [CrossRef]
10. Uto, T.; Akagi, T.; Yoshinaga, K.; Toyama, M.; Akashi, M.; Baba, M. The Induction of Innate and Adaptive Immunity by Biodegradable Poly(γ-Glutamic Acid) Nanoparticles via a TLR4 and MyD88 Signaling Pathway. *Biomaterials* **2011**, *32*, 5206–5212. [CrossRef]
11. Mano, S.S.; Kanehira, K.; Taniguchi, A. Comparison of Cellular Uptake and Inflammatory Response via Toll-like Receptor 4 to Lipopolysaccharide and Titanium Dioxide Nanoparticles. *Int. J. Mol. Sci.* **2013**, *14*, 13154–13170. [CrossRef] [PubMed]
12. McKeown-Longo, P.J.; Higgins, P.J. Integration of Canonical and Noncanonical Pathways in TLR4 Signaling: Complex Regulation of the Wound Repair Program. *Adv. Wound Care* **2017**, *6*, 320–329. [CrossRef] [PubMed]
13. Zaffaroni, L.; Peri, F. Recent Advances on Toll-like Receptor 4 Modulation: New Therapeutic Perspectives. *Future Med. Chem.* **2018**, *10*, 461–476. [CrossRef]
14. O'Hagan, D.T.; Fox, C.B. New Generation Adjuvants—From Empiricism to Rational Design. *Vaccine* **2015**, *33*, B14–B20. [CrossRef]
15. Seydoux, E.; Liang, H.; Dubois Cauwelaert, N.; Archer, M.; Rintala, N.D.; Kramer, R.; Carter, D.; Fox, C.B.; Orr, M.T. Effective Combination Adjuvants Engage Both TLR and Inflammasome Pathways to Promote Potent Adaptive Immune Responses. *J. Immunol.* **2018**, *201*, 98–112. [CrossRef] [PubMed]
16. Gombault, A.; Baron, L.; Couillin, I. ATP Release and Purinergic Signaling in NLRP3 Inflammasome Activation. *Front. Immunol.* **2012**, *3*, 1–6. [CrossRef]
17. Fox, C.B.; Carter, D.; Kramer, R.M.; Beckmann, A.M.; Reed, S.G. Current Status of Toll-Like Receptor 4 Ligand Vaccine Adjuvants. In *Immunopotentiators in Modern Vaccines*; Elsevier: Amsterdam, The Netherlands, 2017; pp. 105–127. ISBN 9780128040195.
18. Duthie, M.S.; Windish, H.P.; Fox, C.B.; Reed, S.G. Use of Defined TLR Ligands as Adjuvants within Human Vaccines. *Immunol. Rev.* **2011**, *239*, 178–196. [CrossRef]
19. Cauwelaert, N.D.; Desbien, A.L.; Hudson, T.E.; Pine, S.O.; Reed, S.G.; Coler, R.N.; Orr, M.T. The TLR4 Agonist Vaccine Adjuvant, GLA-SE, Requires Canonical and Atypical Mechanisms of Action for TH1 Induction. *PLoS ONE* **2016**, *11*, e0146372. [CrossRef]
20. Misquith, A.; Fung, H.W.M.; Dowling, Q.M.; Guderian, J.A.; Vedvick, T.S.; Fox, C.B. In Vitro Evaluation of TLR4 Agonist Activity: Formulation Effects. *Colloids Surf. B Biointerfaces* **2014**, *113*, 312–319. [CrossRef]
21. Orr, M.T.; Duthie, M.S.; Windish, H.P.; Lucas, E.A.; Guderian, J.A.; Hudson, T.E.; Shaverdian, N.; O'Donnell, J.; Desbien, A.L.; Reed, S.G.; et al. MyD88 and TRIF Synergistic Interaction Is Required for TH1-Cell Polarization with a Synthetic TLR4 Agonist Adjuvant. *Eur. J. Immunol.* **2013**, *43*, 2398–2408. [CrossRef]

22. Desbien, A.L.; Dubois Cauwelaert, N.; Reed, S.J.; Bailor, H.R.; Liang, H.; Carter, D.; Duthie, M.S.; Fox, C.B.; Reed, S.G.; Orr, M.T. IL-18 and Subcapsular Lymph Node Macrophages Are Essential for Enhanced B Cell Responses with TLR4 Agonist Adjuvants. *J. Immunol.* **2016**, *197*, 4351–4359. [CrossRef] [PubMed]
23. Chu, L.H.; Indramohan, M.; Ratsimandresy, R.A.; Gangopadhyay, A.; Morris, E.P.; Monack, D.M.; Dorfleutner, A.; Stehlik, C. The Oxidized Phospholipid OxPAPC Protects from Septic Shock by Targeting the Non-Canonical Inflammasome in Macrophages. *Nat. Commun.* **2018**, *9*, 996. [CrossRef] [PubMed]
24. Bochkov, V.N.; Kadl, A.; Huber, J.; Gruber, F.; Binder, B.R.; Leitinger, N. Protective Role of Phospholipid Oxidation Products in Endotoxin-Induced Tissue Damage. *Nature* **2002**, *419*, 77–81. [CrossRef] [PubMed]
25. Di Gioia, M.; Spreafico, R.; Springstead, J.R.; Mendelson, M.M.; Joehanes, R.; Levy, D.; Zanoni, I. Endogenous Oxidized Phospholipids Reprogram Cellular Metabolism and Boost Hyperinflammation. *Nat. Immunol.* **2020**, *21*, 42–53. [CrossRef] [PubMed]
26. Watson, A.D.; Leitinger, N.; Navab, M.; Faull, K.F.; Hörkkö, S.; Witztum, J.L.; Palinski, W.; Schwenke, D.; Salomon, R.G.; Sha, W.; et al. Structural Identification by Mass Spectrometry of Oxidized Phospholipids in Minimally Oxidized Low Density Lipoprotein That Induce Monocyte/Endothelial Interactions and Evidence for Their Presence in Vivo. *J. Biol. Chem.* **1997**, *272*, 13597–13607. [CrossRef] [PubMed]
27. Zanoni, I.; Tan, Y.; Di Gioia, M.; Springstead, J.R.; Kagan, J.C. By Capturing Inflammatory Lipids Released from Dying Cells, the Receptor CD14 Induces Inflammasome-Dependent Phagocyte Hyperactivation. *Immunity* **2017**, *47*, 697–709.e3. [CrossRef] [PubMed]
28. Knapp, S.; Matt, U.; Leitinger, N.; van der Poll, T. Oxidized Phospholipids Inhibit Phagocytosis and Impair Outcome in Gram-Negative Sepsis In Vivo. *J. Immunol.* **2007**, *178*, 993–1001. [CrossRef]
29. Hill, D.L.; Pierson, W.; Bolland, D.J.; Mkindi, C.; Carr, E.J.; Wang, J.; Houard, S.; Wingett, S.W.; Audran, R.; Wallin, E.F.; et al. The Adjuvant GLA-SE Promotes Human Tfh Cell Expansion and Emergence of Public TCRβ Clonotypes. *J. Exp. Med.* **2019**, *216*, 1857–1873. [CrossRef]
30. Duthie, M.S.; Frevol, A.; Day, T.; Coler, R.N.; Vergara, J.; Rolf, T.; Sagawa, Z.K.; Marie Beckmann, A.; Casper, C.; Reed, S.G. A Phase 1 Antigen Dose Escalation Trial to Evaluate Safety, Tolerability and Immunogenicity of the Leprosy Vaccine Candidate LepVax (LEP-F1 + GLA–SE) in Healthy Adults. *Vaccine* **2020**, *38*, 1700–1707. [CrossRef]
31. Orr, M.T.; Beebe, E.A.; Hudson, T.E.; Moon, J.J.; Fox, C.B.; Reed, S.G.; Coler, R.N. A Dual TLR Agonist Adjuvant Enhances the Immunogenicity and Protective Efficacy of the Tuberculosis Vaccine Antigen ID93. *PLoS ONE* **2014**, *9*, e83884. [CrossRef]
32. Fox, C.B.; Barnes, V.L.; Evers, T.; Chesko, J.D.; Vedvick, T.S.; Coler, R.N.; Reed, S.G.; Baldwin, S.L. Adjuvanted Pandemic Influenza Vaccine: Variation of Emulsion Components Affects Stability, Antigen Structure, and Vaccine Efficacy. *Influenza Other Respir. Viruses* **2013**, *7*, 815–826. [CrossRef] [PubMed]
33. Lutz, M.B.; Kukutsch, N.; Ogilvie, A.L.J.; Rößner, S.; Koch, F.; Romani, N.; Schuler, G. An Advanced Culture Method for Generating Large Quantities of Highly Pure Dendritic Cells from Mouse Bone Marrow. *J. Immunol. Methods* **1999**, *223*, 77–92. [CrossRef]
34. Fox, C.B.; Van Hoeven, N.; Granger, B.; Lin, S.; Guderian, J.A.; Hartwig, A.; Marlenee, N.; Bowen, R.A.; Soultanov, V.; Carter, D. Vaccine Adjuvant Activity of Emulsified Oils from Species of the Pinaceae Family. *Phytomedicine* **2019**, *64*, 152927. [CrossRef] [PubMed]
35. Orr, M.T.; Ireton, G.C.; Beebe, E.A.; Huang, P.-W.D.; Reese, V.A.; Argilla, D.; Coler, R.N.; Reed, S.G. Immune Subdominant Antigens as Vaccine Candidates against Mycobacterium Tuberculosis. *J. Immunol.* **2014**, *193*, 2911–2918. [CrossRef] [PubMed]
36. Mariathasan, S.; Weiss, D.S.; Newton, K.; McBride, J.; O'Rourke, K.; Roose-Girma, M.; Lee, W.P.; Weinrauch, Y.; Monack, D.M.; Dixit, V.M. Cryopyrin Activates the Inflammasome in Response to Toxins and ATP. *Nature* **2006**, *440*, 228–232. [CrossRef] [PubMed]
37. Saikh, K.U. MyD88 and beyond: A Perspective on MyD88-Targeted Therapeutic Approach for Modulation of Host Immunity. *Immunol. Res.* **2021**, *69*, 117–128. [CrossRef]
38. Fox, C.B.; Baldwin, S.L.; Duthie, M.S.; Reed, S.G.; Vedvick, T.S. Immunomodulatory and Physical Effects of Oil Composition in Vaccine Adjuvant Emulsions. *Vaccine* **2011**, *29*, 9563–9572. [CrossRef]
39. Danner, R.L.; Joiner, K.A.; Rubin, M.; Patterson, W.H.; Johnson, N.; Ayers, K.M.; Parrillo, J.E. Purification, Toxicity, and Antiendotoxin Activity of Polymyxin B Nonapeptide. *Antimicrob. Agents Chemother.* **1989**, *33*, 1428–1434. [CrossRef]
40. Ohto, U.; Fukase, K.; Miyake, K.; Shimizu, T. Structural Basis of Species-Specific Endotoxin Sensing by Innate Immune Receptor TLR4/MD-2. *Proc. Natl. Acad. Sci. USA* **2012**, *109*, 7421–7426. [CrossRef]
41. Vijayan, V.; Pradhan, P.; Braud, L.; Fuchs, H.R.; Gueler, F.; Motterlini, R.; Foresti, R.; Immenschuh, S. Human and Murine Macrophages Exhibit Differential Metabolic Responses to Lipopolysaccharide—A Divergent Role for Glycolysis. *Redox Biol.* **2019**, *22*, 101147. [CrossRef]
42. Nahori, M.-A.; Fournié-Amazouz, E.; Que-Gewirth, N.S.; Balloy, V.; Chignard, M.; Raetz, C.R.H.; Saint Girons, I.; Werts, C. Differential TLR Recognition of Leptospiral Lipid A and Lipopolysaccharide in Murine and Human Cells. *J. Immunol.* **2005**, *175*, 6022–6031. [CrossRef] [PubMed]
43. Stewart, E.; Triccas, J.A.; Petrovsky, N. Adjuvant Strategies for More Effective Tuberculosis Vaccine Immunity. *Microorganisms* **2019**, *7*, 255. [CrossRef] [PubMed]
44. Reed, S.G.; Scott, P. T-Cell and Cytokine Responses in Leishmaniasis. *Curr. Opin. Immunol.* **1993**, *5*, 524–531. [CrossRef]

45. Akashi, S.; Nagai, Y.; Ogata, H.; Oikawa, M.; Fukase, K.; Kusumoto, S.; Kawasaki, K.; Nishijima, M.; Hayashi, S.; Kimoto, M.; et al. Human MD-2 Confers on Mouse Toll-like Receptor 4 Species-Specific Lipopolysaccharide Recognition. *Int. Immunol.* **2001**, *13*, 1595–1599. [CrossRef]
46. Abhyankar, M.M.; Orr, M.T.; Lin, S.; Suraju, M.O.; Simpson, A.; Blust, M.; Pham, T.; Guderian, J.A.; Tomai, M.A.; Elvecrog, J.; et al. Adjuvant Composition and Delivery Route Shape Immune Response Quality and Protective Efficacy of a Recombinant Vaccine for Entamoeba Histolytica. *Npj Vaccines* **2018**, *3*, 22. [CrossRef]
47. Adeagbo, B.A.; Akinlalu, A.O.; Phan, T.; Guderian, J.; Boukes, G.; Willenburg, E.; Fenner, C.; Bolaji, O.O.; Fox, C.B. Controlled Covalent Conjugation of a Tuberculosis Subunit Antigen (ID93) to Liposome Improved In Vitro Th1-Type Cytokine Recall Responses in Human Whole Blood. *ACS Omega* **2020**, *5*, 31306–31313. [CrossRef]
48. He, W.; Qu, T.; Yu, Q.; Wang, Z.; Lv, H.; Zhang, J.; Zhao, X.; Wang, P. LPS Induces IL-8 Expression through TLR4, MyD88, NF-KappaB and MAPK Pathways in Human Dental Pulp Stem Cells. *Int. Endod. J.* **2013**, *46*, 128–136. [CrossRef]
49. Marr, N.; Turvey, S.E. Role of Human TLR4 in Respiratory Syncytial Virus-Induced NF-KB Activation, Viral Entry and Replication. *Innate Immun.* **2012**, *18*, 856–865. [CrossRef]
50. Lonez, C.; Irvine, K.L.; Pizzuto, M.; Schmidt, B.I.; Gay, N.J.; Ruysschaert, J.-M.; Gangloff, M.; Bryant, C.E. Critical Residues Involved in Toll-like Receptor 4 Activation by Cationic Lipid Nanocarriers Are Not Located at the Lipopolysaccharide-Binding Interface. *Cell. Mol. Life Sci.* **2015**, *72*, 3971–3982. [CrossRef]
51. Wong-Baeza, C.; Tescucano, A.; Astudillo, H.; Reséndiz, A.; Landa, C.; España, L.; Serafín-López, J.; Estrada-García, I.; Estrada-Parra, S.; Flores-Romo, L.; et al. Nonbilayer Phospholipid Arrangements Are Toll-Like Receptor-2/6 and TLR-4 Agonists and Trigger Inflammation in a Mouse Model Resembling Human Lupus. *J. Immunol. Res.* **2015**, *2015*, 369462. [CrossRef]
52. Lancaster, G.I.; Langley, K.G.; Berglund, N.A.; Kammoun, H.L.; Reibe, S.; Estevez, E.; Weir, J.; Mellett, N.A.; Pernes, G.; Conway, J.R.W.; et al. Evidence That TLR4 Is Not a Receptor for Saturated Fatty Acids but Mediates Lipid-Induced Inflammation by Reprogramming Macrophage Metabolism. *Cell Metab.* **2018**, *27*, 1096–1110.e5. [CrossRef] [PubMed]
53. Eisenbarth, S.C.; Colegio, O.R.; O'Connor, W.; Sutterwala, F.S.; Flavell, R.A. Crucial Role for the Nalp3 Inflammasome in the Immunostimulatory Properties of Aluminium Adjuvants. *Nature* **2008**, *453*, 1122–1126. [CrossRef] [PubMed]
54. Mestas, J.; Hughes, C.C.W. Of Mice and Not Men: Differences between Mouse and Human Immunology. *J. Immunol.* **2004**, *172*, 2731–2738. [CrossRef] [PubMed]
55. Fox, C.B.; Baldwin, S.L.; Duthie, M.S.; Reed, S.G.; Vedvick, T.S. Immunomodulatory and Physical Effects of Phospholipid Composition in Vaccine Adjuvant Emulsions. *AAPS PharmSciTech* **2012**, *13*, 498–506. [CrossRef]
56. Calabro, S.; Tritto, E.; Pezzotti, A.; Taccone, M.; Muzzi, A.; Bertholet, S.; De Gregorio, E.; O'Hagan, D.T.; Baudner, B.; Seubert, A. The Adjuvant Effect of MF59 Is Due to the Oil-in-Water Emulsion Formulation, None of the Individual Components Induce a Comparable Adjuvant Effect. *Vaccine* **2013**, *31*, 3363–3369. [CrossRef]
57. Chen, B.-M.; Cheng, T.-L.; Roffler, S.R. Polyethylene Glycol Immunogenicity: Theoretical, Clinical, and Practical Aspects of Anti-Polyethylene Glycol Antibodies. *ACS Nano* **2021**, *15*, 14022–14048. [CrossRef]
58. Ahmad Ruzaidi, D.A.; Mahat, M.M.; Shafiee, S.A.; Mohamed Sofian, Z.; Mohmad Sabere, A.S.; Ramli, R.; Osman, H.; Hamzah, H.H.; Zainal Ariffin, Z.; Sadasivuni, K.K. Advocating Electrically Conductive Scaffolds with Low Immunogenicity for Biomedical Applications: A Review. *Polymers* **2021**, *13*, 3395. [CrossRef]
59. Coler, R.N.; Bertholet, S.; Moutaftsi, M.; Guderian, J.A.; Windish, H.P.; Baldwin, S.L.; Laughlin, E.M.; Duthie, M.S.; Fox, C.B.; Carter, D.; et al. Development and Characterization of Synthetic Glucopyranosyl Lipid Adjuvant System as a Vaccine Adjuvant. *PLoS ONE* **2011**, *6*, e16333. [CrossRef]
60. Seubert, A.; Calabro, S.; Santini, L.; Galli, B.; Genovese, A.; Valentini, S.; Aprea, S.; Colaprico, A.; D'Oro, U.; Giuliani, M.M.; et al. Adjuvanticity of the Oil-in-Water Emulsion MF59 Is Independent of Nlrp3 Inflammasome but Requires the Adaptor Protein MyD88. *Proc. Natl. Acad. Sci. USA* **2011**, *108*, 11169–11174. [CrossRef]

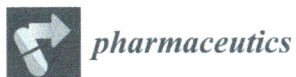 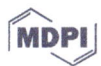

Article

Amphotericin B- and Levofloxacin-Loaded Chitosan Films for Potential Use in Antimicrobial Wound Dressings: Analytical Method Development and Its Application

Ke Peng [1], Mingshan Li [1], Achmad Himawan [1,2], Juan Domínguez-Robles [1], Lalitkumar K. Vora [1], Ross Duncan [1], Xianbing Dai [1], Chunyang Zhang [1], Li Zhao [1], Luchi Li [1], Eneko Larrañeta [1] and Ryan F. Donnelly [1,*]

1 School of Pharmacy, Queen's University Belfast, Medical Biology Centre, 97 Lisburn Road, Belfast BT9 7BL, UK
2 Department of Pharmaceutical Science and Technology, Faculty of Pharmacy, Hasanuddin University, Makassar 90245, Indonesia
* Correspondence: r.donnelly@qub.ac.uk

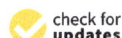

Citation: Peng, K.; Li, M.; Himawan, A.; Domínguez-Robles, J.; Vora, L.K.; Duncan, R.; Dai, X.; Zhang, C.; Zhao, L.; Li, L.; et al. Amphotericin B- and Levofloxacin-Loaded Chitosan Films for Potential Use in Antimicrobial Wound Dressings: Analytical Method Development and Its Application. *Pharmaceutics* 2022, *14*, 2497. https://doi.org/10.3390/pharmaceutics14112497

Academic Editors: Vibhuti Agrahari and Prashant Kumar

Received: 27 September 2022
Accepted: 9 November 2022
Published: 17 November 2022

Publisher's Note: MDPI stays neutral with regard to jurisdictional claims in published maps and institutional affiliations.

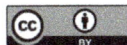

Copyright: © 2022 by the authors. Licensee MDPI, Basel, Switzerland. This article is an open access article distributed under the terms and conditions of the Creative Commons Attribution (CC BY) license (https://creativecommons.org/licenses/by/4.0/).

Abstract: Levofloxacin (LVX) and amphotericin B (AMB) have been widely used to treat bacterial and fungal infections in the clinic. Herein, we report, for the first time, chitosan films loaded with AMB and LVX as wound dressings to combat antimicrobial infections. Additionally, we developed and validated a high-performance liquid chromatography (HPLC) method coupled with a UV detector to simultaneously quantify both AMB and LVX. The method is easy, precise, accurate and linear for both drugs at a concentration range of 0.7–5 µg/mL. The validated method was used to analyse the drug release, ex vivo deposition and permeation from the chitosan films. LVX was released completely from the chitosan film after a week, while approximately 60% of the AMB was released. Ex vivo deposition study revealed that, after 24-hour application, 20.96 ± 13.54 µg of LVX and approximately 0.35 ± 0.04 µg of AMB was deposited in porcine skin. Approximately 0.58 ± 0.16 µg of LVX permeated through the skin. AMB was undetectable in the receptor compartment due to its poor solubility and permeability. Furthermore, chitosan films loaded with AMB and LVX were found to be able to inhibit the growth of both *Candida albicans* and *Staphylococcus aureus*, indicating their potential for antimicrobial applications.

Keywords: amphotericin B; levofloxacin; chitosan film; wound dressing; antimicrobial

1. Introduction

Chronic, difficult-to-heal wounds are at risk of fungal infections and are also at risk of developing bacterial infections. They are generally polymicrobial in nature [1]. Various microorganisms cluster and coexist in their niche, where bacteria (*Staphylococcus spp.*) and fungi (*Candida spp.*) generally predominate the polymicrobial population [2]. Therefore, antibiotics and fungicides must be used in combination to combat those types of polymicrobial wounds [3,4]. Levofloxacin (LVX), a fluoroquinolone antibiotic, is active against a broad range of Gram-positive, Gram-negative and atypical bacteria. It has been widely used in the treatment of various infectious diseases. Although LVX is relatively safe and tolerable, gastrointestinal (GI) disturbances and stimulation of the central nervous system (CNS) have been observed [5]. Topical application of LVX could avoid GI and CNS side effects andLVX has been widely reported in the application of wound dressings [6–8]. Amphotericin B (AMB), a polyene fungicide, has been in clinical use for decades for treating human fungal infections, especially opportunistic systemic fungal infections [9]. It possesses broad-spectrum antifungal activities and rare antifungal resistance [10]. Systemic use of AMB has the potential for significant toxicity, especially nephrotoxicity and electrolyte abnormalities [11]. AMB has been suggested to be used topically to treat wound infections [12–14].

In wound management, topical application is the first choice, but several antibiotics, including AMB, suffer from low wound drug concentrations, which are needed to eradicate infections. A preliminary study reported poor wound penetration of AMB after systemic liposomal AMB administration, risking subinhibitory concentrations of the fungicide at the site of infection [13]. Another case report attempted to administer topical AMB for postoperative mucormycosis with positive outcomes observed from the wound healing process [13,15]. In contrast with AMB, LVX was reported to have good wound penetration, but considering its systemic side effects, the topical route may be beneficial to avoid adverse reactions [16,17].

Wound dressings can be enriched with antimicrobial drugs to better address the risk of developing infections during wound care [18–20]. Two antimicrobial agents can be combined in one preparation to resist the development of resistant pathogens [21,22]. To extend its antimicrobial properties and to better tackle polymicrobial infection, an antibacterial and antifungal drug can be combined into one preparation [3]. In this work, we use LVX and AMB where a synergistic interaction between LVX and AMB has been reported [4].

A novel dual drug-loaded wound dressing using a chitosan film to deliver AMB and LVX was designed in the study with the idea of extending the antimicrobial activities of the chitosan films. Chitosan, a natural cationic polysaccharide obtained by alkaline deacetylation of chitin, is nontoxic, biocompatible, biodegradable, mucoadhesive and antimicrobial [23]. Chitosan exerts its antibacterial activities through the binding of its cationic amino groups to anionic groups of these microorganisms [24]. These properties make chitosan an ideal vehicle for the medical field. Chitosan possesses outstanding film-forming capabilities, which are greatly appreciated in wound dressing systems, and its films are sometimes stated as "bioactive dressings" [23,25]. Moreover, the combined use of AMB and LVX was found to exert synergistic interactions against fungal cells, which may potentially treat concurrent bacterial and fungal infections [4]. Therefore, both bacterial and fungal infections may be treated by using only one pharmaceutical dosage form.

Method development followed by validation is an important step in the development of novel pharmaceutical preparations, especially in combination drug products. Several analytical methods have been reported to analyse AMB and LVX individually but to the best of our knowledge, no analytical method has been reported for the simultaneous quantification of AMB and LVX. Herein, we have developed and validated an HPLC-UV analytical method to fill this gap. The developed and validated method was applied to evaluate the release profile of the film, and antimicrobial performance was studied to demonstrate antimicrobial efficacy.

2. Materials and Methods

2.1. Materials

Amphotericin B (AMB) was purchased from Cayman Chemical Company (purity specification $\geq$ 95%), Ann Arbor, MI, USA. Levofloxacin hydrochloride (LVX) was obtained from Zhejiang Jingxin Pharmaceuticals (Xinchang, China). Plasdone™ K-29/32 (poly(vinylpyrrolidone), PVP) (MW 58 kDa) was donated by Ashland (Kidderminster, UK). Chitosan (low molecular weight), ethylenediaminetetraacetic acid disodium salt dehydrate (EDTA-Na2), dodecyl sodium sulphate (SLS) and HPLC-grade methanol were also supplied by Sigma-Aldrich (Poole, Dorset, UK). Dimethyl sulfoxide (DMSO) was provided by VWR International Limited, Leicestershire, UK. Phosphate buffered saline (PBS) pH 7.4 tablets were acquired from Oxoid Limited, Hampshire, UK. All other chemical reagents were of analytical grade and purchased from Sigma-Aldrich (Dorset, UK) or Fisher Scientific (Leicestershire, UK).

2.2. Film Preparation and Characterization

The films were prepared using the solvent casting method. Chitosan stock solution was prepared by dissolving 3% w/v chitosan in 1 M acetic acid and stirring overnight at 25 °C. This chitosan stock solution (5 g) was mixed with 0.10 g PVP and 0.90 g water to form the film solution. For the films containing AMB and LVX, 25 mg of AMB dissolved in 0.3 mL DMSO and 25 mg of LVX were added to the film solution and mixed using a SpeedMixer™ (DAC 150.1 FVZ-K, FlackTek, Hamm, Germany) at 3500 rpm for 3 min to form a homogenous solution. An aliquot of 250 µL of the resulting solution was added into a circular silicone mould with a diameter of 2 mm and placed in a fume hood to dry overnight. For the blank film, 0.3 mL DMSO was added to the film solution. For films containing only AMB, 25 mg of AMB dissolved in 0.3 mL DMSO was added into the film solution without the addition of 25 mg of LVX. For films containing only LVX, 25 mg of LVX with 0.3 mL DMSO was added to the film solution. The structures of the obtained films were studied by scanning electron microscopy (SEM) (Hitachi TM3030; Tokyo, Japan), a digital microscope (Leica EZ4 D, Wetzlar, Germany) and an optical coherence tomography (OCT) microscope (EX1301, Michelson Diagnostics Ltd., Kent, UK).

2.3. Instrumentation and Chromatographic Conditions

Simultaneous analysis of AMB and LVX was performed with an Agilent Technologies 1260 Infinity HPLC consisting of an Agilent degasser, quaternary pump, auto standard injector and detector (Agilent Technologies UK Ltd., Stockport, UK). Separation was achieved by using a C18 Phenomenex InertClone™ analytical column ODS (3) (250 mm × 4.60 mm internal diameter, 5 µm packing; Phenomenex InertClone™, US). The mobile phase consisted of a mixture of 2.5 mM EDTA-Na$_2$ (mobile phase A) and methanol (mobile phase B). The injection volume was 20 µL, and elution was performed at a constant flow rate of 1 mL/min for 16 min. The column was thermostated at 30 °C. The detection wavelengths were set at 295 nm (for the analysis of LVX) and 406 nm (for the analysis of AMB). The obtained chromatographs were analysed using Agilent ChemStation® software B.02.01.

The stock solutions were prepared by dissolving 10 mg of AMB and 10 mg of LVX together with 10 mL of DMSO and methanol (1:1, v/v), and the standard samples were prepared by diluting the stock solution using methanol. The instrumentation and chromatographic conditions for AMB and LVX are presented in Table 1. These HPLC methods were validated according to the International Council for Harmonisation (ICH) guidelines for Validation of Analytical Procedures Q2 Analytical Validation Revision one (R1) 2005 [26,27].

Table 1. Gradient parameters for simultaneous analysis of AMB and LVX.

Time (min)	Mobile Phase A, % (2.5 mM EDTA-Na$_2$)	Mobile Phase B, % (Methanol)
0	65	35
4	35	65
5	15	85
12	15	85
12.01	65	35
16	65	35

2.4. Analytical Method Validation

2.4.1. Specificity

The specificity of the method was guaranteed by observing potential interferences caused by blank release medium under current chromatographic conditions without the presence of both drugs to evaluate if the matrices have interferences from other components of similar behaviour.

2.4.2. Linearity and Calibration Curve

The linearity of the proposed method was assessed through calibration curves, constructed with eight standard solutions ranging from 0.7 to 5.0 µg/mL to determine the coefficient of correlation, slope and intercept values. The calibration curves were obtained by plotting the peak areas against the corresponding drug concentrations with least squares linear regression analysis using the Analysis ToolPak of Microsoft Excel® (Microsoft Corp., Redmond, WA, USA).

2.4.3. Detection and Quantitation Limits (LODs, and LOQs)

The theoretical LOD and LOQ for the developed methods were calculated using the standard deviation of the response (σ) and slope (S) of the calibration curve according to the following equations:

$$LOD = \frac{3.3 \times \sigma}{S}$$

$$LOQ = \frac{10 \times \sigma}{S}$$

2.4.4. Precision and Accuracy

The precision of the methods was verified using three standard concentrations of each drug (1, 2, 4 µg/mL as low, medium, high concentrations). Accuracy is defined as the closeness of agreement between the measurements and an accepted reference value, expressed as the relative error (RE). The precision is expressed as the closeness of agreement (degree of scatter) between a series of measurements, represented as the relative standard deviation (RSD) [28]. Both RSD and RE were calculated using the following equations. Accuracy and precision were evaluated intraday and interday, and the method was deemed to be accurate and precise if the RSD and RE from all samples fell below 15% [29,30].

$$RSD\ (\%) = \frac{Standard\ deviation}{Mean} \times 100\%$$

$$RE\ (\%) = \frac{Back\ calculated\ value - true\ value}{True\ value} \times 100\%$$

2.5. Application of the Analytical Method to the In Vitro Release Study

The release profiles of both AMB and LVX were investigated as a direct application of the analytical method. The chitosan films were placed in 10 mL of PBS (pH 7.4) with 1% w/v SLS at 37 °C and 40 rpm. SLS was added to increase the solubility of AMB in PBS (pH 7.40) to maintain a sink condition. An aliquot of 1 mL of sample was taken at 1 d, 2 d, 3 d, 4 d, 5 d, 6 d, and 7 d and replaced with a fresh release medium. The release samples were analysed using the validated simultaneous analytical method for AMB and LVX.

2.6. Application of the Analytical Method to Skin Deposition and Permeation Studies in Franz Cells

Skin deposition and permeation experiments were carried out using a glass vertical Franz diffusion cell setup. A piece of excised neonatal full-thickness (500 µm) porcine skin obtained from stillborn piglets was sandwiched between the donor and the receptor compartments with SC facing the donor. The receptor compartment was filled with 12 mL of PBS (pH 7.4) containing 1% w/v SLS and allowed to equilibrate for 1 h at 37 °C. To start the test, 10 µL of water was added to the skin surface, and the chitosan films containing AMB+LVX were put into the donor compartment with close contact with the skin. The receptor compartment was maintained at 37 °C and constantly stirred using a magnetic bar at 600 rpm. At 24 h, samples (1 mL) were withdrawn from the receptor compartment, filtered using a 0.45 µm syringe filter and analysed using HPLC. The AMB and LVX deposited in skin were estimated after the 24 h permeation studies. The skin was carefully removed from the Franz cell, wiped with a paper towel and cut into small pieces using surgical scissors. The skin tissue was further homogenized with 1 mL DMSO using a Tissue Lyser LT (Qiagen, Ltd., Manchester, UK) at 50 Hz for 15 min. The skin homogenate samples were centrifuged at 16,160× g for 20 min to collect the supernatant for further dilution and HPLC analysis.

2.7. Microbiological Assay

A disk diffusion test was performed to evaluate the antibacterial and antifungal properties of the films against *Staphylococcus aureus* NCTC 10788 and *Candida albicans* NCYC 610 from the National Collection of Type Cultures, Central Public Health Laboratory, Colindale Avene, London, respectively. *C. albicans* was grown and maintained on Sabouraud dextrose (SDE) agar (Oxoid, Hampshire, UK) and incubated at 37 °C for 48 h. *C. albicans* was incubated overnight at 37 °C in SDE broth at 100 rpm in an orbital shaker. After growth, *C. albicans* culture was diluted using sterile PBS (pH 7.4) to an OD_{550} value of 0.10 (approx. 6.0×10^5 cfu/mL). Then, 1 mL of the diluted culture was added to 5 mL of soft SDE agar, which had been previously heated to 100 °C before being allowed to cool down to below 55 °C. This composition was then mixed using a vortex and poured onto the surface of an SDE agar plate. Similarly, *S. aureus* was inoculated overnight at 37 °C in lysogeny broth (LB) at 100 rpm in an orbital shaker. The culture was then diluted using PBS to an OD_{550} value of 0.10 (approx. 1.0×10^8 cfu/mL). Subsequently, 1 mL of the diluted culture was mixed with 5 mL of soft Lysogeny agar (LA) and poured on the surface of an LA plate. The chitosan films containing both drugs (AMB+LVX), containing only one drug (AMB or LVX) and blank films were placed in the centre of the inoculated plates. The agar plates containing different film samples were then incubated at 37 °C for 24 h. The whole process was conducted under aseptic conditions, and untreated inoculated plates were used as a control (n = 4).

2.8. Statistical Analysis

The data are shown as the means ± standard deviation (SD) unless otherwise noted. The calculation of means, SD, %RSD, %RE, LOD, LOQ and least-squares linear regression analysis were all performed using Microsoft® Excel 2019 (Microsoft Corporation, Redmond, WA, USA). Unless otherwise noted, $p < 0.05$ was used to indicate statistical significance in all cases.

3. Results

3.1. Preparation and Characterization of Topical Films

Chitosan films can be prepared using the solvent casting method, electrostatic spraying method and dry wet phase separation method, due to the film-forming capabilities of chitosan [31]. Overall, the solvent casting method is the most commonly used and most convenient method [23]. The morphology of the chitosan films we prepared using the solvent casting method was investigated using SEM [32]. As shown in Figure 1B, the films presented a smooth, flat surface without any phase separation, indicating homogenous blending between chitosan, PVP and the drugs. This finding correlates with the report in the literature [33], indicating the film forming capability of chitosan and PVP [34]. At 1000× magnification (Figure 1C), the surface was found to have crystals due to the semicrystalline nature of the polymers and the crystalline nature of the drugs [34]. To further understand the films, OCT was used to visualize the cross-section of the films. OCT is a well-established imaging tool to noninvasively map the variation in reflected light as a function of depth to indicate the cross-section information of samples [35]. As shown in Figure 1D, chitosan films containing AMB and LVX had a homogeneous thickness. The obstruction density of the chitosan films containing AMB and LVX was much higher than that of the blank chitosan films (Figure 1E), indicating a homogenous distribution of drugs inside the films. Additionally, the films were analysed using DSC. AMB is characterized by double broad endothermic peaks at approx. 144 °C and 215 °C during DSC analysis. The endothermic peak at 144 °C could be the melting point of AMB [36]. Additionally, the endothermic peak at 215 °C can be attributed to drug decomposition [37]. This is consistent with previous reports, as AMB has been reported to be a crystalline drug. Moreover, LVX shows an endothermic peak at approx. 90 °C due to the loss of free water and the drug characteristic melting point at approx. 230 °C, which demonstrates good agreement with previously reported values [7,38–41]. It is important to note that, when both drugs were incorporated into the film, these melting points were not observed. Therefore, it can be concluded that both drugs were dispersed homogenously in the film. Chitosan and PVP are stable polymers with high decomposition temperatures. The endothermic peaks observed in the blank and drug-containing films probably contributed to the residual solvent loss, including acetic acid and water, after preparation [42]. This is because chitosan is known to have a strong affinity with water [43] and PVP is hygroscopic in nature [44]. The thermogram also indicates that the films might be amorphous/semi-crystalline in nature, as PVP is known as an amorphous material [45]. PVP is a well-known pharmaceutical ingredient for its nontoxic, bioinert, and hydrophilic properties and has been widely used in wound dressings. The addition of PVP to chitosan has been reported to have little effect on the physical and chemical properties of chitosan, but can improve the mechanical properties of chitosan due to its ability to interact with PVP *via* hydrogen bond formation between the carbonyl group of PVP and the amino or hydroxyl groups of chitosan [46]. Moreover, the addition of PVP to chitosan films lowers the preparation cost, as PVP is a synthetic polymer much more affordable than the naturally occurring polymer chitosan, which requires extraction from crustacean shells [25].

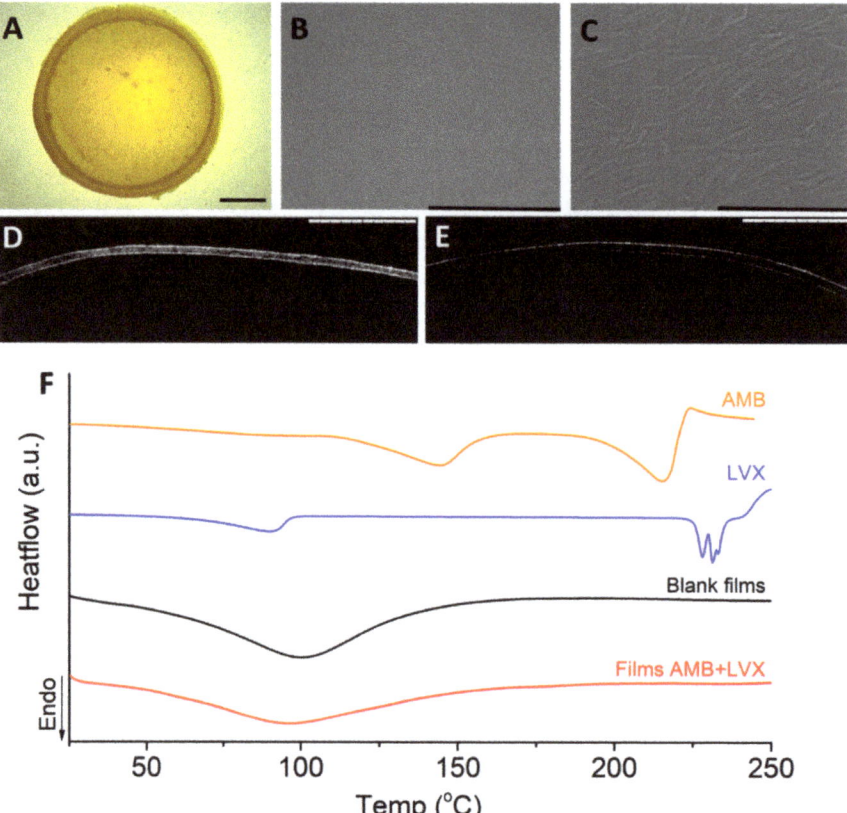

Figure 1. The structure of chitosan films containing AMB and LVX. (**A**) Digital microscopy. Scale bar: 2 mm. (**B**) SEM image. Scale bar, 1 mm. (**C**) SEM image. Scale bar, 100 μm. (**D**) OCT image of chitosan films containing AMB+LVX. Scale bar, 1 mm. (**E**) OCT image of blank chitosan films without AMB and LVX. Scale bar, 1 mm. (**F**) DSC thermograms of chitosan films containing AMB+LVX, blank chitosan films, AMB and LVX.

3.2. Analytical Method Development

A C18 column was chosen in this analytical method due to its adaptability and versatility for a broad range of compounds. The HPLC analysis of AMB reported in the literature generally uses the chelating agent EDTA in the mobile phase, as EDTA could directly compete against AMB for chelation with metal ions possibly from the column packing materials, therefore improving the chromatographic peak shape [47,48]. At the beginning of the method development, an isocratic elution was applied to separate AMB and LVX. However, a high ratio (over 60%) of the aqueous phase was required to retain LVX, in which case the retention time of the AMB was over 30 min. A gradient method was, therefore, developed in this study to achieve a shorter runtime and desired sensitivity for simultaneously analysing AMB and LVX due to the huge difference between these two molecules in polarity. The wavelengths were set at both 295 nm and 406 nm in the analysis based on the maximum absorption wavelengths of individual compounds (406 nm for AMB and 295 nm for LVX) [49–51].

3.3. Method Validation

ICH recommendations were consulted to perform method validation.

3.3.1. Specificity

The retention time for AMB and LVX under the present experimental conditions was 10.028 (at 406 nm) and 4.965 min (at 295 nm), respectively (Figure 2B). The resolution of the two peaks is 3.74, greater than 1.5, indicating that the sample components are well-separated to an extent where the area or height of each peak can be accurately measured [52]. Representative chromatograms of the drug-free release medium (as presented in Figure 2A) showed no peaks at these retention times, demonstrating the specificity of the current analytical method.

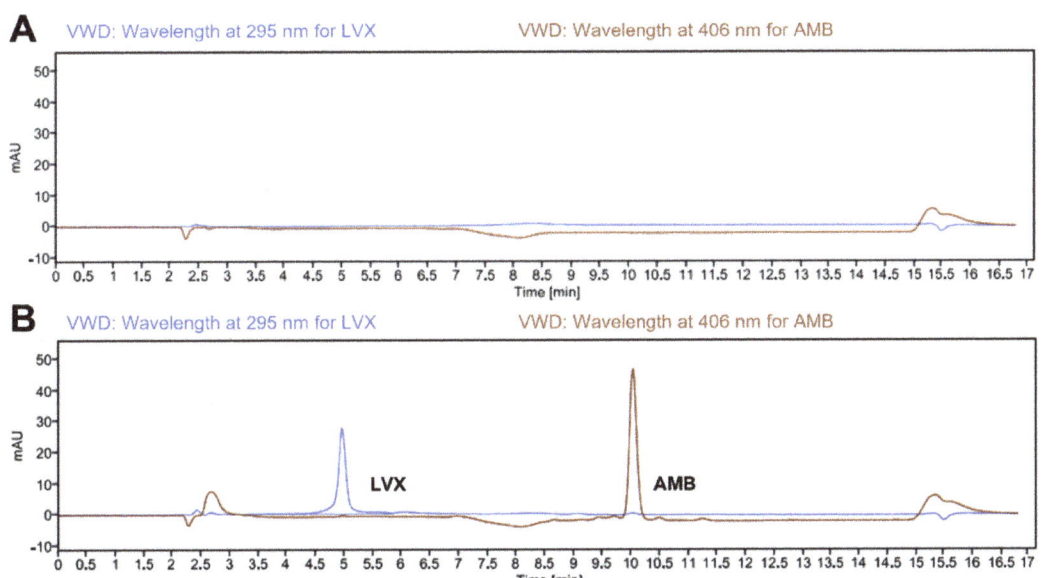

Figure 2. Representative chromatograms of (**A**) blank release medium (PBS pH 7.4 containing 1% w/v SLS); and (**B**) LVX and AMB (4.0 μg/mL for both drugs) in release media.

3.3.2. Linearity and Calibration Curve

The linearity of the proposed method was determined by analysing different concentration levels of both AMB and LVX and determining their integrated peak area. The peak areas were correlated to the corresponding concentrations to plot the calibration curve. Linearity and the parameters of the regression equation are listed in Table 2. The results demonstrate that the calibration curves for both drugs exhibited a linear response with a coefficient of determination (R^2) $\geq$ 0.99 over the concentration range analysed. Additionally, Table 2 shows the LOD and LOQ for both drugs. These values obtained for LVX are lower than previously reported HPLC methods using UV-visible detection for the quantification of the drug in dosage forms [53]. The LOD and LOQ could be reduced by using more sensitive detectors, such as fluorescence detectors or higher-end equipment, such as UPLC [54–56]. However, these methods were developed in many cases for the quantification of LVX in biological fluids requiring low drug concentrations. On the other hand, AMB methods described in the literature are focused on the quantification of the drug on biological matrices and therefore are not suitable for formulation development, as they require complex extraction procedures or the use of high-end equipment such as mass spectrometry [57,58].

Table 2. Calibration parameters and sensitivity of AMB and LVX (n = 3).

Drug	Concentration Range (µg/mL)	Slope	Y-Intercept	Correlation Coefficient (R^2)	LOD (µg/mL)	LOQ (µg/mL)
AMB	0.7–5	123.99	−8.64	0.999	0.20	0.62
LVX	0.7–5	92.16	−16.74	0.999	0.16	0.48

3.3.3. Accuracy and Precision

The accuracy and precision results for the QC samples are reported in Table 3. In terms of accuracy, the values of %RE were found to be within −6.02 to 5.63%, falling within the required limits of 15%, demonstrating that the current analytical method is accurate [29]. In regard to precision, the values of %RSD were found to be within 1.62 to 5.06%, falling within the required limits of 15%, showing that the current analytical method is precise [30,59].

Table 3. Intraday and interday accuracy and precision of AMB and LVX (Means ± SD; n = 3).

Drug	Spiked Concentration (µg/mL)	Calculated Concentration (µg/mL)	Precision (RSD%)	Recovery (%)	Accuracy (RE%)
AMB	intraday				
	1	1.05 ± 0.04	4.08	105.12	5.12
	2	2.03 ± 0.04	2.00	101.55	1.55
	4	3.99 ± 0.17	4.35	99.78	−0.22
AMB	interday				
	1	1.01 ± 0.02	1.77	100.93	0.93
	2	1.98 ± 0.03	1.62	98.91%	−1.09
	4	3.89 ± 0.20	5.05	97.19	−2.81
LVX	intraday				
	1	1.00 ± 0.05	5.06	100.21	0.21
	2	1.91 ± 0.04	2.00	95.31	−4.69
	4	4.23 ± 0.12	2.86	105.63	5.63
LVX	interday				
	1	1.00 ± 0.05	5.02	100.02	0.02
	2	1.88 ± 0.04	2.07	93.98	−6.02
	4	3.92 ± 0.20	5.01	98.11	−1.89

3.4. Release of Topical Films

The release of AMB and LVX from the chitosan films was evaluated and quantified using the analytical method validated above, and the release profiles are shown in Figure 3. The amount of AMB and LVX was kept the same at 1.00 mg per disc to study the release profiles of each drug at the same level. The release of AMB and LVX from chitosan films followed a similar pattern: they were released quickly in the first three days and reached a plateau by seven days. However, compared to AMB, LVX was released more quickly and more completely from the chitosan films. It released 924.8 µg (92%) by the third day and 958.5 µg (96%) by the seventh day. In the case of AMB, its release reached 422.8 µg (42%) by the third day and increased gradually afterward to 567.5 µg (57%) on the seventh day. These similar patterns could be attributed to the same shape and fabrication materials of the films. The different release phenomena could be explained by the different properties of the drugs. LVX is a water-soluble compound that can easily dissolve and enter the release medium by free diffusion, thereby presenting a more complete release after 3 days [60]. However, AMB is practically insoluble in water at neutral pH values. In the PBS environment (pH 7.4), the release of AMB from chitosan films was found to be slow. Similar release profiles have been demonstrated in the literature, with AMB being released slowly from chitosan particles [61].

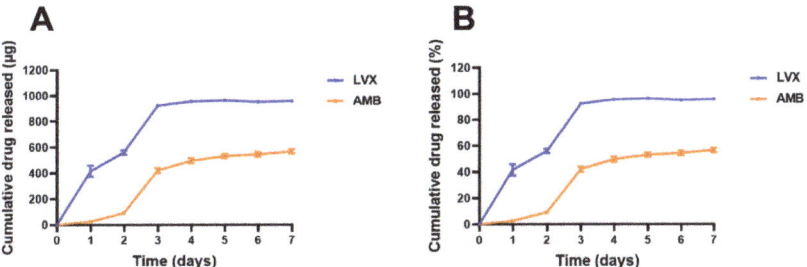

Figure 3. Release profiles of AMB and LVX in PBS (pH 7.4) containing 1% w/v SLS over seven days. Cumulative drug released in µg (**A**) and percentage (**B**). (Means ± SD, n = 5).

3.5. Skin Deposition and Permeation Studies in Franz Cells

Ex vivo skin deposition and permeation experiments were performed on modified Franz cell setup (Figure 4A) using excised neonatal full-thickness porcine skin because of its remarkable similarity in general structure and physical characteristics to human skin [62,63]. Water (10 µL) was added to facilitate adhesion between the film and the skin as well as to mimic the moist environment of the wound tissue. As shown in Figure 4B, after 24-hour of application, 20.96 ± 13.54 µg of LVX was deposited in the skin and approximately 0.58 ± 0.16 µg of LVX could permeate from the skin to the receptor compartment. Approximately 0.35 ± 0.04 µg of AMB was deposited in the skin and little amount of AMB was able to reach the receptor compartment. These data showed a very limited permeation profile of AMB and relatively better profiles of LVX. This has been well documented in the literature [13,16,17]. This could be attributed to the different characteristics of the drugs [64]. LVX is classified as a BCS class I drug, which possesses high solubility and high permeability [65]; while AMB is characterized as a BCS class IV drug, which is notorious for its low solubility and low permeability [66]. The MIC of LVX against *S. aureus* is reported to be in the range of 0.06–0.5 mg/L [67–69] The skin deposition and permeation of LVX from the film was high enough to inhibit the growth of *S. aureus* deep in the skin layer. The MIC of AMB against *Candida* is reported to be mostly around 0.25–1 mg/L [70]. The deposition of AMB reached 0.35 ± 0.04 µg, indicating the applicability of the chitosan films to treat superficial fungal infections. These data indicated that the chitosan films we developed in this study could serve for localized topical use as the systemic exposure (indicated by the permeation data) is likely to be minimal, indicating good safety profiles, especially for toxic drugs such as AMB [71]. Even though there are very limited resources to define concentration toxicity threshold for levofloxacin [72,73], the safety profile of levofloxacin has been widely reported in the literature and a high daily dose of 1000 mg is recommended for patients [74]. The deposition and permeation of LVX from the film (approximately 21.54 µg in total) should be tolerable [75].

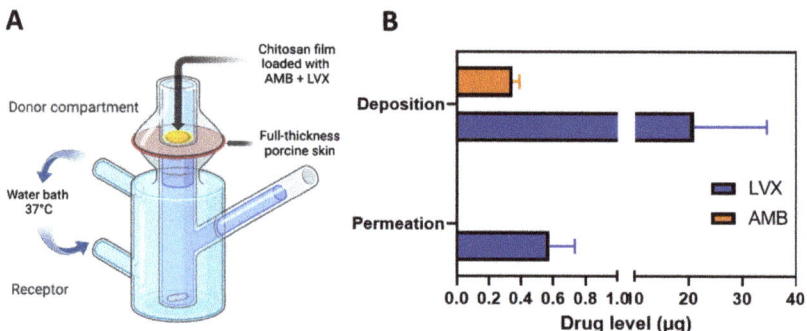

Figure 4. Skin permeation and deposition results. (**A**) Schematic representation of the modified Franz cell setup for the ex vivo skin permeation and deposition study. The chitosan films containing AMB+LVX were placed on top of the full-thickness porcine skin and 10 µL of water was added between the film and skin to facilitate adhesion and mimic the moist environment of the wound tissue. The skin tissue was homogenized to extract the drug deposited and the samples from the receptor compartment were analysed for permeation data. (**B**) Ex vivo permeation and deposition results of AMB and LVX from the chitosan films. (Means + SD, n = 3).

3.6. Antimicrobial Efficacy

Chitosan films, with or without drugs, were evaluated for their antimicrobial effects against both microorganism strains (*C. albicans* NCYC 610 and *S. aureus* NCTC 10788). The disk diffusion test here was used to represent the overall antimicrobial ability of the films and a complementary examination to confirm the release of both drugs. *C. albicans* was used as a representative fungus because it is commonly found on the skin surface and mucous membranes and is the most common cause of invasive fungal infections coinciding with mortality rates as high as 40% [76,77]. Moreover, *S. aureus* is a Gram-positive bacterium that can cause a wide variety of clinical diseases. *S. aureus* is a good example of a pathogen that is involved in both community-acquired and hospital-acquired infections [78,79].

Chitosan films containing both AMB + LVX were found to be effective against both *C. albicans* (inhibition zone of 18.93 ± 1.95 mm) and *S. aureus* (inhibition zone of 38.89 ± 1.76 mm) (Figure 5). Furthermore, chitosan films containing only LVX showed no inhibition against *C. albicans*. However, these samples presented considerable inhibition against *S. aureus* (inhibition zone of 40.10 ± 0.79 mm). Chitosan films containing only AMB drug not only exhibited a clear inhibition against *C. albicans* (inhibition zone of 21.46 ± 2.2 mm) but also against *S. aureus* (inhibition zone of 25.30 ± 2.40 mm). Additionally, although blank chitosan films (no loaded drugs) showed no inhibition against *C. albicans*, these films showed a clear inhibition against *S. aureus* (inhibition zone of 18.15 ± 5.98 mm).

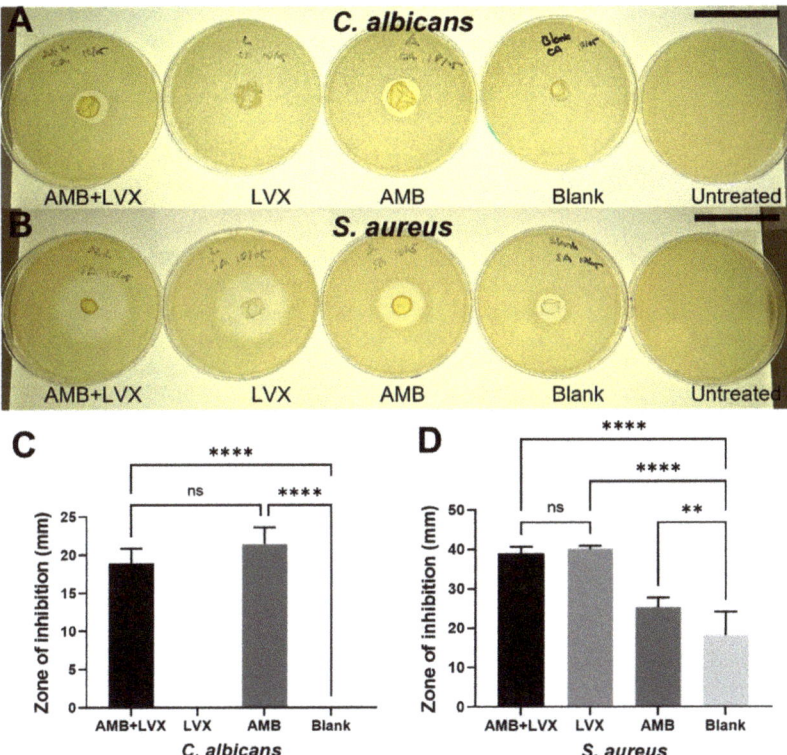

Figure 5. Antimicrobial performances of chitosan films containing AMB and LVX. (**A**) Representative disk diffusion test pictures against *C. albicans* after exposure to chitosan films containing AMB and LVX, chitosan films containing LVX, chitosan films containing AMB, blank chitosan films and untreated control. Scale bar, 5 cm. (**B**) Representative disk diffusion test results against *S. aureus* after exposure to chitosan films containing AMB and LVX, chitosan films containing LVX, chitosan films containing AMB, blank chitosan films and untreated control. Scale bar, 5 cm. (**C**) Disk diffusion test results of chitosan films with or without AMB or LVX against *C. albicans* (means + SD, n = 4). (**D**) Disk diffusion test results of chitosan films with or without AMB or LVX against *S. aureus* (means + SD, n = 4; ns: not significant, ** $p < 0.01$, **** $p < 0.0001$).

With regard to antifungal activities, blank chitosan films and chitosan films containing only LVX failed to inhibit the growth of *C. albicans*. However, AMB-loaded chitosan films, including both chitosan films with AMB+LVX and chitosan films loaded only with AMB, offered substantial antifungal activities, although no significant differences in terms of inhibition zone diameter between these two samples were found ($p > 0.05$). These results demonstrated that LVX, chitosan or PVP had no meaningful effect on inhibiting the growth of *C. albicans*, and thus AMB was the main cause of the fungicidal activities from AMB-loaded chitosan films. Chitosan has well-known antibacterial activities against bacteria. However, its effects on fungal cells depend on several factors, including molecular weight, the length of the polymeric chains and variations in pH and concentration [80–82]. It has been reported that blank chitosan films did not show any inhibitory effects on the *Candida* species, including *C. albicans*, *Candida tropicalis* and *Candida parapsilosis* tested in the study conducted by Oliveira et al. [81].

In terms of their antibacterial activities, chitosan films themselves presented a modest reduction in *S. aureus* growth. This antibacterial behaviour could also be attributed to the possible existence of acetic acid in the formulation. The antibacterial ability of acetic acid has been widely applied in wound management for a long time as a disinfected and antiseptic agent [83]. Although corrosive at concentrations between 10%–30%, acetic acid is considered harmless below concentrations of 5% [84]. The residue acetic acid should be within the safety range after evaporation overnight as demonstrated by the DSC result in Figure 1F: no obvious endothermic peak is present at 118 °C at the melting point of acetic acid. Furthermore, AMB-loaded chitosan films showed an inhibition zone of 25.30 ± 2.40 mm against *S. aureus*, which presented a significant difference ($p < 0.01$) compared with the results found for blank chitosan films. Therefore, these results indicate that AMB may have notable bactericidal effects against *S. aureus*, which is consistent with the results found in the literature [85]. Moreover, both chitosan films containing only LVX or containing LVX in combination with AMB showed the greatest zone of inhibition against *S. aureus* and no significant differences were found between these two film samples ($p > 0.05$). To summarize, chitosan films containing both AMB+LVX were able to inhibit the growth of both microorganisms, *C. albicans* and *S. aureus*, tested in this study.

4. Conclusions

This study developed, for the first time, a chitosan film loaded with AMB and LVX for wound dressing. A simultaneous quantification method for AMB and LVX using HPLC-UV was developed, validated and found to be accurate, precious and linear based on ICH guidelines. The in vitro release profiles were examined using the validated method over seven days. Ex vivo skin deposition and permeation studies were performed to further understand the utility of the film and the applicability of the method. Antimicrobial tests demonstrated the antibacterial and antifungal effects of the chitosan films containing both drugs. This study provides some insightful and preliminary foundation for the combined formulation of these two well-established drugs.

Author Contributions: K.P.: Conceptualization, Investigation, Methodology, Formal analysis, Writing—original draft, Writing—review and editing. M.L.: Investigation, Methodology, Formal analysis, Writing—review and editing. A.H.: Investigation, Methodology, Writing—review and editing. J.D.-R.: Investigation, Methodology, Writing—review and editing. L.K.V.: Writing—review and editing. R.D.: Methodology, Writing—review and editing. X.D.: Investigation, Methodology, Writing—review and editing. C.Z.: Investigation, Methodology. L.Z.: Methodology. L.L.: Investigation. E.L.: Conceptualization, Supervision, Methodology, Writing—review and editing. R.F.D.: Supervision, methodology, Resources, Funding acquisition, Writing—review and editing. All authors have read and agreed to the published version of the manuscript.

Funding: This research was funded by Wellcome Trust grant number WT094085MA.

Institutional Review Board Statement: Not applicable.

Informed Consent Statement: Not applicable.

Data Availability Statement: Not applicable.

Acknowledgments: We are also thankful to the School of Pharmacy, Queen's University Belfast, Northern Ireland, United Kingdom, for their technical support and for providing research facilities.

Conflicts of Interest: The authors declare no conflict of interest.

References

1. Brogden, K.A.; Guthmiller, J.M.; Taylor, C.E. Human Polymicrobial Infections. *Lancet* **2005**, *365*, 253–255. [CrossRef]
2. Pruitt, B.A.; McManus, A.T.; Kim, S.H.; Goodwin, C.W. Burn Wound Infections: Current Status. *World J. Surg.* **1998**, *22*, 135–145. [CrossRef] [PubMed]
3. Thattaruparambil Raveendran, N.; Mohandas, A.; Ramachandran Menon, R.; Somasekharan Menon, A.; Biswas, R.; Jayakumar, R. Ciprofloxacin-and Fluconazole-Containing Fibrin-Nanoparticle-Incorporated Chitosan Bandages for the Treatment of Polymicrobial Wound Infections. *ACS Appl. Bio Mater.* **2019**, *2*, 243–254. [CrossRef] [PubMed]
4. Stergiopoulou, T.; Meletiadis, J.; Sein, T.; Papaioannidou, P.; Tsiouris, I.; Roilides, E.; Walsh, T.J. Comparative Pharmacodynamic Interaction Analysis between Ciprofloxacin, Moxifloxacin and Levofloxacin and Antifungal Agents against Candida Albicans and Aspergillus Fumigatus. *J. Antimicrob. Chemother.* **2009**, *63*, 343–348. [CrossRef] [PubMed]

5. Lipsky, B.A.; Baker, C.A. Fluoroquinolone Toxicity Profiles: A Review Focusing on Newer Agents. *Clin. Infect. Dis.* **1999**, *28*, 352–364. [CrossRef] [PubMed]
6. Valizadeh, A.; Shirzad, M.; Pourmand, M.R.; Farahmandfar, M.; Sereshti, H.; Amani, A. Levofloxacin Nanoemulsion Gel Has a Powerful Healing Effect on Infected Wound in Streptozotocin-Induced Diabetic Rats. *Drug Deliv. Transl. Res.* **2020**, *11*, 292–304. [CrossRef]
7. Pásztor, N.; Rédai, E.; Szabó, Z.-I.; Sipos, E. Preparation and Characterization of Levofloxacin-Loaded Nanofibers as Potential Wound Dressings. *Acta Medica Marisiensis* **2017**, *63*, 66–69. [CrossRef]
8. Siafaka, P.I.; Zisi, A.P.; Exindari, M.K.; Karantas, I.D.; Bikiaris, D.N. Porous Dressings of Modified Chitosan with Poly(2-Hydroxyethyl Acrylate) for Topical Wound Delivery of Levofloxacin. *Carbohydr. Polym.* **2016**, *143*, 90–99. [CrossRef]
9. Nasiri, M.I.; Vora, L.K.; Ershaid, J.A.; Peng, K.; Tekko, I.A.; Donnelly, R.F. Nanoemulsion-Based Dissolving Microneedle Arrays for Enhanced Intradermal and Transdermal Delivery. *Drug Deliv. Transl. Res.* **2022**, *12*, 881–896. [CrossRef]
10. Obayes AL-Khikani, F.H. Amphotericin B, the Wonder of Today's Pharmacology Science: Persisting Usage for More Than Seven Decades. *Pharm. Biomed. Res.* **2020**, *6*, 173–180. [CrossRef]
11. Pendleton, R.A.; Holmes IV, J.H. Systemic Absorption of Amphotericin B with Topical 5% Mafenide Acetate/Amphotericin B Solution for Grafted Burn Wounds: Is It Clinically Relevant? *Burns* **2010**, *36*, 38–41. [CrossRef] [PubMed]
12. Wang, K.; Jacinto, J.; Davis, A.; Hetman, A.; Kumar, A. A Case Report: Utilization of Topical Amphotericin in Postoperative Mucormycosis. *HCA Healthc. J. Med.* **2021**, *2*, 3. [CrossRef]
13. Akers, K.S.; Rowan, M.P.; Niece, K.L.; Graybill, J.C.; Mende, K.; Chung, K.K.; Murray, C.K. Antifungal Wound Penetration of Amphotericin and Voriconazole in Combat-Related Injuries: Case Report. *BMC Infect. Dis.* **2015**, *15*, 1–7. [CrossRef] [PubMed]
14. Sanchez, D.A.; Schairer, D.; Tuckman-Vernon, C.; Chouake, J.; Kutner, A.; Makdisi, J.; Friedman, J.M.; Nosanchuk, J.D.; Friedman, A.J. Amphotericin B Releasing Nanoparticle Topical Treatment of Candida Spp. in the Setting of a Burn Wound. *Nanomedicine Nanotechnology, Biol. Med.* **2014**, *10*, 269–277. [CrossRef]
15. Chavda, V.P.; Apostolopoulos, V. Mucormycosis - An Opportunistic Infection in the Aged Immunocompromised Individual: A Reason for Concern in COVID-19. *Maturitas* **2021**, *154*, 58–61. [CrossRef]
16. Giordano, P.; Weber, K.; Gesin, G.; Kubert, J. Skin and Skin Structure Infections: Treatment with Newer Generation Fluoroquinolones. *Ther. Clin. Risk Manag.* **2007**, *3*, 309–317. [CrossRef]
17. Oberdorfer, K.; Swoboda, S.; Hamann, A.; Baertsch, U.; Kusterer, K.; Born, B.; Hoppe-Tichy, T.; Geiss, H.K.; von Baum, H. Tissue and Serum Levofloxacin Concentrations in Diabetic Foot Infection Patients. *J. Antimicrob. Chemother.* **2004**, *54*, 836–839. [CrossRef]
18. Hamedi, H.; Moradi, S.; Hudson, S.M.; Tonelli, A.E. Chitosan Based Hydrogels and Their Applications for Drug Delivery in Wound Dressings: A Review. *Carbohydr. Polym.* **2018**, *199*, 445–460. [CrossRef]
19. Pang, Q.; Zheng, X.; Luo, Y.; Ma, L.; Gao, C. A Photo-Cleavable Polyprodrug-Loaded Wound Dressing with UV-Responsive Antibacterial Property. *J. Mater. Chem. B* **2017**, *5*, 8975–8982. [CrossRef]
20. Adhikari, U.; An, X.; Rijal, N.; Hopkins, T.; Khanal, S.; Chavez, T.; Tatu, R.; Sankar, J.; Little, K.J.; Hom, D.B.; et al. Embedding Magnesium Metallic Particles in Polycaprolactone Nanofiber Mesh Improves Applicability for Biomedical Applications. *Acta Biomater.* **2019**, *98*, 215–234. [CrossRef]
21. Lin, M.; Liu, Y.; Gao, J.; Wang, D.; Xia, D.; Liang, C.; Li, N.; Xu, R. Synergistic Effect of Co-Delivering Ciprofloxacin and Tetracycline Hydrochloride for Promoted Wound Healing by Utilizing Coaxial PCL/Gelatin Nanofiber Membrane. *Int. J. Mol. Sci.* **2022**, *23*, 1895. [CrossRef] [PubMed]
22. Tabbene, O.; Azaiez, S.; Di Grazia, A.; Karkouch, I.; Ben Slimene, I.; Elkahoui, S.; Alfeddy, M.N.; Casciaro, B.; Luca, V.; Limam, F.; et al. Bacillomycin D and Its Combination with Amphotericin B: Promising Antifungal Compounds with Powerful Antibiofilm Activity and Wound-Healing Potency. *J. Appl. Microbiol.* **2016**, *120*, 289–300. [CrossRef] [PubMed]
23. Radha, D.; Lal, J.S.; Devaky, K.S. Chitosan-Based Films in Drug Delivery Applications. *Starch/Staerke* **2022**, *74*, 2100237. [CrossRef]
24. Ravi Kumar, M.N.V. A Review of Chitin and Chitosan Applications. *React. Funct. Polym.* **2000**, *46*, 1–27. [CrossRef]
25. Hasan, A.; Waibhaw, G.; Tiwari, S.; Dharmalingam, K.; Shukla, I.; Pandey, L.M. Fabrication and Characterization of Chitosan, Polyvinylpyrrolidone, and Cellulose Nanowhiskers Nanocomposite Films for Wound Healing Drug Delivery Application. *J. Biomed. Mater. Res. Part A* **2017**, *105*, 2391–2404. [CrossRef]
26. Stewart, S.A.; Waite, S.; Domínguez-Robles, J.; McAlister, E.; Permana, A.D.; Donnelly, R.F.; Larrañeta, E. HPLC Method for Levothyroxine Quantification in Long-Acting Drug Delivery Systems. Validation and Evaluation of Bovine Serum Albumin as Levothyroxine Stabilizer. *J. Pharm. Biomed. Anal.* **2021**, *203*, 114182. [CrossRef]
27. Ramöller, I.K.; Abbate, M.T.A.; Vora, L.K.; Hutton, A.R.J.; Peng, K.; Volpe-Zanutto, F.; Tekko, I.A.; Moffatt, K.; Paredes, A.J.; McCarthy, H.O.; et al. HPLC-MS Method for Simultaneous Quantification of the Antiretroviral Agents Rilpivirine and Cabotegravir in Rat Plasma and Tissues. *J. Pharm. Biomed. Anal.* **2022**, *213*, 114698. [CrossRef]
28. Farrance, I.; Frenkel, R. Uncertainty of Measurement: A Review of the Rules for Calculating Uncertainty Components through Functional Relationships. *Clin. Biochem. Rev.* **2012**, *33*, 49–75.
29. Anjani, Q.K.; Utomo, E.; Domínguez-Robles, J.; Detamornrat, U.; Donnelly, R.F.; Larrañeta, E. A New and Sensitive HPLC-UV Method for Rapid and Simultaneous Quantification of Curcumin and D-Panthenol: Application to In Vitro Release Studies of Wound Dressings. *Molecules* **2022**, *27*, 1759. [CrossRef]
30. Bansal, S.; DeStefano, A. Key Elements of Bioanalytical Method Validation for Small Molecules. *AAPS J.* **2007**, *9*, E109–E114. [CrossRef]

31. Vora, L.K.; Moffatt, K.; Tekko, I.A.; Paredes, A.J.; Volpe-Zanutto, F.; Mishra, D.; Peng, K.; Raj Singh Thakur, R.; Donnelly, R.F. Microneedle Array Systems for Long-Acting Drug Delivery. *Eur. J. Pharm. Biopharm.* **2021**, *159*, 44–76. [CrossRef] [PubMed]
32. Peng, K.; Wu, C.; Wei, G.; Jiang, J.; Zhang, Z.; Sun, X. Implantable Sandwich PHBHHx Film for Burst-Free Controlled Delivery of Thymopentin Peptide. *Acta Pharm. Sin. B* **2018**, *8*, 432–439. [CrossRef] [PubMed]
33. Rosova, E.; Smirnova, N.; Dresvyanina, E.; Smirnova, V.; Vlasova, E.; Ivan'kova, E.; Sokolova, M.; Maslennikova, T.; Malafeev, K.; Kolbe, K.; et al. Biocomposite Materials Based on Chitosan and Lignin: Preparation and Characterization. *Cosmetics* **2021**, *8*, 24. [CrossRef]
34. Kumar, R.; Mishra, I.; Kumar, G. Synthesis and Evaluation of Mechanical Property of Chitosan/PVP Blend Through Nanoindentation-A Nanoscale Study. *J. Polym. Environ.* **2021**, *29*, 3770–3778. [CrossRef]
35. Donnelly, R.F.; Garland, M.J.; Morrow, D.I.J.; Migalska, K.; Singh, T.R.R.; Majithiya, R.; Woolfson, A.D. Optical Coherence Tomography Is a Valuable Tool in the Study of the Effects of Microneedle Geometry on Skin Penetration Characteristics and In-Skin Dissolution. *J. Control. Release* **2010**, *147*, 333–341. [CrossRef] [PubMed]
36. Kim, Y.T.; Shin, B.K.; Garripelli, V.K.; Kim, J.K.; Davaa, E.; Jo, S.; Park, J.S. A Thermosensitive Vaginal Gel Formulation with HPγCD for the PH-Dependent Release and Solubilization of Amphotericin B. *Eur. J. Pharm. Sci.* **2010**, *41*, 399–406. [CrossRef]
37. Peng, K.; Vora, L.K.; Tekko, I.A.; Permana, A.D.; Domínguez-Robles, J.; Ramadon, D.; Chambers, P.; McCarthy, H.O.; Larrañeta, E.; Donnelly, R.F. Dissolving Microneedle Patches Loaded with Amphotericin B Microparticles for Localised and Sustained Intradermal Delivery: Potential for Enhanced Treatment of Cutaneous Fungal Infections. *J. Control. Release* **2021**, *339*, 361–380. [CrossRef]
38. Jalvandi, J.; White, M.; Gao, Y.; Truong, Y.B.; Padhye, R.; Kyratzis, I.L. Polyvinyl Alcohol Composite Nanofibres Containing Conjugated Levofloxacin-Chitosan for Controlled Drug Release. *Mater. Sci. Eng. C* **2017**, *73*, 440–446. [CrossRef]
39. Nugrahani, I.; Laksana, A.N.; Uekusa, H.; Oyama, H. New Organic Salt from Levofloxacin-Citric Acid: What Is the Impact on the Stability and Antibiotic Potency? *Molecules* **2022**, *27*, 2166. [CrossRef]
40. Islam, N.U.; Umar, M.N.; Khan, E.; Al-Joufi, F.A.; Abed, S.N.; Said, M.; Ullah, H.; Iftikhar, M.; Zahoor, M.; Khan, F.A. Levofloxacin Cocrystal/Salt with Phthalimide and Caffeic Acid as Promising Solid-State Approach to Improve Antimicrobial Efficiency. *Antibiotics* **2022**, *11*, 797. [CrossRef]
41. Bandari, S.; Dronam, V.R.; Eedara, B.B. Development and Preliminary Characterization of Levofloxacin Pharmaceutical Cocrystals for Dissolution Rate Enhancement. *J. Pharm. Investig.* **2017**, *47*, 583–591. [CrossRef]
42. Ferrero, F.; Periolatto, M. Antimicrobial Finish of Textiles by Chitosan UV-Curing. *J. Nanosci. Nanotechnol.* **2012**, *12*, 4803–4810. [CrossRef] [PubMed]
43. Harish Prashanth, K.V.; Kittur, F.S.; Tharanathan, R.N. Solid State Structure of Chitosan Prepared under Different N-Deacetylating Conditions. *Carbohydr. Polym.* **2002**, *50*, 27–33. [CrossRef]
44. Rumondor, A.C.F.; Taylor, L.S. Effect of Polymer Hygroscopicity on the Phase Behavior of Amorphous Solid Dispersions in the Presence of Moisture. *Mol. Pharm.* **2010**, *7*, 477–490. [CrossRef]
45. Shahenoor Basha, S.K.; Sunita Sundari, G.; Vijay Kumar, K.; Rao, M.C. Optical and Dielectric Properties of PVP Based Composite Polymer Electrolyte Films. *Polym. Sci. Ser. A* **2017**, *59*, 554–565. [CrossRef]
46. Li, J.; Zivanovic, S.; Davidson, P.M.; Kit, K. Characterization and Comparison of Chitosan/PVP and Chitosan/PEO Blend Films. *Carbohydr. Polym.* **2010**, *79*, 786–791. [CrossRef]
47. Euerby, M.R.; Johnson, C.M.; Rushin, I.D.; Tennekoon, D.A.S.S. Investigations into the Epimerisation of Tipredane Ethylsulphoxide Diastereoisomers during Chromatographic Analysis on Reversed-Phase Silica II. The Involvement of Metals in Commercially Available C18 Silicas. *J. Chromatogr. A* **1995**, *705*, 229–245. [CrossRef]
48. Chang, Y.; Wang, Y.H.; Hu, C.Q. Simultaneous Determination of Purity and Potency of Amphotericin B by HPLC. *J. Antibiot. (Tokyo)* **2011**, *64*, 735–739. [CrossRef]
49. Zhou, Z.L.; Yang, M.; Yu, X.Y.; Peng, H.Y.; Shan, Z.X.; Chen, S.Z.; Lin, Q.X.; Liu, X.Y.; Chen, T.F.; Zhou, S.F.; et al. A Rapid and Simple High-Performance Liquid Chromatography Method for the Determination of Human Plasma Levofloxacin Concentration and Its Application to Bioequivalence Studies. *Biomed. Chromatogr.* **2007**, *21*, 1045–1051. [CrossRef]
50. McAlister, E.; Dutton, B.; Vora, L.K.; Zhao, L.; Ripolin, A.; Zahari, D.S.Z.B.P.H.; Quinn, H.L.; Tekko, I.A.; Courtenay, A.J.; Kelly, S.A.; et al. Directly Compressed Tablets: A Novel Drug-Containing Reservoir Combined with Hydrogel-Forming Microneedle Arrays for Transdermal Drug Delivery. *Adv. Healthc. Mater.* **2021**, *10*, 2001256. [CrossRef]
51. Santoro, M.I.R.M.; Kassab, N.M.; Singh, A.K.; Kedor-Hackmam, E.R.M. Quantitative Determination of Gatifloxacin, Levofloxacin, Lomefloxacin and Pefloxacin Fluoroquinolonic Antibiotics in Pharmaceutical Preparations by High-Performance Liquid Chromatography. *J. Pharm. Biomed. Anal.* **2006**, *40*, 179–184. [CrossRef] [PubMed]
52. Czyrski, A.; Sznura, J. The Application of Box-Behnken-Design in the Optimization of HPLC Separation of Fluoroquinolones. *Sci. Rep.* **2019**, *9*, 1–10. [CrossRef] [PubMed]
53. Maharini, I.; Martien, R.; Nugroho, A.K. RP-HPLC-UV Validation Method for Levofloxacin Hemihydrate Estimation in the Nano Polymeric Ocular Preparation. *Arab. J. Chem.* **2022**, *15*, 103582. [CrossRef]
54. Dabhi, B.; Parmar, B.; Patel, N.; Jadeja, Y.; Patel, M.; Jebaliya, H.; Karia, D.; Shah, A.K. A Stability Indicating UPLC Method for the Determination of Levofloxacin Hemihydrate in Pharmaceutical Dosage Form: Application to Pharmaceutical Analysis. *Chromatogr. Res. Int.* **2013**, *2013*, 1–5. [CrossRef]

55. Toker, S.E.; Kızılçay, G.E.; Sagirli, O. Determination of Levofloxacin by HPLC with Fluorescence Detection in Human Breast Milk. *Bioanalysis* **2021**, *13*, 1063–1070. [CrossRef] [PubMed]
56. Czyrski, A.; Szałek, E. An HPLC Method for Levofloxacin Determination and Its Application in Biomedical Analysis. *J. Anal. Chem.* **2016**, *71*, 840–843. [CrossRef]
57. Campanero, M.A.; Zamarreño, A.M.; Diaz, M.; Dios-Vieitez, M.C.; Azanza, J.R. Development and Validation of an HPLC Method for Determination of Amphotericin B in Plasma and Sputum Involving Solid Phase Extraction. *Chromatographia* **1997**, *46*, 641–646. [CrossRef]
58. Pippa, L.F.; Marques, M.P.; da Silva, A.C.T.; Vilar, F.C.; de Haes, T.M.; da Fonseca, B.A.L.; Martinez, R.; Coelho, E.B.; Wichert-Ana, L.; Lanchote, V.L. Sensitive LC-MS/MS Methods for Amphotericin B Analysis in Cerebrospinal Fluid, Plasma, Plasma Ultrafiltrate, and Urine: Application to Clinical Pharmacokinetics. *Front. Chem.* **2021**, *9*, 998. [CrossRef]
59. Asma, N.; Maddeppungeng, N.M.; Raihan, M.; Erdiana, A.P.; Himawan, A.; Permana, A.D. New HPLC-UV Analytical Method for Quantification of Metronidazole: Application to Ex Vivo Ocular Kinetic Assessments Following the Administration of Thermosensitive Ocular in Situ Gel. *Microchem. J.* **2022**, *172*, 106929. [CrossRef]
60. Chen, R.; Xu, C.; Lei, Y.; Liu, H.; Zhu, Y.; Zhang, J.; Xu, L. Facile Construction of a Family of Supramolecular Gels with Good Levofloxacin Hydrochloride Loading Capacity. *RSC Adv.* **2021**, *11*, 12641–12648. [CrossRef]
61. Riezk, A.; van Bocxlaer, K.; Yardley, V.; Murdan, S.; Croft, S.L. Activity of Amphotericin B-Loaded Chitosan Nanoparticles against Experimental Cutaneous Leishmaniasis. *Molecules* **2020**, *25*, 4002. [CrossRef]
62. Tekko, I.A.; Vora, L.K.; Volpe-zanutto, F.; Moffatt, K.; Jarrahian, C.; Mccarthy, H.O.; Donnelly, R.F. Novel Bilayer Microarray Patch-Assisted Long-Acting Micro-Depot Cabotegravir Intradermal Delivery for HIV Pre-Exposure Prophylaxis. *Adv. Funct. Mater.* **2021**, *32*, 2106999. [CrossRef]
63. Summerfield, A.; Meurens, F.; Ricklin, M.E. The Immunology of the Porcine Skin and Its Value as a Model for Human Skin. *Mol. Immunol.* **2015**, *66*, 14–21. [CrossRef] [PubMed]
64. Li, M.; Vora, L.K.; Peng, K.; Donnelly, R.F. Trilayer Microneedle Array Assisted Transdermal and Intradermal Delivery of Dexamethasone. *Int. J. Pharm.* **2022**, *612*, 121295. [CrossRef] [PubMed]
65. Koeppe, M.O.; Cristofoletti, R.; Fernandes, E.F.; Storpirtis, S.; Junginger, H.E.; Kopp, S.; Midha, K.K.; Shah, V.P.; Stavchansky, S.; Dressman, J.B.; et al. Biowaiver Monographs for Immediate Release Solid Oral Dosage Forms: Levofloxacin. *J. Pharm. Sci.* **2011**, *100*, 1628–1636. [CrossRef] [PubMed]
66. Ghadi, R.; Dand, N. BCS Class IV Drugs: Highly Notorious Candidates for Formulation Development. *J. Control. Release* **2017**, *248*, 71–95. [CrossRef]
67. Drago, L.; De Vecchi, E.; Mombelli, B.; Nicola, L.; Valli, M.; Gismondo, M.R. Activity of Levofloxacin and Ciprofloxacin against Urinary Pathogens. *J. Antimicrob. Chemother.* **2001**, *48*, 37–45. [CrossRef]
68. Licata, L.; Smith, C.E.; Goldschmidt, R.M.; Barrett, J.F.; Frosco, M. Comparison of the Postantibiotic and Postantibiotic Sub-MIC Effects of Levofloxacin and Ciprofloxacin on Staphylococcus Aureus and Streptococcus Pneumoniae. *Antimicrob. Agents Chemother.* **1997**, *41*, 950–955. [CrossRef]
69. Schmitz, F. Relationship between Ciprofloxacin, Ofloxacin, Levofloxacin, Sparfloxacin and Moxifloxacin (BAY 12-8039) MICs and Mutations in GrlA, GrlB, GyrA and GyrB in 116 Unrelated Clinical Isolates of Staphylococcus Aureus. *J. Antimicrob. Chemother.* **1998**, *41*, 481–484. [CrossRef]
70. Ellis, D. Amphotericin B: Spectrum and Resistance. *J. Antimicrob. Chemother.* **2002**, *49*, 7–10. [CrossRef]
71. Hamill, R.J. Amphotericin B Formulations: A Comparative Review of Efficacy and Toxicity. *Drugs* **2013**, *73*, 919–934. [CrossRef] [PubMed]
72. Lewis, S.J.; Chaijamorn, W.; Shaw, A.R.; Mueller, B.A. In Silico Trials Using Monte Carlo Simulation to Evaluate Ciprofloxacin and Levofloxacin Dosing in Critically Ill Patients Receiving Prolonged Intermittent Renal Replacement Therapy. *Ren. Replace. Ther.* **2016**, *2*, 1–11. [CrossRef]
73. Canouï, E.; Kerneis, S.; Morand, P.; Enser, M.; Gauzit, R.; Eyrolle, L.; Leclerc, P.; Contejean, A.; Zheng, Y.; Anract, P.; et al. Oral Levofloxacin: Population Pharmacokinetics Model and Pharmacodynamics Study in Bone and Joint Infections. *J. Antimicrob. Chemother.* **2022**, *77*, 1344–1352. [CrossRef] [PubMed]
74. Setiawan, E.; Abdul-Aziz, M.H.; Cotta, M.O.; Susaniwati, S.; Cahjono, H.; Sari, I.Y.; Wibowo, T.; Marpaung, F.R.; Roberts, J.A. Population Pharmacokinetics and Dose Optimization of Intravenous Levofloxacin in Hospitalized Adult Patients. *Sci. Rep.* **2022**, *12*, 1–11. [CrossRef]
75. Norrby, S.R. Levofloxacin. *Expert Opin. Pharmacother.* **1999**, *1*, 109–119. [CrossRef]
76. Ashrafi, M.; Bayat, M.; Mortazavi, P.; Hashemi, S.J.; Meimandipour, A. Antimicrobial Effect of Chitosan–Silver–Copper Nanocomposite on Candida Albicans. *J. Nanostructure Chem.* **2020**, *10*, 87–95. [CrossRef]
77. Peng, K.; Vora, L.K.; Domínguez-Robles, J.; Naser, Y.A.; Li, M.; Larrañeta, E.; Donnelly, R.F. Hydrogel-Forming Microneedles for Rapid and Efficient Skin Deposition of Controlled Release Tip-Implants. *Mater. Sci. Eng. C* **2021**, *127*, 112226. [CrossRef]
78. Park, J.Y.; Seo, K.S. Staphylococcus Aureus. In *Food Microbiology: Fundamentals and Frontiers*; ASM Press: Washington, DC, USA, 2019; pp. 555–584. ISBN 9781683670476.
79. Domínguez-Robles, J.; Utomo, E.; Cornelius, V.A.; Anjani, Q.K.; Korelidou, A.; Gonzalez, Z.; Donnelly, R.F.; Margariti, A.; Delgado-Aguilar, M.; Tarrés, Q.; et al. TPU-Based Antiplatelet Cardiovascular Prostheses Prepared Using Fused Deposition Modelling. *Mater. Des.* **2022**, *220*, 110837. [CrossRef]

80. Peña, A.; Sánchez, N.S.; Calahorra, M. Effects of Chitosan on Candida Albicans: Conditions for Its Antifungal Activity. *Biomed Res. Int.* **2013**, *2013*. [CrossRef]
81. Oliveira, V.d.S.; da Cruz, M.M.; Bezerra, G.S.; E Silva, N.E.S.; Nogueira, F.H.A.; Chaves, G.M.; Sobrinho, J.L.S.; Mendonça-Junior, F.J.B.; Damasceno, B.P.G.d.L.; Converti, A.; et al. Chitosan-Based Films with 2-Aminothiophene Derivative: Formulation, Characterization and Potential Antifungal Activity. *Mar. Drugs* **2022**, *20*, 103. [CrossRef]
82. Verlee, A.; Mincke, S.; Stevens, C.V. Recent Developments in Antibacterial and Antifungal Chitosan and Its Derivatives. *Carbohydr. Polym.* **2017**, *164*, 268–283. [CrossRef] [PubMed]
83. Ryssel, H.; Kloeters, O.; Germann, G.; Schäfer, T.; Wiedemann, G.; Oehlbauer, M. The Antimicrobial Effect of Acetic Acid-An Alternative to Common Local Antiseptics? *Burns* **2009**, *35*, 695–700. [CrossRef] [PubMed]
84. Bjarnsholt, T.; Alhede, M.; Jensen, P.Ø.; Nielsen, A.K.; Johansen, H.K.; Homøe, P.; Høiby, N.; Givskov, M.; Kirketerp-Møller, K. Antibiofilm Properties of Acetic Acid. *Adv. Wound Care* **2015**, *4*, 363–372. [CrossRef]
85. Akbar, N.; Kawish, M.; Khan, N.A.; Shah, M.R.; Alharbi, A.M.; Alfahemi, H.; Siddiqui, R. Hesperidin-, Curcumin-, and Amphotericin B- Based Nano-Formulations as Potential Antibacterials. *Antibiotics* **2022**, *11*, 696. [CrossRef] [PubMed]

MDPI
St. Alban-Anlage 66
4052 Basel
Switzerland
www.mdpi.com

Pharmaceutics Editorial Office
E-mail: pharmaceutics@mdpi.com
www.mdpi.com/journal/pharmaceutics

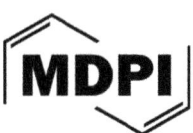

Disclaimer/Publisher's Note: The statements, opinions and data contained in all publications are solely those of the individual author(s) and contributor(s) and not of MDPI and/or the editor(s). MDPI and/or the editor(s) disclaim responsibility for any injury to people or property resulting from any ideas, methods, instructions or products referred to in the content.

www.ingramcontent.com/pod-product-compliance
Lightning Source LLC
LaVergne TN
LVHW070430100526
838202LV00014B/1563